Women's Leadership in Peace Building

Women's Leadership in Peace Building:
Conflict, Community and Care

International Colloquium on Women in Peace-building
From Monrovia (2009) to Harare (2014)

=============❖=============

Edited by:

Mirjam van Reisen,

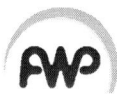

AFRICA WORLD PRESS
TRENTON | LONDON | CAPE TOWN | NAIROBI | ADDIS ABABA | ASMARA | IBADAN

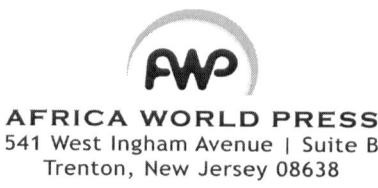

AFRICA WORLD PRESS
541 West Ingham Avenue | Suite B
Trenton, New Jersey 08638

Copyright © 2015 Mirjam van Reisen

All rights reserved. No part of this publication may be reproduced, stored in a retrieval system or transmitted in any form or by any means electronic, mechanical, photocopying, recording or otherwise without the prior written permission of the publisher.

Book and cover design: Lemlem Taddese
Front cover picture courtesy of Milly Buchanan
Copy Editors: Simon Stocker and Catherine Schook

In Acknowledgment of the generous support from Cordaid

Cordaid
BUILDING FLOURISHING COMMUNITIES

ISBN: 978-1-59221-994-0 (PB)

TABLE OF CONTENTS

FOREWORD XI
Ellen Johnson Sirleaf

INTRODUCTION XIII
Mirjam van Reisen

PART I – WOMEN'S LEADERSHIP IN COMMUNITY PEACE BUILDING IN AFRICA

CHAPTER 1. TO OFFER A GLASS OF MILLET-MILK IS TO OFFER YOU MY PEACE: THE RELATIONAL RELEVANCE OF FOOD IN ORGANIZING COMMUNITY PEACE 3
Primrose Nakazibwe

CHAPTER 2. WOMEN'S PROTECTION AND MECHANISMS OF CONFLICT RESOLUTION IN ANKORE FAMILIES 17
Clementia Neema Murembe

CHAPTER 3. UBUNTU AND PEACE: WITHOUT A MOTHER, THERE IS NO HOME 37
Gertjan van Stam

CHAPTER 4. WOMEN HAVE ALWAYS HAD THEIR SPECIAL PLACE IN HISTORY AS PEACE-MAKERS: WOMEN AND PEACE BUILDING IN THE GREAT LAKES REGION 55
Pamela K. Mbabazi

CHAPTER 5. THE POLITICS OF THE BODY IN CONFLICT: FOLLOWING WOMEN'S FOOTSTEPS: A HOLISTIC RESPONSE TO END SEXUAL VIOLENCE 65
Ruth Ojiambo Ochieng and Sandra Tumwesigye

CHAPTER 6. AGEING AND CHANGING COMMUNITY DYNAMICS IN AFRICA 83
Antony Ong'ayo Otieno

PART II – WOMEN'S POLITICAL LEADERSHIP

CHAPTER 7. THE STRUGGLE OF THE SOUTH SUDANESE WOMEN 99
Betty Achan Ogwaro

CHAPTER 8. REVOLVING REVOLUTIONS: THE INCLUSION OF WOMEN IN PEACE BUILDING IN NEPAL AFTER THE WAR 113
Susan Sellars-Shrestha and Leena Rikkila Tamang

CHAPTER 9. TOUGH CHOICES, LIMITED SPACES AND CONFLICTED LOYALTIES: WOMEN'S LEADERSHIP IN GOVERNANCE IN AFRICA TODAY: THE KENYAN EXPERIENCE 131
Stella Maranga

PART III – GENDER IN THE CONTEXT OF SECURITY CHALLENGES

CHAPTER 10. "BRING BACK OUR GIRLS": CONFLICT AND INSURGENCY IN NIGERIA 147
Obadiah Mailafia

CHAPTER 11. OF MULLAHS, RADIO AND RELIGION: THE TALIBAN AND TRIBAL SWAT'S WOMEN IN PAKISTAN 181
Syed Manzar Abbas Zaidi

CHAPTER 12. NATIONAL SECURITY: NAVIGATING THE COMING ROUGH SEAS BETWEEN THE USA AND CHINA ... 197
Andre Zaaiman

PART IV – WOMEN'S LEADERSHIP IN RE-INVENTING A GLOBALIZED WORLD

CHAPTER 13. TECHNOLOGY AND THE POWER TO CONNECT: PARTICIPATION OF WOMEN IN SUPPORTING ACTIVITIES THROUGH INTERNET COMMUNITIES 213
Gerard van Oortmerssen

CHAPTER 14. WOMENLEADERS4PEACE: FINDING AN AUTHENTIC AND MEANINGFUL CONTRIBUTION IN A CONFLICTED AND SEXIST GLOBALIZING WORLD 229
Ineke Buskens

CHAPTER 15. A RELIGIOUS DEDICATION TO COMMUNITY: THE LASTING PROMISE OF THE CONCEPT OF CARITAS IN A PLURALIST WORLD 249
Erik Borgman

CHAPTER 16. DIGNITY AS A BASIS FOR THE POST-2015 DEVELOPMENT AGENDA: THE RELEVANCE OF THE LEGACY OF MARGA KLOMPÉ FOR A UNIVERSAL POVERTY ERADICATION PROGRAMME 261
Mirjam van Reisen

PART V – WOMEN'S LEADERSHIP IN GLOBALISED COMMUNITIES AS PEACE-BUILDERS

CHAPTER 17. REDEMPTION IN SINAI: A STORY OF SLAVERY TODAY 279
Mirjam van Reisen

CHAPTER 18. DESERTS, HIGH SEAS AND HOPE 289
Selame Kidane

CHAPTER 19. A PLACE CALLED HOME: THE MARGINALISATION OF ZIMBABWEAN WOMEN 301
Grace Kwinjeh

CHAPTER 20. "GIRLS MAKE MUSIC, WOMEN CREATE CHANGE": ALTERNATIVE APPROACHES TO FIGHTING FOR A LIVING WAGE IN LONDON 313
Robyn Stocker

CHAPTER 21. HOME-BASED CARE: THE POWER OF WOMEN TO CONNECT VULNERABLE MEMBERS OF THE COMMUNITY 321
Catherine Schook

PART VI – A REFLECTION ON THE CHALLENGES OF REBULDING POST-CONFLICT LIBERIA

CHAPTER 22. INTERNATIONAL SOCIAL RESPONSIBILITY ... 331
Ellen Johnson Sirleaf

CHAPTER 23. LAUDATIO 337
Mirjam van Reisen

PART VII – THE PRAXIS OF ENGAGING WITH WOMEN'S AGENCY IN PEACE BUILDING

CHAPTER 23. "SHOW ME YOUR FRIENDS, AND I WILL TELL YOU WHO YOU ARE": THE ROLE OF REHABILITATION PROGRAMMES IN REDUCING RECIDIVISM AMONG PRISON INMATES 343
Vickie Wambura

CHAPTER 25. THE HAND THAT ROCKS THE CRADLE IS THE HAND THAT RULES THE WORLD: WOMEN'S ROLE IN IMPROVING COMMUNITY SECURITY 353
Agnes Dinkelman

CHAPTER 26. CHALLENGING THE STATUS QUO AND UNLEASHING THE HIDDEN POWER OF WOMEN: THE ZIMBABWEAN EXPERIENCE 363
Chikomborero Mafuriranwa

CHAPTER 27. ONE HAND CANNOT TIE A BUNDLE: PEACE BUILDING IN SECULAR AND FAITH-BASED COMMUNITIES IN UGANDA 371
Angeline Nguedjeu-Momekam

CHAPTER 28. CONFLICT, CONTRADICTION AND CONSCIOUSNESS: AN ARTIST'S EVOLUTION 377

CHAPTER 29. COMPREHENSIVE COMMUNITY CARE IN RURAL REALITIES THROUGH THE LENS OF JANNEKE VAN DIJK 379
Mirjam van Reisen

ABOUT THE AUTHORS 389

FOREWORD

Due to the magnificent vibrancy and positive spirit of Liberians, my country has been rebuilt since the civil war, which had destroyed it and in which many Liberians were killed or made destitute. The great country that Liberia is, has now been in peace for over a decade. It had just begun to pick up its economic recovery, with the enterprising spirit of my fellow countrymen. Sadly, we are now facing another magnificent challenge, which is rocking the fabric of our society: the ebola epidemic.

This fast-spreading disease is ravaging the communities, not only of Liberia, but also of its neighbours, Sierra Leone, and Guinea. Our women, the natural caregivers within our families and communities are at the frontline of this mammoth battle. The danger that this health crisis poses to the peace in our communities is now recognized in the United Nations Security Council Resolution 2177 (2014) "Urging Immediate Action, End to Isolation of Affected States". I urge the international community to stand by my country, by our neighbours and by all countries equally challenged.

As human beings, we are not fighting to die, but to live. We invoke the spirit of communities, of all men, women and children of Liberia, of Africa and of the world to stand together. If we care about our communities we can resolve conflict, overcome the hardest challenges and rebuild our peace. We know that when God brings us to it, he will help us through it.

Ellen Johnson Sirleaf
President of Liberia

INTRODUCTION

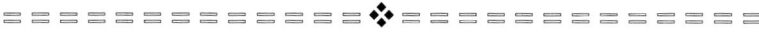

Mirjam van Reisen

I.

A war on a virus.

The Ebola virus is taking its deathly toll, spreading along vulnerable communities and taking governments unprepared, killing health workers, mothers and wives, attending to dying patients, while they are trying to stop the spread of the virus. A virus, killing women, men, children, sparing no-one. A threat to one person is a threat to all.

A virus, causing conflict between authorities, who are trying to define the measures to take to contain the spread of the disease. A people in fear, revolting, breaking through the military established closed quarantined areas, to collect their dying and loved ones. Statistics of inadequate numbers of body-bags. A Health Ministry weighing up the risks of large-scale use of certain medicines. Airlines closing their services. Neighbouring countries closing their borders. This is Liberia today, Liberia, which has led the way on women's leadership in peace-building in Africa and in the world. Once a country of freedom, a country that proudly built its independence on (the struggle to liberate itself) from slavery. Liberia, is now left in dire isolation.

A deadly virus. This is the only certainty we have. Death can overtake our efforts at any time and destroy our vulnerable common world.

II.

The old philosophies teach us that existence requires non-existence. This leads us to the deep human truth that existence depends on otherness. This is the essence of the understanding of the African philosophy of Ubuntu: I exist because you do. This brings us back to the only certain knowledge that we have: in isolation of other matter, of other people, we cannot exist and our existence has no meaning. Hence, the profound self-interest is the need to recognize the other in his or her otherness. We all depend on it. In recognising the other and in being recognized by the other, I belong and therefore I exist.

This book testifies to the bonds of families, communities, elderly parents, husbands, wives, partners, sisters, brothers, friends or neighbours. Bonds are sustained in a shared common world, nearby, or over long distances, in which we care. In her article, Catherine Schook highlights the unseen female informal care providers, a working force that has thinned out but is ever greater in demand worldwide. These are brought out in stories, such as those narrated by Schook, and in the pictures by medical doctor, Janneke van Dijk, based in Harare. They give us a glimpse of how identities of children, parents and elderly, develop and change in a globalised world, with the need for care as a constant reminder of the bonds between them. Even when people are living in worlds apart, they care, sustaining elderly parents and vulnerable family members. As part of this caring bond, different perspectives, responsibilities and concerns are shared. Even when people are living physically in one place and virtually in another, they do, as described by Geresu Tufa in this volume. Worries between refugees and people at home are shared by internet, chatrooms and mobile phones, and money is exchanged through MoneyGram or Western Union, creating new common places for people physically living in different countries and even continents. Women look after their family in their country of residence, as well as for their families back at home, with responsibilities shouldered on them to find solutions for the many problems communicated in real time.

Grace Kwinjeh describes how refugees may find that they "jumped out of the frying pan into the fire." She illustrates the challenges of diaspora women and men from Zimbabwe. The importance of inclusion in a common world is brought out in this article. Refugees often feel insufficiently recognised and may feel excluded from the political affairs at home. She also explores the situation of women who end up in the diaspora, working as care-workers or nurses in the UK. They become engaged in activities of professional care, which may have profound repercussions on relations within families. Antony Otieno Ong'ayo discusses another aspect of international links of care. He focuses on the challenges of global ageing in terms of care for the elderly. He discusses how emerging labour migration leaves care gaps in communities of origin of the care-workers.

This common place is a world, where one belongs, not because of sameness, but because of difference. The common world can only exist because each occupant is situated in a different place and lives with a different perspective from anyone else in the common space. Because people are different they can give one another something, they can be a gift to one another. Gertjan van Stam discusses how Ubuntu as an African worldview treats peace and women's leadership in it. He emphasises that peace-building requires the recognition of local communities, and women who nurture bonds in local communities: "Without a woman, there is no home." Peace-building is the creation of a common home, a space of belonging for everyone, premised on the importance of recognising 'otherness' as the basis of a common world.

The natural condition of life is necessarily based in otherness. Otherness makes the one valuable for the other, but otherness also means a constant potential for conflict. Peace is therefore not the absence of conflict, but the recognition of conflict as an essential component of the common world we occupy. It is changing the potential in an opportunity to belong together.

Ineke Buskens focuses on women's leadership in peace-building. This requires a process of women freeing themselves from the conditions, which may constrain their contribution, as they may be trapped in a patriarchal society. She discusses the importance of creating understanding and confidence of what women can contribute through leadership so that it enhances a natural orientation to promote cooperation and assert those attributes of providing direction based on care. Milly Buchanan, Liberian diplomat and artist, depicts this strength of women in her art.

III.

Where possible, families eat together. The knowledge of belonging to a world where food is given, produced and harvested, has linked humanity to the nurturing aspect of creation in the image of the mother, who feeds and cares for her children, the dependency of a creation based in the material world that sustains us. This is what, in old societies and modern cities, sharing of a meal may do: link us in this common bond, revive the understanding that we need to sustain the common with the limited means available. So that we will not forget that our existence depends on the other. That we need to feed ourselves as well as the other, that life itself depends on nurture and care.

In her contribution, Primrose Nakazibwe researches the relationship between peace and food. Women in rural communities know that peace on empty stomachs is not possible. She describes how old traditions, associated with food, help peace-building within communities. She argues that these traditions may still have a meaningful application today.

IV.

"Shit happens." Sekai Holland is the former Minister of National Healing, Reconciliation and Integration in Zimbabwe. Courageously, she took leadership for peace-building under President Mugabe, despite having been severely tortured and left to die by thugs operating under government orders, aiming to spread fear.

"Forgive me the rude language" she says with a chuckle, to then repeat: "Shit happens." She takes a long reflective pause. "But you see, we have created civil ways of dealing with it. We have constructed toilets, sewers and other infrastructure to remove it and to prevent it from spreading disease." She looks around the room. "Conflict is like shit. It is an essential part of life, but it needs to be channelled, to be removed to a place where it can decompose so that it cannot infect and spread. Decomposed it can be a fertile basis for growth."

In a conversation with Sekai Holland on the achievements of the Zimbabwe peace process, she describes the institutions set up for peace-building. Traditional healing practices may help bring persecutor and victims together and are crucial for a transformation of society away from cyclical violence: "An eye for an eye makes Zimbabwe blind." Women have an important part to play in providing leadership in communities, to allow healing and to create security for all members of the community. By demanding peace, women all over the world, have forced fighting to stop, calling upon their authority and critical role in the family, in the community and society at large.

Betty Ogwara discusses the difficult situation in South Sudan, and the importance of women's presence in peace-building and the relevance and need of their political inclusion. Post conflict situations can provide openings for women's increased participation, but is by no means guaranteed. The increased participation of women in governance does not just benefit women, but society in general. Susan Sellars-Shrestra and Leena Rikkila-Tamang analyse the contribution of women in the transformations from a feudal society to a parliamentary democracy in Nepal, and the challenges that still remain. Stella Maranga discusses the negotiations to increase political participation of women in Kenya, the gains made and the difficulties encountered.

The recognition of the other can awaken aspirations to be as the other. Gender-analysis depends on the recognition of difference between the sexes and the contributions they make to society: men are simply not women. They have to be recognized not in how they should be or what they should do, but in what they are and what they do. Many contributors in this book point to the capacities of women in mediation, in diplomacy, in negotiations between warring factions, in information gathering and communication, in decision-making and leadership. Women appear as good peace-builders, military strategists and security analysts. Women emerge confident and competent.

V.

Many chapters in this book discuss the unspeakable reality of Gender-Based Sexual Violence used as a weapon in conflict and war, or used just randomly, as part of a violence embodied in conditions of patriarchal domination. The women's body becomes the place where war is carried out.

After rape, young girls and women are shunned by communities, left to deal with the consequences, without support. The medical attention needed is lacking, and the complications, such as fistula, resulting from the violence are often left unattended, creating continued suffering, isolation and shame. Yet, even pregnant from rape, women still give birth, raise the child, even care and love their child born under such circumstances. The power of a caring community, the will to care is there.

Clementia Neema Murembe analyses the situation of Gender Based Violence in the home and how women have found strategies to protect themselves and coping with it. Indeed, even a Good Samaritan sometimes cannot be trusted and may use and abuse a child, as reflected in the sad story, told by Chikomborero

Mafuriranwa, illustrating the vulnerability of care, the potential of abuse in care, and the weaknesses of a caring community.

The severity of the trauma that women endure, and the impact on their lives is described in several contributions to this book. Much greater attention needs to be given to the long-term impact of such trauma and resources are needed for mental health care to support women who have been traumatized. Pamela Mbabazi discusses women's leadership in peace-building strategies in communities in East Africa. It is critical that women have access to support in medical, mental and spiritual healing. The importance of healing, and also the challenges associated with it, are set out in the contribution by Ruth Ojiambo Ochieng and Sandra Tumwesigye based on extensive experience. Ngeudieu compares secular and faith-based initiatives to support women in post conflict communities in North Uganda. Agnes Dinkelman describes her experience with communities and security forces, such as the police and military, to empower women to demand measures that support their own security.

Mirjam van Reisen and Selam Kidane discuss the dramatic situation of human trafficking in Sinai and how African women are tortured and violated. One of the mothers, given birth to her child while in chains, named her baby Redemption. Selam Kidane describes the importance of hope. Hope, the new beginning, the new creation of life, under unspeakable circumstances, women stubbornly continue to live, give life, nurse and care.

VI.

Looking at hope, Erik Borgman investigates what the story of the Good Samaritan means for caritas in today's globally connected and technologically advanced world, at a deep level associated with the worldview of Ubuntu, arguing that the concept of caritas is directed towards a community of people aware of the fact that we depend on one another and that we are responsible for each other's wellbeing. Mirjam van Reisen addresses how notions of the social world influence the common agenda's agreed at international level and how women, such as the first Dutch female Minister, Marga Klompé, who translated her experience of war in advocating for universal mechanisms to help deal with conflict. Van Reisen critically analyses how a global programme for universal eradication of poverty combined with approaches of peace-building can be conceptualised.

Gerard van Oortmerssen explores how an ever rapidly evolving technology may or may not serve people in participating meaningfully in society, the unknown challenges and uncontrollable nature of these developments and the conflicts emerging from it and how women participate in this. Local groups, combating violence against women, use social media to seek protection and this also may help in raising public awareness and mobilize international support. Access to social media is a particularly effective way to reach youth and mobilise them in campaigns against gender-based violence.

This book includes several inspiring chapters of young women, who provide leadership to demand greater inclusion of people living on the margins of society. Vicky Wambura examines how the lack of opportunities for young people lead to crime and how the harsh conditions in the Kenyan prison system fail to provide the support needed for inmates to build an alternative future. Robyn Stocker addresses the challenges of young women in Brixton, London, who live as creative music artists but are exploited trying to make a living, without even being paid a minimum living wage by some service industries.

The thought that perhaps we can control our own creation, and our own death, the ever-increasing development of science and technology, has lead our thinking to confide in a new god; man as its own creator. We thought this god would lead us to independence and security. Free from everything and everyone. In fact, it has connected humanity much closer across continents and rooted us deeper in the universe. Globalisation has decreased our dependency on food or medicine produced in our own immediate environment, but increased our dependency on people on the other side of the world, and on the fruit of their labour. It has enlarged the family to a common space of connectivity, dependence and community that is now truly global. This has also increased the risks of conflict associated with global dependency on resources, as some of the chapters illustrate. International competition over key economic resources will play out in Africa, argues André Zaaiman. Conflicts rooted in religious extremism and linked to international terrorism can spread globally too and both Obadiah Mailafia and Manzar Zaidi show how extremism and jihadism result in increased tensions in their respective regions in the West African Sahel and the Pakistani South East Asia region. Both authors argue how this poses serious challenges to progress in gender equality and may threaten the participation of women in public and in the common world. Both argue that this is to be a priority for the international community to address.

VII.

In 2009, Liberia celebrated its peace. The International Colloquium rooted in the UN Security Council Declaration 1325 based on the African experience and on the notion that peace-building starts at home, in communities. Liberia invited the world's political leaders and opened a large market-place so that all women of Liberia could attend the festivities. As the first female President of Africa, Ellen Johnson-Sirleaf, who authored with Elisabeth Rehn in 2002 the book "Women, War and Peace", showed Africa leading the way on women's leadership in peace-building. The "International Colloquium on Women's Empowerment, Leadership Development, International Peace and Security" adopted the Monrovia Declaration. Our globalised common world needs shared aspirations and commitments to help guide our collective existence.

This book brings together reflections in the context of the International Colloquium in Liberia of 2009. Authors met at various occasions. An expert meeting held in October 2014 in Naivasha, Kenya, under the auspices of UNWomen, looked at the inclusion of peace-building and women's leadership in the Post-2015 Development Agenda. Five years after the Liberia Colloquium a meeting was organised by the Association of Women's Clubs in Zimbabwe to look at the results of peace-building in this country. This meeting was followed by the International Colloquium held in Leiden at the Africa Works! Conference. This meeting emphasized the positive contribution Africa makes to the international social and economic development for well-being of the world's citizens. It explored common priorities for the Post-2015 Development Agenda, in the area of peace-building.

The negotiations on the Post-2015 Agenda express a global and public understanding that this world is a common place, where resources need to be shared and negotiated as a basis for continuous peace-building. Peace – seen through the negotiation of different interests, is a vital foundation for the maintenance of the common good. As is argued by several contributors, UN SCR 1325 is a crucial framework for the Post 2015 Agenda and it should be integrated together with the emphasis on vulnerable countries, such as Liberia, brought together in the New Deal. Financing arrangements and budgets of these three frameworks should be integrated to give government the best scope to bring together crucial areas of government: in health, education, trauma support and women' empowerment. The importance of an integrated coherent support is poignantly shown by the Ebola virus, as it has wiped away the efforts of years of investment.

This book argues in different ways that women's leadership in homes, in small communities, in government or at global level, is essential for processes aiming to strengthen the potential for peace. In the first part of this Volume the contribution of African tradition and philosophy to peace-building are explored. In the second part the experience gained in conflict-resolution and peace-building enhancing women's leadership is examined. The third part of this book discusses the contribution women make to governance and the obstacles they encounter in participating in leadership at national governance level. The fourth part identifies global developments and how they interact with peace in the international arena. The fifth and final part gives the floor to the women and men who are practitioners in peace-building in small and in big ways. Their stories relate in a different way, what has been examined in this book.

VIII.

We thank those that made it possible to publish this book and to organise the meetings that prepared for it, especially the Dutch development organisation, Cordaid, the European Commission as well as UNWomen and Oxfam Novib. We thank our collaegues from Africa Works! providing us with a space to celebrate the International Colloquium. We recognise the partnership with the Midlands State University, Liberia University, Mbabara University and Tilburg University to create the academic foundation to deepen peace-education and women's leadership education.

IX.

The threat of the further spreading of the deadly ebola virus seems sometimes to inspire attempts to quarantine the whole country. As if we can ever say that anything is only 'their problem'. No problem, no people confronted with a problem can be isolated in our globalized world. The ebola crisis requires therefore a concerted international response that lifts Liberia's isolation in combating the virus. The world must stand in solidarity and spare no means to solve this emergency in one of the world's poorest countries. This book calls on international agencies, bilateral development partners and the private sector to assist Liberia, and its neighbouring countries Sierra Leone and Guinea, in their attempt deal with the virus and the danger it embodies.

H.E. Ellen Johnson-Sirleaf has marked the international understanding of how local women are at the core of peace-building. She has given us access to a new understanding of Africa, as the continent from which a worldview emerges that gives hope, and that may help the entire world to cope with conflict inherent to the many globalised challenges. President Sirleaf has demonstrated women to be outstanding capable leaders and strategists, and above all has shown the potential of women as peace-builders at all levels.

The achievements of President Sirleaf have been recognised by many awards; we have published the speeches held at Tilburg University where she received an honorary doctorate in 2012 to honour her contribution to women's leadership in peace-building.

We pay tribute to the legacy of the Liberia Colloquium in the spirit of the Monrovia Declaration, five years later. It is important to mark the ongoing importance and relevance of the International Colloquium and express the wish that the Monrovia Declaration will provide a basis for a strong inclusion of women's leadership in peace building in the Post-2015 Development Framework.

PART I – WOMEN'S LEADERSHIP IN COMMUNITY PEACE BUILDING IN AFRICA

CHAPTER 1. TO OFFER A GLASS OF MILLET-MILK IS TO OFFER YOU MY PEACE: THE RELATIONAL RELEVANCE OF FOOD IN ORGANIZING COMMUNITY PEACE

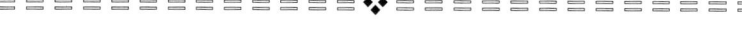

Primrose Nakazibwe

Introduction

This chapter seeks to address the way in which food has been used as a tool or symbol of community-peace in Ankore. Ankore region, as it is known today, was among the main kingdoms that were amalgamated to become Uganda. The other name for the region is "Karo karungi" meaning the "beautiful land" that makes the people who live in it proud of its geographical features and acts as the source for their livelihood (Kirindi, 2008). The land that the residents refer to as the 'land of milk and honey' was known to be land of food where each and every person had enough to eat and share with others. In this region referring to a person as a "Mushaija" (meaning a man) literally included other attributes including not telling lies, not stealing and causing no trouble to others. But most importantly, a "Mushaija" was not expected to 'eat alone' and was supposed to entertain his clansmen (Mushanga, 2011). This expression of a man in the Ankore setting revealed the importance of food in defining a peaceful community. Food was central in ensuring community peace through building peaceful relationships among members of the community. Since community peace building was predominantly social and structural, food played a big role in the social elements of peace.

Community peace is a participatory bottom-up approach, which was founded on the premise that people are the best resource for building and sustaining peace (Waldman, 2008:5). Community peace building is entrenched in community-based approaches that put people at the centre of the development discourse (people-centred development). These approaches have been upgraded to include community peace approaches used by many societies for a very long period of time. Community-based peace-building interventions always seek to change relationships through cooperating with a wide range of actors within and from outside the community which links to broader peace strategies (Haider, 2009:5). Thus, trust, safety, and social cohesion within and between communities are the core aims of community peace-building. These strengthen social and cultural capacities to resolve disputes and conflict and to promote inter-ethnic and inter-group interaction and dialogue (Waldman, 2008:5). It should be noted that community peace, both in traditional and contemporary contexts, aims at preventing conflict through the promotion of community values of peace and tolerance as ideal behaviours among its members.

Many studies that have attempted to address the linkage between food and peace have concentrated much on the role of conflict in exacerbating food insecurity (Robertson, 2012:2; Simmons, 2013), thus ignoring the role of food in creating peaceful relationships in communities. This chapter reviews the thinking and practice around the ability of food (its production and consumption practices) in organizing community peace. Traditionally, food has always been at the centre of peace processes (conflict prevention, management and resolution) and has been used as a way to maintain harmony in the society. This has been particularly so in rural areas, where the main livelihood was derived from food production. The core values of traditional food production: sharing, cooperation and respect for others are consistent with the values of peace. Producing food as a group in a community helps empower those involved – both women and men - through enhanced resiliency, self-esteem and connections with others, which are key for maintaining peace within the community. This study assesses the role of food in building peaceful relationships in Uganda: a case of Ankore. This is done by assessing both the traditional and modern approaches of peace building in Ankore and identifying how these can be adopted today to safeguard community peace.

This ethnographic study was carried out in Mbarara District, which lies at the heart of the Ankore region in western Uganda. The district consists of Kashari and Rwampara Counties and one Municipality [Mbarara Municipality]. It boarders Ibanda and Kiruhura Districts in the north, Kiruhura and Ishingiro Districts in the East, Shema District in the west and Isingiro and Ntungamo Districts in the south (Mbarara District Planning

Unit, 2011). The district is mainly comprised of the Banyankore tribe who constituted Ankore Kingdom (a social and political kingdom before the coming of the colonialists). The Banyankore speak Runyankore, a Bantu language, although with education many of them also speak English as well, particularly those living in urban communities. The Banyankore are divided into two small ethnic groups namely the Bahima and the Bairu. The Bairu were mainly farmers who traditionally grew millet and occupied the western region; the Bahima (pastoralists) occupied the eastern region of the district. Traditionally the relationship between the Bahima and Bairu was a master-servant relationship with the former ruling the latter in the traditional kingship. Food was a central aspect in the relationship between the two groups. Karugire noted "the economic activities of both Bairu and Bahima were complementary and were based on interdependence through mutual exchange" (Karugire, 1971:22). The Bahima and Bairu traded amongst themselves and the main items of exchange were millet and beer for the Bairu and milk and butter for the Bahima. Millet was also used as an item for the payment of taxes to the local leaders before and after the coming of colonialists in the kingdom. The discussion in this chapter draws examples from the two economic systems adopted by the two ethnic groups in Ankore. A detailed interview with two focus groups (which constituted both men and women) as well as five individual interviews with key informants (including religious, opinion and local leaders) provided the information used in this chapter. The participants' own voices reveal how communities in Ankore used food as a tool for peace. The words of the people are important because they offer facts and reveal their perspectives on the researched issues (Hymes, 1964:375).

Food For Peace

> ...Giving someone a good bull which would produce good cows was used to gain friendship and bring us together for team work and to strengthen relationship. When someone fell in love with a beautiful girl, he would give beautiful cows as dowry. ... We used to hold meetings in the milking area after milking. We would call for meetings and advice one another during these meetings (Kirindi, 2008:7).

Traditionally, food was produced for personal use and also used as a symbol of peace among the members of the community. This involved growing food together as a community and also supporting each other in individual farms. One's relationship with the community would be tested in the way he or she participates in the production of crops such as millet where a lot of labour was required. It was a sign of individualism for one to grow such crops without seeking the support from the community, for which labour was supposed to be reciprocated. All the activities of millet production were supposed to be done communally. Every category of people knew their role in the production of millet and there was no overlapping of those roles, which observed respect and hierarchy of the individual in the society. Produce was shared among the families in the same community as a way of supporting each other in times of need. Today women, more especially those living in rural areas, have used food production to keep or seek peace with others through group production and sharing the produce with others. The respondents in this study explained the different peaceful gestures associated with traditional millet production in Ankore.

One of the respondents interviewed in this study indicated that:

> … in Ankore, traditionally, we grew millet to be able to give to friends and neighbours when they have festivals but also in times of need, say during prolonged dry spells or droughts. We call it 'Otahirira Obugyenyi (food support given to others when they have a function). When you don't give out to others in times of need, then you are not worth a friend or neighbour. During a funeral, when the news of death comes around, the first action one must take is to look for food to take to the bereaved family. Even today, families that buy food during such hard times are questioned!! Their relationships with others are doubted and this means that the community must intervene to find out what is the problem. If it was found that the family in question does not associate with others, they were supposed to pay a fine (goats or beer) as a way of accepting them back in the community.

Another respondent also said that:

> … Millet porridge (entackweka) is a traditional recreational drink, which must be served during ceremonies like 'Kuhingira' (a traditional giveaway ceremony where the parents of the girl give the groom gifts (emihingiro) to help him start a family) as a sign that the visitors are welcome. If someone came to visit you and you don't serve them with this porridge then it means they are not welcome. During marriages, it is not served until the two families agree to the bond of marriage for their children. It is served as gestures that that the two families are joined by the marriage and that each of the two families will thereafter serve each other the drink on each visit.

Another male respondent explained that:

> … No woman with good relations with her in-laws would eat millet without sharing it with her in-laws. Actually, it was an obligation for a wife to keep good relations with her mother-in-law, who traditionally was supposed to do the first harvest from the daughter in law's garden to establish if the millet was ready for harvest. In situations where the father-in-law was still alive, he was supposed to eat the first meal of harvested millet by the daughter-in-law. This meant that the daughter-in-law had to keep a healthy relationship with her in-laws to avoid rejection of her food. Even today, it is a good sign for us as men for our wives to relate well with our families. But when you see a woman taking all the harvest without reserving some for her in-laws, then you just know that there is trouble. [Pauses] By the way, it also keeps respect between wife and husband, because even when I am not at home, I don't

expect my wife to eat all the millet harvested without keeping some for 'Nyineka' (head of a home). Eeeehhhh!! Or else she tells me who has taken over my position!! (Laughter!.

According to one of the key informants:

>...In Ankore, food such as millet and milk was used to settle fines by those whose behaviours were considered unacceptable to the rest of the community. If a child conflicted with his parents, as a punishment, he/she would be required to pay a fine of either millet for the case of Bairu or a cow for the Bahima. Among the Bairu, food items were emphasized so that they are eaten and not kept to maintain the grudge. The food was eaten by the group so that the people involved forget the conflict and move on.

From these excerpts, it is clear that peace building was not a duty of an individual alone, but the whole community. Food was used as a tool for conflict resolution as well as a tool for peaceful co-existence in the society. This was a responsibility for every individual to ensure that they produced enough food so that in situations where the need for food arose, they would be able to comply. This not only contributed to food security but also created peace in the community as conflicts resulting from food insecurity such as theft were controlled. Food for peace also created obligations on individuals as society placed expectations on them regarding food production and sharing, which brought forth values for peaceful communities.

Role of food in the creation of peaceful communities

Food production, processing and consumption played a key role in building peaceful relationships among people living in the same community. Production, whether done individually or in groups, demonstrated the relational engagements of individuals in their communities. Farming, whether by male or female, was done with community involvement in one way or another, which meant that failure to get support sent a different message to the rest of the community.

The Banyankore used food as a medium of exchange to acquire resources that they would not have otherwise. The Banyankore used millet beer to get land from their kings (Omugabe) who were the custodians of land on behalf of the people. According to Mwanahebwa (2006:3), in order for an individual to get land from the king, one would give a gourd of beer in return for land. This showed that food was important to all regardless of whether one owned land or not. This fostered peace in the community. For example, food items such as millet were also used to pay for 'protection' in the form of what was known as 'okutoija' from their leaders.

Millet and milk were used as symbols in rituals such as the traditional ceremonies of blood brotherhood (Omukago), which was a symbol for peace among men in a particular society. Among the Bahima, Omukago would be established by simply giving each other a calf (the best calf in the kraal) to cement such a relationship. When the colonialists first came to Ankore, they underwent the practice as a way of keeping peace with the local leaders in the Kingdom. When Captian Fredrick Lugard (the first British colonial agent) came to Ankore, he underwent the custom of blood brotherhood with several chiefs, the most prominent being the representative of King Ntare (Mwanahebwa, 2006:9). The rationale of the practice was to ensure that the two parties undertaking the ritual would not fight against each other again since it bonded the two parties into brotherhood. Death was the punishment for violation of this oath.

An elderly respondent narrated that:

> In most cases the practice was done out of will of two individuals whose friendship had reached a point of being brothers. Because these were not blood brothers by birth, they opted to instead just eat the blood as a way of compensating for unborn blood links. Sometimes, after the conflicting parties reached an agreement, the mediators subjected them to this bond as a way of keeping a long time or sometimes lifetime brotherhood. The ethnic divide between the Bahima and Bairu were also checked through this symbolized union, which was accepted by the two groups. The practice of brotherhood among the Banyankore involved men usually of different clans coming together to share their blood (cut from each man) which they mixed with local tree species, millet (Bairu) or milk (Bahima) and swallowed.

The bonds created by the two parties involved, involved other family members, lasting for generations. Some of these bonds reached a limit of forbidding family members from marrying each other as they were thought to be blood sisters and brothers. The conflicting families would even exchange their children to grow up in the two different families. Thus food became the core of such peaceful symbols and in this context also applied as symbols of ethnic identity.

The Banyankore used their own local dialect to express the importance of food in ensuring better relationships amongst themselves and also support each other in times of scarcity. They supported each other during times of hunger instead of fighting and causing trouble between each other. People depended on food to keep good relationships between themselves more especially when need arose. An old Ankore proverb of "akaibo kaza owanyamugarura" meant that a basket goes to someone who can refill it. Even when one would be begging, one had to demonstrate that they are capable of giving themselves, before being given. According to Mwanahebwa (2006:3), "In case of famine, one took a small basket of millet and beans to distant relatives. In turn one would be given large baskets of food to take home".

The Banyankore used millet or milk to facilitate a peaceful process through which unmarried men found spouses. The traditional marriage known as 'Okuteera Oruhoko' involved use of millet between the Bairu or milk between the Bahima to initiate marriage. The practice used young men who had been rejected by girls to force them into the Bahima to get marriage-partners without the consent of girls. "Okuteera oruhoko" was done by smearing millet flour on the face of the girl whom the boy has admired or been suggested for marriage. The boy waited for an opportunity to find the girl grinding millet and then he used some of the flour from the basket and smeared it on her face. Then the man ran away which pushed the relatives of the girl to make arrangements for her marriage. The Bahima used milk instead of millet to sprinkle on the girls face during milking. Such boys were charged a double bride price and it was never returned even when the girl divorced.

Food and justice systems

In many African societies food was used as an item of compensation and reconciliation in order to restore peace among the offended parties. If one would be found guilty, she/he would be asked to give food to the offended to settle the conflict and to reconcile with the mediators involved. In Ankore, the food items were supposed to be perishable so that the offended person has no option but to eat it or share it with others so that the case is ended. Thus food was a key item in restorative justice within the community. The offender was supposed to bring enough food so sometimes friends and relatives contributed, so that all the members of the community could take part in celebrating the achieved justice and peace. Thus, the mediator and the neighbours as witnesses all partook in the celebration of the resolved conflict. The aspect of sharing a meal and drinking Milk (for Bahima) or Millet Beer (for Bairu) was very important as a way of concluding reconciliation processes and relaxing the minds and hearts of the conflicting parties.

One of the respondents for this study indicated that:

> for us as Banyankore, that was a sincere and an inward humble way of asking for pardon, mercy, forgiveness and repentance from the offender and acceptance from the offended in order to facilitate reconciliation and co-existence (Key Informants interview.

Food items such as animals and birds were also key in the traditional convents of peace known as "Okukaraba" (Mushanga, 2011). One of the elderly key respondents explained that:

> When a person committed an offence which was regarded to cause ritual danger, such as killing accidently another person, to avoid a bad omen on the family and even the entire clan, a ritual cleansing ceremony was organized in which the culprit and the family would be involved to ensure

that the future generation did not suffer the consequences of the act. This ritual was done by slaughtering a sheep or chicken in the middle of the cross roads (aha ntangatangiro y'emihanda), for reasons that the bad omen associated with the offense would remain stranded in middle of the cross roads and would not follow anyone after the ceremony, or on a special species of tree known as a 'ekyiko' (known to house all bad omen) and each member of the group would wash their hands in the blood collected from the animals while reciting the oath that whatever was done would not be repeated and the offended party would never long for revenge. This event was only organized when the two parties involved had agreed to forgive one another. Abuse of the covenant was associated to death.

The traditional legendary stories that were told also depicted the importance of food as a tool for implementing justice and resolving conflict. The mythical story of Kairu, Kakama and Kahima as told by one of the key respondents demonstrated how the Ruhanga (the creator) used pots of milk to create the stratification of the different classes among the Banyankore, which were intended to create a peaceful environment among the brothers (Doornbos, 1978:20). The story runs as:

> Ruhanga was the God of the Banyankore who came from the skies to earth with his three sons; Kairu, Kakama and Kahima. Fearing that his return to heaven may end up bringing conflict amongst his sons, Ruhanga decided to give them a test, which would simplify his hard decision of choosing the heir to the throne. The king decided to use milk to carry out his test. He gave each of his sons a pot full of milk to keep on their laps throughout the night. As sleep took its toll on the youngest (Kakama), he spilled his milk and had to ask his brother to help him refill his pot. The two brothers filled his pot again. Shortly after, the elder brother also slept and spilled his milk and his brothers could not help him out and by morning he had an empty pot. By morning, Kakama the youngest had passed the test, followed by Kahima the second youngest and Kairu the oldest came last. The elder brothers (Kairu and Kahima) were left to serve their younger brother Kakama. Kairu was declared a servant of the two brothers and Kakama become a herdsman for his young brother (Key Informant, 2014).

Food and peace building in modern times

Talking to people about peace today means so many things beyond absence of conflict. The description of peace by Martin Luther King that "peace is not absence of tension, but presence of justice" (Karen, 1990:3) has given a new understanding of peace to include many things. Those working on peace studies no longer focus on the simplistic view of peace as the product of the end of war but have included the notion of its positive content which looks at the need for justice in relations between societies and the acknowledgement all people are of equal worth (Rodriguez and Natukunda-Tagboa, 2005). Thus looking at peace from a political perspective has become a narrow view to those seeking to understand peace from an individual perspective. During one of the focus group discussions, one of the female respondents questioned the relevance of national political peace when she argued that:

> Peace which does not bring food to the table does not make sense to an ordinary person. Peace should stem from within the household where we live and should be felt in our hearts. I feel more peaceful when my family eat and sleep, than sleeping on hungry stomach because there is peace in the country!! I feel more peaceful when I can dictate things around my life and that is why people here associate gaining weight to peaceful leaving. But how can you gain weight without eating!! To me, food is peace!!

The arguments raised by this female respondent not only draws us to the new meaning of peace in society today, but also brings on board the discussion of peace from a holistic perspective. This involves looking at the person as a whole including his or her public and private life. The private part of a peaceful person rotates around their welfare, which in many cases depends on the person's livelihood. During one of the focus group discussions, another respondent raised a question that stirred debate on the relevancy of peace on individual welfare. She asked: "has anybody ever eaten peace?" To her peace was something she could only associate with a satisfied person. She noted that: "you can only feel peace when you have eaten and absence of food not only disturbs the body, but also steals away the peaceful mind".

Reaching and maintaining peace involves recognition and valuing relationships among people that foster long-term co-operation through the creation of institutions as useful resource for conflict resolution in the community. Food production has been key in creating such relationships among different people in rural areas today. One of the key informants noted that "the current trends of community peace are embedded in farmer groups which are created by members of particular communities". These groups of farmers have been created to boost agricultural production and also play a key role in ensuring that communities live in harmony with each other. Members are encouraged to join the groups for both social and economic reasons. These groups have provided delineated structures, roles, and rules within which group members operate (Colletta and Cullen, 2000:19). The farmer groups are based at various levels from the village to the district.

They have been able to encompass individuals left out of development initiatives for a long time such as women and people of low social caste. These groups have been able to include women giving opportunities to participate in the group's activities, including around leadership. They provide avenues for women's empowerment, through increased involvement in decision making both at household and community levels. A new perspective gaining recognition asserts that the empowerment of women is the only way to achieve lasting peace (Rodriguez and Natukunda-Tagboa, 2005). Group food production has played a key role in empowering rural women in Uganda, which has had a positive impact on reducing conflicts, especially at the household level. Women have been able to speak to each other about the conflicts in their households and have found support from other women to deal with them. They have also been able to raise money to address their relatives or sometimes their own husbands with respect to any injustices surrounding them. One of the female respondents noted that:

> Being in this group has given me a new meaning of the notion of peace. I know for sure now that peace means freedom from many things. A poor person can never have peace and can never say farewell to conflicts. I feel more peaceful now because I am free from violence, I can access basic needs without any hassle; I command mutual respect from my family members and community. I have total command of my body and spirit.

Women have taken a lead in mobilizing community based farmers groups that contribute greatly to community peace building. Women community production groups have been promoting food security, a key element in community peace building as a state without food is a state of conflict. These groups have mobilised women against community-based violence as they give women a new face before the community. They provides solutions to causes of domestic violence related to production and income management. Women have used these groups to find mechanism to deal with conflicting situations in their households, as well as with conflict with members of the community.

Women have been able to contribute to community peace through ensuring that there is enough nutritious food in their homes, which creates happy homes. Husbands gain some economic freedom by managing surplus production. This not only facilitates individual peace, but also community peace. One of the respondents explained that; "a peaceful community is made by food and women are food". There was consensus among the respondents that a community without women cannot eat and a hungry mind is the genesis of conflict. Another respondent said that;

> during the era of Amin (President of Uganda from 1971-1979), there were general tensions in the country and a lot of insecurity. The government instituted compulsory cotton production for each and every home, which was supervised by the local chiefs (Mayumba kumi). Men thus transferred all their production time to cotton production leaving food production to women. The women supported their homes by ensuring that there was a constant food supply which controlled the conflict from reaching the household level.

Conclusions

Migration and other social and economic challenges remain major limitations in adopting the traditional methods of justice. Drawing from the contributions made by the MatoOput (which means drinking the herb of the Oput tree) and nyouo tong gweno (which means stepping on an egg over opobo twig) which was re-adopted by the Acholi, in Gulu, Northern Uganda after the Kony insurgence and the Gacaca System in Rwanda after the 1994 genocide, it is clear that traditional justice systems are still relevant in administering justice to create peaceful communities, particularly in rural areas,

Food supports endogenous approaches of building community peace. In Ankore, the "Okukaraba" approach was useful in creating peaceful living among the people of Ankore. Wherever these traditional practices have been used, such communities have enjoyed peace and avoided conflicts. The traditional approaches to justice contribute to the healing of the community and parties involved and also build social trust.

The Banyankore say, "eka yenjara tebura nduru" (meaning a family besieged with hunger is always in quarrels and fights). This is an indication that food is the source of peace in a family and once it is lacking it is every body's concern. The absence of food in Ankore is blamed on a woman who is expected to ration food to ensure that her family has a full supply of food throughout the year. This places the duty of ensuring a peaceful home in the hands of the woman. The story of the Banyankore of the mother who cooked stones for her family demonstrates the woman's strategy to keep a peaceful home even in situations of food crisis. The story goes that; " once in a while during a famine in the history of Ankore, a mother who had nothing to give her children decided to cook stones to keep her hungry children hopeful that food was about to come. They dozed off one by one, thinking that their mother would wake them up as soon as food was ready" (key informant). She was able to keep her home calm despite the fact that the members of the family were hungry. This helped her to sort herself out later in the morning as the Ankore proverb says that 'agwayosha, guhuha empoza' (meaning that a postponed case gives you time for an alternative solution). Thus the role of women in peace building, particularly at household level cannot be doubted as they undertake their role of food providers.

Women as managers of food at household level ensured that their families did not end up in crisis and thus ensure that they were consulted on every decision made in regard to food use. Men would therefore, not make any decisions without consulting their wives whom they referred to as 'nyina bwenge' (meaning the mother of wisdom). This dependency on women for answers in relation to family management was translated into other aspects of life including conflict resolution. It was a common practice for a man faced with a challenge of mediating conflicting situation to ask for some time to 'sleep over' the problem. This meant that men needed to get time to consult their wives whose confidence could only be established in her ability to keep her family together using food.

The wife in any home had a final say on the whether the visitor would get a glass of millet/milk as a gesture of peace at the household level. Much as husbands owned homes, the duty of expression of peaceful gestures remained in the hands of the woman. She would decide to offer 'her' millet to the people she was pleased to give otherwise, the man would not want to shame himself and would find an excuse to see off the visitor. Thus a peaceful home was managed by a woman and food was the power she used to perform this role. Much as many things have changed in modern homes, this role has not changed and instead has moved from home to public places where secretaries or office messengers, jobs that are usually done by women, took up this role in public places like offices. Thus the role of women in peace building should not be undermined and efforts invested in empowering women to ensure food security should also extend to the notion of community peace building. Those who have perceived women as victims of conflict have not realized that women are also victims of peace. They need to be involved in the peace making processing to which they contribute greatly through their innovations in food security and household management. Thus, their capacities and contribution to food security should be drawn upon in community peace building.

References

Colletta, N. and Cullen, M. (2000) *The Nexus between Violent Conflict, Social Capital and Social Cohesion: Case Studies from Cambodia and Rwanda*, World Bank, Washington DC.

Doornboss, M. (1978) *Not All the King's Men: Inequality as a Political Instrument in Ankore Uganda*, Mouton Publishers, The Hague.

Haidar, H. (2009) *Community-based Approaches to Peacebuilding in Conflict-affected and Fragile Contexts,* Issues Paper, International Development Department, University of Birmingham.

Hymes, D. (1998). *"When is Oral Narrative Poetry? Generative Form and its Pragmatic Conditions ",* International Pragmatics Association (4): pp. 475-500.

Karugire, S. (1970) Relations between the Bairu and the Bahima in the Nineteenth Century Nkore, *Tarikh*, vol. 13, no. 2, pp. 22-33.

Kirindi, P. (2008) *History and Culture of the Kingdom of Ankore*, Fountain Publishers, Kampala.

Mbarara District Planning Unit (2011) *Higher Local Government Statistical Abstract: Mbarara District*, Republic of Uganda.

Morrison, K. (1990) *Education for Human Rights*, Longman, Namibia

Mushanga T. (2011) *Criminal Homicide in Uganda,* Law Africa Publishing (U) Ltd, Kampala.

Mwanahebwa, A. (2009) *Bribery: An Exploration of Uganda Perspectives*, Éthiqueet Économique/Ethics and Economics, 4 (2).

Robertson, A. (2012) *Enabling Agricultural Extension for Peace Building; Special Report 320*, United States Institute for Peace.

Rodriguez, D. and Natukunda-Tagboa E. (2005) *Gender and Peace Building in Africa*, University of Peace, Costa Rica.

Simmons, E. (2013) Harvesting Peace: Food Security, Conflict and Cooperation *Environmental Change & Security Report* Vol. 14, Issue 03, Woodrow Wilson International Center for Scholars, Washington DC.

Waldman, M. (2008) *Community Peace Building in Afghanistan: The Case of a National Strategy*, OXFAM International Research Report.

CHAPTER 2. WOMEN'S PROTECTION AND MECHANISMS OF CONFLICT RESOLUTION IN ANKORE FAMILIES

Clementia Neema Murembe

Introduction

Gender discrimination and the subordinate position of women to men has not only attracted worldwide attention but also influenced policies and guidelines, to empower and improve gender relations at international, national, local and family levels. (European Commission 2012; UNDP 2012)While this study focuses on women's empowerment and gender relations in decision-making in Ankore families, gender inequality is a global problem. Women's empowerment therefore, is advocated as a crucial intervention strategy for transforming worldwide gender inequality and discrimination. (UN 1979, 2013)

The Ugandan government has adopted inclusion of women into political and policy decision-making positions to enhance gender equality. (Tamil 1993, 2003) Gender-sensitive strategies like amendments in land policy were included in the national planning programmes in the 1995 Ugandan Constitution and the 1997 Local Government Act (Republic of Uganda 2010; 2011) granting women CSOs and NGOs such as Fida-U an autonomous working environment. (Tripp 2001; Tripp et al 2009) Fida-U is a non-governmental association that is privately run by women lawyers who intervene in family problems through advocacy and interpretation of the law. Government institutions specifically constituted for the protection of women's rights (such as the Family Protection Unit in the police, Family Courts and Probation Offices at district level), were all put in place. The Government institutionalised local councils as local courts to bring law and justice close to the people. (Mushemeza 2009)

Despite strategies put in place to empower women, gender inequalities in decision-making are still evident at household level. Women's decision-making power in family resource use, control and ownership capacity, are still relatively low compared to men. This chapter examines whether the existing strategies and institutions have improved gender relations at household level in Ankore families. Women's empowerment is evaluated from the participants' perspectives of married women's social wellbeing in terms of their protection and success in family conflict resolution. The focus is on married women's awareness, use of established institutions, gender parity and women's protection in Ankore family relations. The evaluation of women's empowerment is based on a survey of 240 married people, 20 separated women, 50 elderly and institutional leaders' key informants and 11 Focus Group Discussions (FGDs) of married men and women who shared their own personal opinions and experiences.

Causes and mechanism to resolve family conflicts in traditional Ankore families

There is a saying in Ankore: "people that live together cannot avoid quarrelling", meaning that family relations where husband, wife and their relatives co-exist, conflicts are bound to happen. Marital and family conflicts occur in practically all families, but with differences in context, magnitude, frequency and the intervention mechanisms for resolving them. Marital and family conflicts are understood and expressed in different words or phrases, referring to different situations occurring in the day-to-day life of the people in Ankore. These include:

- obuteikirizana (disagreements),
- oburyaane (conflicts),
- okurwanagana (fights),
- omuhondano (non-compromising),
- oburemeezi (difficult relations)
- okugumizana omumaka (Creation of difficult environment for each other).

These situations involve couples' frequent quarrels, fights, withdrawal, silence, victimisation and abuse of their children. The result is transferred anger, evasion of family obligations, desertion of the family, refusal to eat and denial of sex. Some of these conflicts can be resolved internally by the couples themselves, while others require an intervention of mediators like parents, relatives, friends, neighbours, religious leaders or courts of law. In situations of extreme conflict, or failure of the couple or mediators to resolve the problems, some people opt for separation or divorce. Traditional causes of family conflicts in Ankore, (problems such as lack of basic needs, childlessness, hereditary diseases and wife-beating), are identified and discussed. Escalating poverty, financial constraints, dependency syndromes, time constraints, work-related stress and differences of religion, tribes and education, were identified as new challenges facing family relations today. Some of these problems are explained in detail below:

Lack of basic needs of life or cases of irresponsibility

The respondents in this study confirmed what has been cited by various authors (European Commission 2012; Butamanya 1992; Mubangizi 1963) that the mode of life in pre-colonial traditional Ankore families was relatively egalitarian, more or less dependent upon nature. The population was still very small compared with the available resources hence the basic needs of life, such as shelter, food or clothing (made out of skins and bark cloths) were available locally. The number of items per person depended on the wealth of the family. However, over time, these basic needs have been changing in quality and quantity. Traditionally marital conflicts resulting from lack of basic needs were relatively few and in cases where husbands failed to provide clothing and proper shelter for their families, other family members or friends intervened to help out. This would be the result of the wife reporting it to her relatives, principally her in-laws and particularly the mother-in law). The natal home of the wife only came in to support the family in question when the husband's family was unable. However, such situations were avoided as it brought shame to the husband and his family. The interventions from family and friends included giving food and other household needs as well as disciplining and fining of the husband by fellow kinsmen as a corrective measure against him. The fines would include a goat and/or a pot of local beer, depending on the gravity of the matter. For fear of stronger measures, such as being beaten or ex-communicated from family membership, he would abide by and cater to his family's needs. In scenarios where the husband had physical or psychological ill health, the 'extended' family members would take on the responsibility to provide and protect the wife and the children. The role of family members or friends in Ankore was thus very important in marital conflict resolution, hence the Ankore proverb 'abeinekiramura tibeitana', (those who have advisers cannot fail to be corrected or those with interveners cannot kill each other).

Childlessness

In Ankore families a childless marriage was not recognised as marriage in the traditional setting and it was unbearable for a man to acknowledge and be known as impotent and childless. On the other hand, a woman would live with barrenness but she could look after her husbands' children from other women. It was acceptable for a man to divorce a childless wife, especially if she had other problems with the family members. The participants emphasised that problems hindering procreation called for the concerted attention of the family, to avoid the most feared after-effects of someone dying childless (enfanabujune). (It was believed that if someone died childless, his or her spirit would haunt those left behind). In situations where the family of the impotent man did not have male relatives to produce children with his wife, it was acceptable for a woman to divorce her husband and for the enjugano (bride price) to be returned, so allowing her to get some other man. Some of the traditional mechanisms that were applied to solve childlessness and to save the marriage included the use of diviners or traditional healers, marrying another wife, or allowing the wife to produce with her in-laws enabling the couple to get children. Although the mechanism of wife sharing by brothers or relatives was said to be disappearing among the elites in urban areas, it is still maintained among rural families, especially among unschooled and pastoralist-bahima families. The participants argued that wife-sharing mechanisms not only left the impotent husband and wife psychologically and physically happy but also kept family secrets, which kept the family relationship stable.

Comparing traditional mechanisms to the modern handling of childlessness, the elderly key informants explained that modern society today regards childless women as 'Ebiifeera' (worthlessness or useless persons). They explained that unlike the traditional approach of secretiveness to sexual problems, modern society handles such problems inappropriately in the public forum. They said that it is not only improper but also unhelpful for a woman to publicly reveal sexually related issues to non-partisan members. They argued that barrenness or impotence should never be openly revealed, as the public doesn't have solutions for childlessness and the resulting conflicts. There were culturally acceptable means of knowing secret problems and addressing them privately. Family members could detect the likelihood of conjugal problems affecting their newly married family members and find solutions within the family. A Runyankore proverb that 'the eye of an elder is decisive' explains how elders had the skills to observe and interpret signals of a problem without asking or being told by the concerned person. Hence, the problem would be dealt with even without the whole family knowing, for instance, the wife-sharing mechanism.

Hereditary diseases or habits

Chronic diseases are costly, have an impact on a family's happiness and a source of family conflict. To avoid such problems precautionary secret and open investigations were carried out prior to and in the process of choosing a marriage partner. The emphasis on the matter was expressed by use of the Runyankore proverb translated as 'the one who intends to marry or to be married should always make precautionary investigations and consultations about the person and the family they wish to marry or get married to". Families with hereditary diseases tended to marry each other. In recent times, however, the principle of consultations before marriage has been dishonoured and ignored, primarily among the elite and co-habiting spouses. Although there would be no guarantee of knowing and avoiding every disease and behavioural practice, traditional enquiries were said to have minimized the spread of certain diseases and habits in families that did not have them previously. The hereditary diseases that were said to be avoided include epilepsy, cancer, leprosy, elephantiasis, propensity to madness, suicidal tendencies, night dancing, witchcraft practices, cannibalism, barrenness, separation or divorce tendencies. Due to the fact that such hereditary problems disrupted family relations, avoiding them was a great mechanism for protecting family members and relations.

Problems of drunkenness

Prior to formal employment and the advent of the money economy brought by the colonial government in Uganda, drunkenness was not a problem in Ankore. Alcohol products were prepared at home and freely taken by family members and neighbouring families in the evenings; for example 'amaarwa' (alcohol beverage made out of sorghum and millet). A few isolated cases of drunken men who fought with their wives were noted. Such men were given sanctions such as being denied free social drink. The social sanctions of isolation by the family and community members used to protect the wife and children against mistreatment by their drunken husbands. The gender perspectives in the traditions of social drinking indicated that women were expected to drink moderately in their homes or their immediate neighbourhood. Whilst the drunkenness of a man would be tolerated, that of a woman would disrupt marital and family relations and could lead to marriage breakup.

Wife beating

Wife beating was common among the Bairu and Bahima, it being condoned in Ankore traditional families. Women were not allowed to scream or fight back during such fights. to keep such fights private not to cause more anger from the husbands. One of the female key informants explained that: "when a wife would be beaten, she would not fight back or flee yelling outside the homestead; instead she was expected to run to the inner-room or back yard, where she would either be thoroughly beaten or be left free. The advice was that a woman should never scream, run away or fight back her husband".

Although wife-beating was presented as a habit, sometimes it happened as a consequence of some other problems existing in the home which could include unwelcoming wives, neglecting in-laws, mistrust and suspiciousness, arrogance of wives, a nagging personality, poor hygiene, sexual dissatisfaction, rumour-mongering, and witchcraft. Today more causes of fights among the couple were listed to include drunkenness, extra-marital affairs, inferiority or superiority complex and disagreements about the use and control of family resources. To sustain family relations in such situations Ankore family values dictate that women should be tolerant and compromising so as to remain in their marriages. In a few instances, a wife would decide to fight her husband to defend herself and if she proved a match, or even stronger than the husband, the practice of wife-battering either reduced or stopped. When the children (mostly boys) of a recurrently beaten mother grew up, they would intervene to protect their mother. In such circumstances, the child could be punished for the unbecoming act of beating up the parent. It was reported that wife beating has now reduced in modern society. Several reasons for this include the rule of law that criminalize open fights, increased levels of education, the impact on social status, and protection of their public image,.

Traditional strategies to combat and protect women against domestic violence

This section presents the indigenous mechanisms of combating domestic violence against women and promoting better family relations in Ankore. These mechanisms included temporary separation and involvement of kinsmen, traditional arbitration, beating up the brother-in law, silence and consultation of diviners and herbalists. All these are discussed in detail below.

Temporary separation and kinsmen involvement

When wife beating became extreme, the wife needed to seek the intervention of her natal family or community by leaving her marital home temporarily. This is known as 'okwangana' (wife protesting the way she is being treated). There were also scenarios where husbands forced their wives to go back to their natal family - known as 'okubinga omukazi' (dismissing the wife). However, this was differentiated from okushenda (divorce and return of bride price) that usually came as the last resort. Temporary separation would facilitate the healing process of reconciliation. Absence from each other was a moment for self-reflection, for the couple to realise the worthiness of being together in the home, hitherto taken for granted. Separation itself would naturally heal the relationship and there would be no need for arbitration procedures. It would give parents and concerned relatives on both sides an opportunity to examine the couple's problems and enough time to address them amicably. Temporary separation was a learning experience for the couple on how to better handle their differences and appreciate importance of each other.

Traditional arbitration and process

After staying for a while at her natal home, the traditional arbitration meeting (composed of natal and marital parents, relatives and trusted community members, especially the elders) would be convened. Each party would be given a chance to present the issues responsible for their misunderstanding. The guiding principle during the 'eishazi' (traditional arbitration meeting) was to listen and observe emotions carefully, in order to interpret the given information, which in most cases remains implicit. From the traditional Ankore perspective, the intention was not to suppress or hide evidence in order to win or lose the presented case. There was effort to ensure the couple did not lose their tempers and say what should have been left unsaid, to safeguard their integrity and family secrets. The sanctions imposed on the offender integrated counselling and reconciliation. The Ankore arbitration process encouraged dialogue between the conflicting parties while other family and society members listened, allowing the aggrieved partners to air their differences as they narrated their plight. In most instances the verdict made through such reconciliation mechanisms of family meetings and intervention, was accepted and family relations restored. It was mentioned that, although the mechanism is still in use, conflicting spouses nowadays generally tend not to adhere to the reconciliation process and resolutions made by family members.

Beating by the brother-in-law

Beating up of the husband by a brother-in-law, though rarely used, was acceptable and used by some of the people in Ankore as a way of punishing a cruel man. This was often used in situations where other mechanisms had failed. The relatives of the woman would consider it demeaning to her for the husband to continue mistreating their sister even after caution. The brother(s)-in-law would trap the husband of their sister either on the way into the drinking place or when he came to negotiate for the usual reconciliations, and there beat him thoroughly. Although its contribution to protection of family relations was confirmed, the respondents reported that further wife beating tended to persist. This practice is slowly dying out due to widespread rule of law against fights for revenge.

Silence

Silence was expected of a married woman as a tool, a sign of compromise, to avoid wrath and violent confrontations from her husband. The respondents explained that, normally, husbands became impatient of, and intolerant to, argumentative wives especially when they were stressed, infuriated or under the influence of alcohol. Hence, they expected such women to be quiet. It was therefore argued that "a wise" woman normally sensed those moods and avoided being irksome to the already-disturbed husband. There is a famous story known to most people in Ankore, which was repeatedly shared by married woman interviewees, which illustrates the value attached to silence as a mechanism to avoid or minimise marital and family conflicts. It was explained that this story is usually told to advise nagging women who may not know why they are always being beaten by their husbands. An English version of the story is below.

> One day a woman decided to consult a diviner to control her husband's hot temper and restore peace at home. She informed the medicine man that her husband comes home quarrelling and is very furious with everyone; and that whenever she tries to question him, the beating starts immediately. From the composure and manner of speaking, the medicine man suspected the 'pesky' behaviour of the woman. He gave her coloured water, as medicine, in a container. She was to take a mouthful and keep it in her mouth for a while whenever her husband came home, which she did. Because she could not talk with water in her mouth she did not get trouble with her husband for the whole week. When she updated the diviner on the progress of the treatment, the medicine man gave her more doses of coloured water for over a month and by the end of it a new improved relationship had been formed in the family.

Rather than the water, other study participants spoke of a herbal weed leaf which was meant to be stored under her tongue. When the woman went to thank the medicine man later, he became parental and revealed to her that there was no medicine involved but the leaf under her tongue or water in the mouth controlled her speech. However, some forms of silence were deemed to have resulted in worsening marital and family conflicts, especially when it was interpreted as being arrogant or demeaning to a husband. Actually, the elite and urban participants expressed silence as a sign of defeatism and acceptance of subordinate position.

Consultation of diviners and herbalists

Although consultation of diviners and herbalists is associated with paganism, (Mubangizi 1963) the respondents in this study maintained that every single event that happened to an individual or community was never ignored and assumed to be alright. Although Christianity in Africa criticised traditional beliefs and practices as satanic, the practice of consulting diviners has continued where it has been deemed necessary. (Kasenene 1993) Traditionally any unusual event had to be understood, especially with the help of 'omuhangwa' (a person who is thought to have gifts of interpreting events and if need be, offer solutions to rectify the situation before hand). (Karwemera 1994; Kasenene 1993) So families also consulted these diviners to establish why a particular family experienced such misfortunes as their daughters and sons have unstable marriages. The herbalist would then provide medicine or other traditional remedies to guard against the bad spirits that would be responsible for breaking families.

Divorce

It was both unfortunate and disgraceful when divorce took place in Ankore, not only for the married woman but also for her family. When divorce happened frequently among the girls of particular families, it would be used as a measure of their daughters' stability in their marital and family relations. Consequently, in the enquiry process of searching for a wife, the trait of 'failing to make homes' would be used against the other girls, casting doubt on their credibility and stability in marriage. Considering the value attached to marriage in the Ankore families, married women endured bitter relations to safeguard against such remarks and consequences. However, some of the respondents explained that, rather than insisting on irreconcilable partners staying together, the traditions of Ankore provided for dissolution of fatal marriage relations. Ankore family traditions opted for divorce (okutaana or okushenda) as the way out, so that a couple could escape a hostile and risky relationship. It was emphasized that divorce was the only way to nullify the existing legal customary marriage and set the woman free for re-marriage, although a man could marry other wives without any hindrances.

It should be noted however that, as material needs in Ankore families kept increasing and changing over of time, family problems as well as conflicts and mechanisms for resolving them were also transformed. There has been a transition from traditional approaches in conflict resolution to more modern approaches. However, due to changes in the nature of family problems and trust in some of the traditional approaches, people in Ankore still generally use both traditional and conventional legal mechanisms to resolve conflicts in families. Figure 1 illustrates the situational analysis of changes in marital and family problems in Ankore family relations.

Figure 1. Analysis of changes in marital and family problems, applied mechanisms and implications on position of women

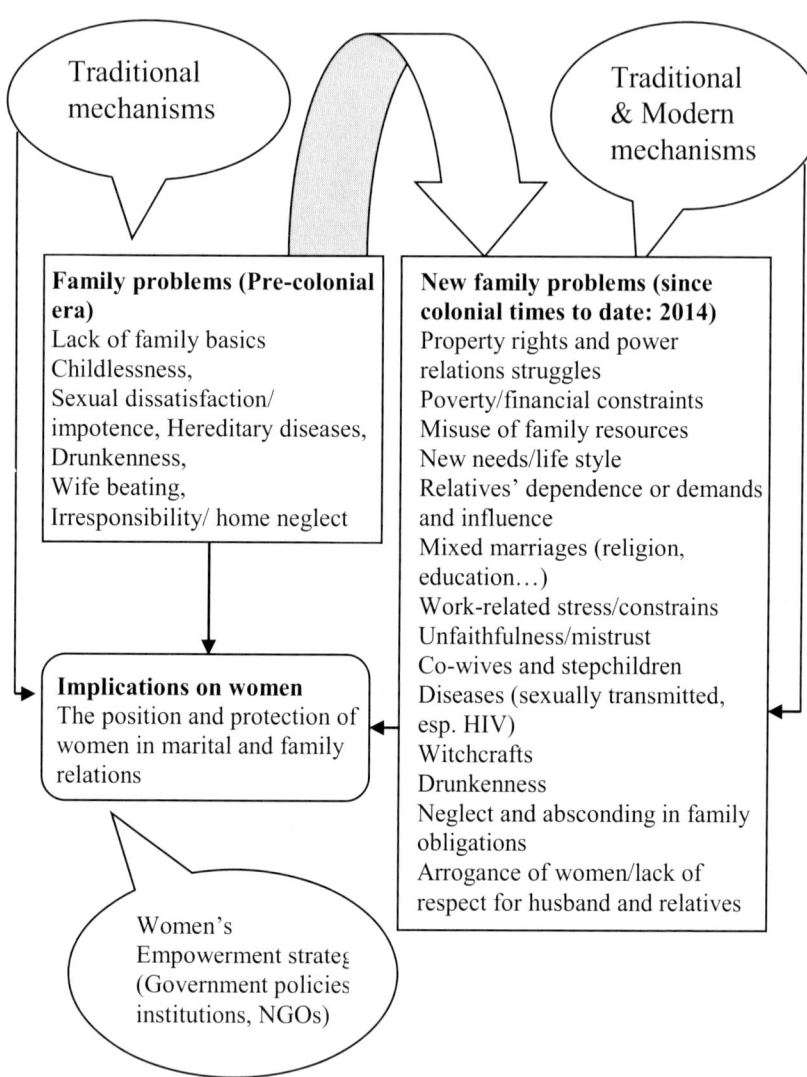

Source: Designed from collected field data (Neema, 2014)

Figure 1 shows a spread out of traditional problems and resolution mechanisms into the current families' situation. Consequently, figure 1 indicates that traditional conflict resolution mechanisms as well as new mechanisms are in use, and apparently, more often than not, the two systems operate in contradiction of each other, as will be discussed. According to the participants, in that situation there are various outcomes to and implications of both systems on the protection of women in family relations.

Current problems, mechanisms and implications on women in family relations

This section analyses the new problems associated with families that result in conflicts and how the new mechanisms of rule of law and their outcomes impact on the protection of women in Ankore family relations. The new problems identified and discussed in this section include poverty and financial constraints, affluence and its challenges, struggle and control over family resources, workloads and conjugal obligations, drunkenness and poor communication system and gaps.

Poverty and financial constraints

Poverty or the inability to satisfy increasing family needs was identified as a main cause of conflict with the family. The increasing financial demand from the needs of family and relatives strains husbands. This usually results in quarrels adversely affecting relations within the family. Husbands' relatives tend to blame their daughters in-law for being responsible for the limited support they get from their sons. The relatives' demands create financial constraints on family resources and consequently the couple's relationship. The basic needs and other necessities of life such as education costs, medical care and standards of living in homes are becoming increasingly hard to obtain and sustain. A family beset by poverty is never free of quarrels and conflicts.

Affluence and its challenges

Issues of money and the quest for affluence have created conflict, especially in relation to its use, control and ownership. Abundance, especially in the hands of husbands, has led to luxury drinking with casual friends or having extra-marital affairs. Such behaviour potentially leads to other problems relating to health (such as sexually transmitted diseases, including HIV/AIDS), infidelity, financial costs, rivalry of co-wives and stepchildren which have often cause marital and family conflicts. On the one hand, in cases where a wife has a better-paying job and has more money than her husband, inferiority complexes of husbands or superiority complexes of women have also caused marital and family conflict. Respondents explained that in male headed households the change in responsibilities where women do much to provide for the household needs undermines husbands who feel placed in a secondary role. Women have improved their economic power through taking jobs outside the home and taking on much of the welfare cost of the household.

On the other hand, men are finding it increasingly difficult to get better paying jobs to meet all the financial obligation of their families. This situation results in dependency on the woman's income. These two scenarios have caused conflict in families that adhere to the mentality that the men should have higher incomes and total control of women's income. It also came out clearly that respondents believed it would be better in the home if a man had a higher income than his wife. They argue that when the man earns more he keeps the headship position giving him psychological and physiological satisfaction, thus enabling married women to peacefully keep the home.

Power struggle and control of family resources

Male control over family properties, including their wives (as part of a husband's property), causes conflict in Ankore homes. Power struggles in the home are exacerbated by misinterpretations of the western approach to women's emancipation, which is locally understood to mean uplifting the status of women over men in the competitive development agendas. Women's empowerment is seen as 'copying and pasting' foreign practices without discerning what is suitable or acceptable in Ankore family relations. Consequently, it attracts opposition and resistance from husbands. Men respond to women's empowerment by manipulation, exploitation, withdrawing contributions to family requirements or drinking, among other habits. These result in more conflicts.

Workload Burdens and conjugal obligations

It is hard to balance the demands of income-generating activities with domestic work and conjugal obligations. The majority of married women said that they have hired full-time housemaids to do most of the domestic work. Husbands expressed disappointment at the increasing number of married women who are not only resigning from domestic work and leaving it to the house maids but are also sacrificing their conjugal obligations in pursuit of income-generating activities (money-making). The married women also explained that being out-of-home for longer hours brought challenges of entrusting their homes to the housemaids, and declining sexual desire, due to busy work schedules and tiredness. With multiple responsibilities, most women revealed that they are usually too torn apart and worn out to attend to their husbands and family obligations.

Drunkenness

Traditionally, drinking was for social gatherings in the evenings, but today drinks can be obtained any time of the day. Drunkenness was reported to be increasing and problematic in marital and family relations. For instance, a drunken husband comes back late at night and makes inconvenient sexual demands, no matter what the wife's health condition may be. He also demands hot food past midnight, or warm water for bathing, even when there are no facilities in the home to ensure such services at that time. Participants noted that drunkard men usually do not want to bath and clean their mouth before going to bed. Furthermore, it was mentioned that, sometimes, women who complain about their husband's hygiene meet violence or are forced out of the house for assuming too much 'power' in the home. It was explained that drinking acts lead to other family problems, especially poverty, misappropriation of family resources, failure to meet family needs, lack of guidance for children, open domestic violence and unfaithfulness, the last of which makes the couple susceptible to health risks, especially HIV/AIDS.

Poor communication systems and gaps

Although 90% of participants identified the need for clear communication and a flow of information as being important in marital and family relations, it was noted there is a tendency amongst married couples to hide information from one another. The participants explained that lack of communication results in rumours, mistrust and conflict. It was reasoned that because informants feel that they have to report some sort of information, they sometimes tell lies, which always exacerbates family problems.

Mechanisms currently used in family conflict resolutions

This section presents mechanisms that couples currently apply in resolving family conflict and also provides a critique of the traditional mechanisms that were used.

Resilient traditional methods

Within Ankore culture parents, especially the father-in-law, are respected as the head of the family or clan. It is therefore the responsibility of family heads to convene meetings to resolve conflict within their families. Bypassing such protocol, especially in families having a strong network and cohesion, is interpreted as undermining family relations. This usually results in criticism of the behaviour of the married woman, regardless of whether or not she is wronged by the husband. Married women that live far away in urban places explained that they tend to consult friends or workmates for resolving their family problems due to the absence of their parents or kinsmen. Traditional mechanisms are used as a way of cooling the temper of their partners in order to amicably overcome their differences. They are mostly used by women. Women who seek other mechanisms were criticised for forgetting the traditions of silence, compromising their views and transferring socio-economic and politically attained status into marital homes to demean their husbands.

Some men also compromise their views and interests to avoid open conflicts. For instance, elderly key informants, referred to the cultural advice given to men in the proverb 'when a man is perturbed, he should resort to his smoking pipe'. The message behind it was that the pipe was a diversion from the angered husband's mind to prevent him taking inappropriate action. The informants explained that one cannot talk seriously with something in the mouth. Besides tobacco being a sedative would eventually soothe the mind to reduce the anger. Currently, while some men may still smoke, others may take a walk away from home, stay longer at the place of work or have a social drink with friends till late in the night to find the wife already asleep or having forgotten. The compromising traditional approach for husbands and wives is in line with the silence strategy Parpart & Kabeer (2010).

Legal institutions and mechanisms of family conflicts resolution

Some married women, particularly those living in urban areas, had used legal courts of law to resolve domestic conflicts. A few rural women also mentioned that they used the legal system (police, the International Federation of Women Lawyers (FIDA) or the Probation Office), having realised that parents and relatives are either the cause of their family problems or are unable to objectively assist in resolving their problems. Women use courts of law when traditional mechanisms become subjective and doubtable, or when such procedures have been exhausted without ending the conflict. Although the extent to which the legal offices are used in addressing marital and family conflicts was small among the sampled respondents, some couples find them helpful as alternative mechanisms for family conflict management. Nevertheless, elderly key informants expressed reservations and resentment towards married women who resort to legal institutions.

Since the constitutional provision for the protection of women's rights, and the use of the legal court system to achieve this goal, is not connected to traditional family values and customs, this has had regrettable consequences for women who sought redress through legal institutions. The process of reaching verdicts by courts of law to protect married women does not consider the underlying risks they face under customary law, such as being exposed to brutal violence and loss of marriage. There is an increasing number of cases of domestic violence reported in the region, although the rate of those brought to a conclusion is very low. Records at the Rwizi-South Western Regional office for 2012 revealed that out of the 369 cases reported to different police stations in the region, 366 were still under investigation and only 3 cases were forwarded to court (Regional office records, 2013).

Recommended mechanisms

Both traditional and Western legal methods have been shown to have weaknesses, yet family conflicts are an accepted part of human existence. While there were differences between participants attitudes towards using traditional of legal mechanisms, they still tended to recommend the same alternatives for dealing with home conflicts) They recommended that married people should live a responsible life and share family obligations as much as they can without force or waiting for external intervention. Others mentioned family discussions and agreement in decision-making as options. It was noted that in the family meetings and discussion, there is also self-counselling and reflections, although others suggested a need to consult or train counsellors in the field of family therapy.

Through 'people initiatives', study participants mentioned that village-institutions and self-help organisations to which they belonged not only played a role in relation to income-generating activities and social support but also for reconciliation purposes. These groups work independently of local council systems and offer each other counselling. They also offer reconciliation sessions to conflicting spouses whose problems affect the participation of their membership. One chairperson of a self-help organisation revealed that they had successfully resolved some 25 family disputes since the initiation of their group in 2006, having realised that courts of law and relatives were causing division.

Conclusions

The colonial administration adopted new systems of western legal mechanisms to address social and family problems concurrently with the traditional mechanisms that were in place, irrespective of cultural differences, and this has remained so to date. The study findings indicate there are weaknesses in both the traditional rule of people and western legal systems of rule of law. The study participants noted that as material demands increased for basic needs in Ankore families, the problems and mechanisms of conflicts resolutions have altered. Although there is resilience in traditional systems for conflict resolution, the social transformation has changed the issues confronting families from traditional problems to more economy-related ones. The study deduces that there is no single mechanism that successfully works in improving marital and family relations. Although high-profile married spouses tend not to use legal courts and traditional mechanisms, the other women in rural areas mostly use any of the existing mechanisms that seem to offer solutions for their protection.

From the comparative analysis of traditional and western legal approaches of family conflict resolution, the study notes that Ankore families have an inbuilt traditional system of resolving family conflicts which is adhered to by family members. There is resilience in the indigenous mechanisms of consulting parents, relatives, friends and trusted married people in community for family conflict management. Married couples who live or work outside their home environment still use indigenous mechanisms of marital and family conflicts resolution. Traditional practices are still used but do not fit easily with the rule of law. Traditional family conflict resolution mechanisms are based on the rule and will of the people and are built on societal values, which generally leaves conflicting partners willing to accept the verdict reached. Such outcomes and agreed consensus resolutions are said to have protected women in their marital and family relations more than those resulting from the rule of law in the adopted western legal system.

The contradictions in the operation of traditional approaches with those of the western legal system undermine and weaken each other. The resistance of indigenous traditional systems to which people in Ankore still seem to be strongly attached undermines legal mechanisms. Being an imported and imposed foreign system, the legal system is not fully understood, accepted or seen as appropriate for respecting the secrecy and privacy attached to family relations. As such my study notes that in most cases, the legal guidelines have remained well intentioned and documented, without helping the intended beneficiaries, the women subjected to gender-based violence. At the same time, traditional mechanisms, including the local council systems, are undermined by the legal system, and are equally incompetent in addressing contemporary issue, leaving married women dissatisfied with the process of family conflict resolution. Participants in the study noted that both legal and traditional systems are inefficient and ineffective in the protection of married women in family relations. Finally, my study concludes that neither the existing legal institutions nor the traditional mechanisms have necessarily enabled married women to attain equality with men, nor have they granted them protection in Ankore family relations.

Table 1. Comparative analysis of indigenous and Western legal mechanisms of family conflict resolution

Characteristics	Traditional Approach [TA]	Western Approach [WA]	Participants' opinions
Mediators and their qualifications	• Family members form a council/*eishaazi*. • Clan leaders/*ekika*, • Community respected elders and neighbors of both sexes, • Diviners, healers and herbalists, • No formal training • Use of experience	• Trained professionals • Lawyers • Police • Judges and magistrates • Local Councils (mostly not trained) • Religious leaders	• Mediators and the conflicting family members in TA know each other unlike in the WA where they are strangers to each other. • There is a sense of trust in TA and mistrust or fears in WA. • Family members in TA are sometimes the causes of conflicts; they have become subjective and thus lose neutrality in finding solutions. • WA is usually corruptible.
Venue and attire	• Sit in a house or compound of • Rivaling couples • Parents of the husband or of the wife • Casual wears	• Sit at established courts of law • Room is reserved for arbitration • Official court attires or vestments	• Familiar environment in TA is conducive for family discussions • Official attire and room in WA makes the setting judgmental and artificial
Procedures	• Informal hearing from conflicting partners who sit among mediating relatives or community members • Each case is uniquely handled • No record	• Conflicting people have their own place in the courtroom. • Recorded rules and policies required as references to solve current cases. • Records or	• Conflicting parties in TA remain part of the families which gives them hope and sense of security, unlike condemned isolation in WA. • Tension of recording what is being said, yet that reference can be changed or easily manipulated in WA. No idea of whether

	keeping • Feedback/resolution given there and then • Use of local, familiar and understood language • No interpreter • Personal presentation and ownership of cases • No fee is required •	writings are made. • Feedback given later after studying written notes. • Several journeys to the courts are usually required • Use of English and interpreter, though sometimes use of local language in LC courts. • Cases argued by lawyers. • High court fee is always required together with transport costs • Takes longer time to get verdict	they are writing what you are saying. In TA, each case is handled uniquely on its own, through listening and observation. • Justice delayed is justice denied in WA which may take years. • English/interpreters rouse mistrust and misrepresentation on resolutions made. • Hired lawyers deprive ownership of the case by concerned parties in WA. • Local council courts are composed of husbands' relatives or colleagues who tend to cover up the truth • WA are financially and timely costly • Most women lack money for costs associated. • There is high corruption rate in the WA
Penalties	Affordable items of sharing • Goats/sheep • Meal sharing Drinks • No court fee is paid	Depending on the magnitude of the problem and decision of the court • Money • Imprisonment • Beating and manual work	• TA asks for affordable local items, relevant for healing relations. • Strenuous penalties in WA widen the relations further and attract revenge. Penalties are not connected to the wrongs done for which the person is being punished. Besides, public labour does not benefit the conflicting family members

Source: Designed by the researcher (2012) with information from conducted interviewees and FGDs

References

European Commission (2012) *ESF Empowerment Handbook: Learning Network on Empowerment and Inclusion*. European Commission, Belfast.

Mushemeza, E. (2009) Contributions of Women in Influencing Legislation and Policy Formulation and Implementation in Uganda 1995-2005. *African Development, xxxiv* (3&4), pp 167-206.

Karwemera, F. (1994) *Emicwe n'Emigyenzo y'Abakiga [Practices and Rituals of Bakiga]*. Fountain Publishers, Kampala.

Kasenene, P. (1993) *Religion and Politics in Nkore*. Spot Publishers, Mbabane-Zwaziland.

Parpart, J. & Kabeer, N. (2010) *Choosing Silence: Rethinking Voice, Agency, and Women's Empowerment*. Gender and Development. Available at: www.gencon.msu.edu (accessed 14 August 2014).

The Republic of Uganda (2010) *National Development Plan: 2010/2011 - 2014/2015*. Government of Uganda, Kampala.

The Republic of Uganda (2011) *The Uganda National Land Policy*. Final Draft. The Government of Uganda, Kampala.

Tamale, S. (1993) Law Reform and Women's Rights in Uganda. *East African Journal of Peace and Human Rights, 1*(2), pp 164-194.

Tamale, S. (2003a) Introducing Quotas in Africa: Discourse and Legal Reforms in Uganda. *Paper presented at the The Implementation of Quotas: African Experiences*, Pretoria.

Tripp, A. (2001) The Politics of Autonomy and Cooptation in Africa: The Case of the Ugandan Women's Movement, *Modern African Studies*, 39(1), pp 101-128.

Tripp, A., Casimiro, I., Kwesiga, J. and Mugwa, A. (2009) *African Women's Movements: Transforming Political Landscapes*. Cambridge University Press, Cambridge.

UNDP (2012) *Women Entity for Gender Equality and the Empowerment of Women: Making a Difference in Women's Lives*. UNDP, New York, NY.

United Nations (1979) *Convention on the Elimination of All Forms of Discrimination against Women*. Available at: www.thegreatinitiative.com/wp-content/uploads/2010/CEDAW.pdf (accessed 14 August 2014).

CHAPTER 3. UBUNTU AND PEACE: WITHOUT A MOTHER, THERE IS NO HOME

Gertjan van Stam

Introduction

> "Our culture guides us in how to behave so we can survive in our land. The culture from Europeans helps them how to survive in their land. We cannot depend on a foreign culture to teach us how to survive in our land, we must use our own culture."[1]

The quotation above gives a clear-cut rational of the value of the contemporary African understanding of current challenges. The African understanding that 'when mother is not kumusha (in the village), there is no home' prompts us to search for a Mother in the 'home of peace'. For this search, we review the concurrency of Ubuntu, peace and women. The first two components and their interaction are relatively buoyant with a literature base. However, literature on the interaction of Ubuntu and women seems to be remarkably scarce. Conversations on women and Ubuntu also seem limited, discouraging the opportunity to discuss possible consequences of their interaction in other fields such as peace.

From my personal observations of being in Africa since 1987 and living full time since 2000, I am proposing that

---

1 Interaction in Harare, Zimbabwe, July 2014

'without Ubuntu there is no peace in Africa.'

This chapter looks into the understanding and meaning of Ubuntu:

- How does Ubuntu give rise to peace becoming present?
- How does Ubuntu provide instruments for reconciliation?
- Does Ubuntu help define the role of women and men in these processes?

Peace Challenges

Peace is not the absence of conflict. Wherever people gather, differences exist. However, the challenge of peace practitioners is to find ways in which communities can resolve such differences without physical violence (Burton, as mentioned in (Cortright, 2008, 7)).

I analyse Ubuntu through a review of behaviour and literature. My observations are framed within a post-colonial critique. Such a critique addresses modernity from a perspective emerging from the Global South (Mignolo, 2000). A post-colonial critique contrasts with a post-modern critique with the latter representing a Eurocentric critique of Eurocentrism. A post-colonial critique strives to give a voice to 'sub-alternity'; the group that is socially, politically, and geographically disenfranchised of hegemonic power, mostly rendered without agency (Grosfoguel, 2011).

A post-colonial critique is necessary; Western philosophy and academia remains steeped in colonialism and imperialism and does very little to incorporate the epistemological and theoretical implications of an epistemic critique coming out of African locations (Mazrui, 2003, Grosfoguel, 2011, Ndlovu-Gatsheni, 2013b). Most African universities were established during colonial times and continue to derive their epistemology from former colonial masters. Even today, the academy remains a colonised space (Davies et al., 2003, Mignolo, 2000, Stam, 2012).

Most academic knowledge continues to be produced from the viewpoint of the Western man (Grosfoguel, 2011). This complicates our endeavour. Much (most?) literature implicitly relies on a paradigm revering the blessings of global capitalism and the hegemonic world-system, where freedom, liberal democracy and the free market are considered self-explanatory virtues. Academic concepts remain in need of de-colonization, which can be achieved through confrontation with a de-colonial epistemology that overtly assumes a de-colonial geopolitics and body-politics of knowledge as points of departure (Anzaldua, 1987, Fanon, 1963).

Both the opening quotation and feminist scholars remind us of the value of positionality, context and local culture. As we always speak from a particular location, we are subject to the power structures in that location (Moraga & Anzaldua, 1983). Knowledge is always situated (Haraway, 1988).

Contemporary African reality is often depicted as dualistic, where traditional African and Western modes of thought are part of a battle of the mind. Du Bois (1994) recognised the battle of the mind in his studies of African Americans and theorised the existence of a double consciousness. With this term, he referred to the challenges of reconciling African Heritage with European education. The need to recognise this battle of the mind is supported by US-based black feminist scholars who call for inputs from an 'Afro-centric epistemology' (Collins, 2000).

The textual expressions of the underlying philosophies tell only a part of the story (Hountondji, 1996, 66). African philosophy literature is not aligned with the history of Western philosophy, nor does it represent the same purpose, meaning or value. It is often apologetic by nature, addressing a non-African audience (Hountondji, 1996). In African conception, the reality consists of the physical, the non-physical and the union of the two (Chimakonam, 2012). Much of the knowledge is stored in orality, not in textuality, often kept by gatekeepers whose livelihood depends on this knowledge. Gatekeepers are people authorised or initiated to know. Knowledge is seldom based upon textual discussions, and is therefore inherently difficult to access and reference from an academic perspective. This representation and content of knowledge challenges a classical (Western) logic and paradigm that regards knowledge to be absolutistic. So African knowledge is relegated, almost per definition, to sub-alternity: thus the need for participatory, trans-disciplinary interaction and studies that take a transcendental approach to reality.

Pan-Africanism

African philosophy, if such could be depicted, does not adhere to the history of Western philosophy. To understand African thought and to untangle the perspective of its philosophy and resulting epistemology is a crucial task for a post-colonial contribution to peace practice. The modern (= Western focused) dominant philosophy is at variance with other philosophies. Fanon saw it to be a body-politics of knowledge (Fanon, 1967). It must be understood that every society has its own way of peace practising, aiming at sustaining the integrity and social fabric of its own particular society.

Thus, 'peace studies' are also subject to positionality. They adhere to the power structures from which they emerge (Moraga & Anzaldua, 1983). Peace processes and interventions that emerge from a foreign culture harbour foreign meanings and understandings, and, therefore, are not necessarily recognised as a fruitful way of purposeful interaction by all involved (Adebajo, 2011).

Culture – as a provider of a sense of meaning – plays a vital role in engendering peace and social order within communities and nations (Murithi, 2006). From an African point of view and through the lenses of post-coloniality, there is need to critique the class, sexual, gender, spiritual, linguistic, geographical, and racial hierarchies of the modern/colonial capitalist/patriarchal world-system. Western philosophy and sciences tend to de-couple the ethnic/racial/gender/sexual epistemic location from the subject that speaks. Grosfoguel (2011) shows how the resulting myth of universal knowledge conceals the context, the geo-political and body-political epistemic location and the power/knowledge location from where the subject speaks. As we speak about Africa and peace, such peace should be understood and addressed from the African position and its cultural approaches need to be explored and understood.

Methodology

This chapter is based on the long-term, participatory action research of the author, lived out in an African environment. Community interactions include numerous travels through Africa beginning in 1987, and from living full-time in rural Zimbabwe (2000-2003), rural Zambia (2003-2012), and (urban) Zimbabwe since 2013. The observations include all aspects in 'the lived environment,' encompassing all dynamics of life, including conflict. The author understands practitioning to involve a sequence of thinking, practise, and progress, and discerning of outcomes to involve processes of community engagement, workforce development, and thought leadership (Bets et al., 2012, Stam, 2013a).

In the lived environment, the author positions himself as a curious observer. This involves an attitude of sympathy for any situation, searching for what it feels like for the local actor to behave the way he/she does. This curiosity is exercised with caution, so as to not fall into the trap of contempt, where the rural activities could be regarded as less developed, or – the opposite – practice would be viewed in a romantic reverence.

Phenomenology informs the description and interpretation of the observation. Such an approach does not seek to analyse and measure objective attributes of a phenomenon, but tries to unearth the underlying subjectivity. All aspects of communications inform the research process: for instance, the record of evanescent sound and all non-verbal communication including season, place, sun position, mental state of the people present, the seating arrangement, and somatic information such as gestures and facial expressions (Stam, 2013b). The researcher assumes a critical attitude while assessing field observations, involving – as far as possible – an intentional attitude of impartiality. Inductions involve a holistically and trans-disciplinary weighing of all aspects of realities observed. Derived outcomes add to the knowledge base as a progressing understanding of how realities are understood within the environment.

Textualisation introduces severe challenge. Readers in different cultures will have different views on how to understand a particular textual representation of the observation. The understanding of the 'truth of the situation' is thus a contemplative understanding. Although pragmatic or instrumental outcomes might be deduced, they are most valid for that instant only – as if freezing time – due to constant flux of the community, with shifting world-views, ethics, culture and systems. Such deductions could be valuable as input for sensitisation (Bets et al., 2012).

Ubuntu

Ubuntu is crystallised African philosophy. Ubuntu stands for the 'essential unity of humanity' and emphasises the importance of constantly involving empathy, sharing and co-operation in the pursuit of peace (Murithi, 2006). The word Ubuntu is derived from Nguni languages. It is a literal translation for 'collective personhood and collective morality' (Mbigi, 1997). Most research on Ubuntu focuses on South Africa. However, the concept exists throughout Africa. One encounters the term Ubuntu all over: for instance in the names 'Centre Ubuntu, a Laboratoire d'Analyse et d'Action' in Burundi and 'Ubuntu Campus' in Macha, Zambia.

The definition of Ubuntu is not uniform: it encompasses a range of interpersonal interactions and behaviour. Examples are co-operation, relationship, reciprocity, orality, and dialogue (Gade, 2012), or all what Ndlovu-Gatsheni (2013a) refers to as positive African values.

Khoza (2005) explains Ubuntu as signifying that 'an individual's humanity is expressed through a person's relationship with others and theirs in turn through recognition of the individual's humanity'. Ubuntu considers the needs of the group first, believing that in so doing, individual needs and desires will be met. As a result, within Ubuntu, team rewards take precedence over individual rewards.

Mangaliso and Mzamo (2001, 24) defined Ubuntu as: 'humaneness – a pervasive spirit of caring and community, harmony and hospitality, respect and responsiveness – that individuals and groups display for one another'. They continue to state that 'Ubuntu is the foundation for the basic values that manifest themselves in the ways African people think and behave towards each other and everyone else they encounter' (ibid).

Mbiqi and Maree (2005) define Ubuntu as the sense of solidarity or brotherhood which arises among people within 'marginalized' or 'disadvantaged' groups'.

Louw (2002) sees Ubuntu as a response to multi-culturalism. With specific reference to South Africa, he defines Ubuntu as 'an African or African-inspired version of an effective de-colonising assessment of the other'.

Colson (2006) shows how Ubuntu involves respect for religiosity, agreement, and the necessity of a dialogue of beliefs. Her extensive works among the Tonga in Southern Zambia give insight into the sheer complexity of the arena of religiosity, and the pivotal role of understanding African religion in its unique worldview, culture, and behaviour.

From these writers it becomes clear that Ubuntu is not set in absolutism, neither does it resorts to relativism. My deduction from observation is that Ubuntu is considered being present in the tangible when good moral behaviour is displayed. Ubuntu is an integral part of an Africa paradigm, within which Ubuntu can be recognised as a virtue to be displayed by the living. Within Ubuntu people are expected to behave well: to show Ubuntu. In that thinking, not to behave in such a way is illogical. Without Ubuntu, one cannot be (recognised as) a whole person. In that sense, Ubuntu is considered to be a universal and inclusive trait, which is shown through active behaviour in line with Ubuntu. Acts of oppression, for instance through colonialisation, are considered inhuman. Gade (2012, 498) quoted Mfuniselwa John Bhengu to say: "The moment you go outside the boundaries of ubuntu, you actually begin to be labeled as an animal [by the community] 'kintu'[2] [animal] as opposed to ubuntu. Once you are at this level, even your community, they just reject and repel [you]". All this is to show that a person subscribing to the paradigm involving Ubuntu will have great difficulty understanding people who do not behave with Ubuntu in mind. As Ubuntu is a self-explanatory part of a paradigm, questioning about Ubuntu involves a response involving reflectiveness towards the one asking.

Ubuntu and peace

Ubuntu shows itself in the lived realm, with expressions and transfer of its substance through orality. Due probably to its oral base and its practice mainly within disenfranchised communities, there is not much literature exploring the practical implications of Ubuntu for peace. Furthermore, much of the literature on Ubuntu has been authored by people of European descent (Gade, 2012).

The pivotal value of Ubuntu is validated by being cited in the epilogue to the South African interim Constitution. In this key document, it was stated:

> there is a need for understanding but not for vengeance, a need for reparation but not for retaliation, a need for ubuntu but not for victimisation (Government of Republic of South Africa, 1993, after section 250).

Neglecting Ubuntu can be a source of disharmony and strife in the daily-lived, African environment (Mangaliso & Mzamo, 2001).

Ubuntu encapsulates orality as the prime means of communication. In that setting, story telling plays a pivotal role (Colff, 2003, Stam, 2013b). In an

---

2 The translation of 'kintu' can also be 'thing'

interview, Modise asked Nelson Mandela the following:

> Many people regard you as a personification of Ubuntu. What do you understand Ubuntu to be?

Nelson Mandela responded in a storytelling way, typical of communication of meaning in orality: "In the old days, when we were young, a traveller through our country would stop at a village and he didn't have to ask for food or for water. Once he stops, the people give him food, entertain him. That is one aspect of Ubuntu, but it will have various aspects"[3].

Gade (2012) in his research of South Africans of African descent about the question "What is Ubuntu?" found many telling him stories too. In his assessment, he recognized two clusters of answers:

- people defining Ubuntu as a moral quality of a person
- people defining Ubuntu as a phenomenon according to which persons are interconnected (for instance a philosophy, an ethic, African humanism, or a worldview)

Healthy relationships with the other support peace. Ubuntu focuses on being together through on-going contact and interaction with others (Ndaba, 1994, 14). It builts a collective and subjective consciousness typified by an 'on-goingness of dialogue' spanning both relationship and distance, while preserving the other in her/his otherness and uniqueness, without letting the person slip into the distance (Louw, 1998). Interest in - and respect for - the historicality of the other person, through mutual exposure of lives lived, especially facilitates a process of building, restoring and growing of an open-ended becoming, an aligned future.

Ubuntu and strife

Ubuntu does not line up with settings enshrining virtues of individuality. It contradicts the Cartesian conception of individuality in which the individual, or self, can be viewed in separation from "the other" (Louw, 1998). In a modernic perspective, both individualism and collectivism are expressions based upon an atomistic, separate, solitary human entity – the individual. Ubuntu, however, defines an individual as a derivative of the community, in terms of relationships with others. In this perspective, an individual is a plural, connected, responding human entity. Therefore, Ubuntu does not align with self-interest focused on self-sufficiency, on private accumulation, or on competitive drive (Sheneberger & Stam, 2011). Ubuntu is not

---

3   http://www.youtube.com/watch? v=ODQ4WiDsEBQ

congruent with an economic assumption that puts self-interest as the ultimate determinant of human behaviour. It does not agree with satisfaction from labourers earning as much as possible whilst contributing as little as possible (Mangaliso & Mzamo, 2001). Actually, the consequences of rewarding individuals in the setting of Ubuntu can result in social punishment and sabotage of performance (April & Ephraim, 2006).

Colonialism – the practice of domination, which involves the subjugation of one people to another – brought a generalised presentation of Africa through a presentation of essentialistic perspectives. Such a perspective loses sight of intangibles like teachings from linguistic analysis. Kaoma (2010, 212) shows how Bantu languages incorporate the message that humans and non-humans are connected in the realm of *being*. This linguistic connection[4] paints a picture of how humans and nonhumans are intrinsically interdependent. Thus, when colonialists act, they act outside of Ubuntu itself, negatively impacting African life as a whole by reducing humanity (Kaoma, 2010, 169).

Khoza (2005) sees Ubuntu as crucial for leadership and management. Mangaliso and Mzamo (2001) record how the omission of Ubuntu in management results in strife. They and other scholars like Mbiqi (1997) go so far as to regard the integration of Ubuntu in the practice of leadership and management as crucial for Africa and beyond:

> Incorporating Ubuntu principles in management hold the promise of superior approaches to managing organizations. Organizations infused with humaneness, a pervasive spirit of caring and community, harmony and hospitality, respect and responsiveness will enjoy more sustainable competitive advantage (Mangaliso & Mzamo, 2001, 32).

Ubuntu, power and colonialism

From my observations over decennia in Africa – through good times and bad – I have deduced that in Ubuntu, leadership involves a presence that often communicates through codified interactions. Such interactions sustain reciprocity, where a leader can only be leader when honouring his/her relationship with the community. In that sense, in Ubuntu, leadership emerges from the community.

Unfortunately, colonialism imposed leadership from the outside. That leadership took political and economic control over a dependent territory in a dominating relationship, establishing a bridgehead as a centre-of-the-

---

4 'Ntu' is the universal force, the Original Being, and is part (or manifested) in Muntu (human being), Kintu (thing/animal), Hantu (place and time) and Kuntu (modality) (Janheinz, 1961)

periphery-nation (cP) with the centre-of-the-centre-nation (cC) (Galtung, 1971). Institutionalised in systems, benefits emerge from international relationships in a co-dependent setting, presumably through a harmony of interest benefiting évoluée in cP and those of the centre nations (mainly people in cC). However, none of these benefits are embedded within Ubuntu and are irrelevant to the local and regional community relationships.

Leadership arriving from the outside carry a worldview sustained by coloniality explicitly, not in Ubuntu. Thus, by definition, such leadership is positioned apart of Ubuntu, and those people involved thus hold a position apart from the community. In the community, potential évoluée are well aware of this situation, and when they aim for, and succeed in assuming such position, they know the consequences. When embracing imperialistic management processes and institutionality, along with the material benefits they bring, they position themselves at that time outside of Ubuntu and are likely to be shunned by the community. Such persons becomes part of 'them' instead of a part of 'us'.

Accepting the colonial system of gaining power seems to involve a (sub)conscious decision in which the advantages (e.g. being able to link to financial streams) are weighed against the disadvantages (exclusion from community). As this is painful, and complicates relationships – for instance within the extended family – it is often the case that such leadership sustained in coloniality will be accepted, but the person will relocate outside of the person's own community.

This process is even more complicated in deep rural areas. Leadership based within coloniality creates, defacto, a centre-of-the-periphery-of-the-periphery (cpP). Naturally, such leadership aspires to a harmony of interest with the centre-of-the-periphery (cP). However, cP is focused on a harmony of interest with cC and a potential relationship with cpP complicates matters significantly. Therefore, a harmony of interest between cP and cpP remains mostly a one-sided longing from cpP. Thus, there is a double rejection of cpP leadership: first a rejection by the Ubuntu-based community, and a second rejection from cP-based peers. Therefore, such leadership appears to be trapped: accepting the indigenous Ubuntu methods could mean losing power, and the rejection by cP represents a glass ceiling preventing integration into the elite in cP. This situation can result in cpP leadership that utilises all means of colonial oppression to remain in power, often with impunity. The community suffers greatly, for leaders stay and remain in place for long periods, possibly for decennia. Such autocratic leadership is mostly found in rural institutions implemented during colonial and post-colonial times. This leadership struggles to contribute in peace processes since they necessarily rely on foreign structures, mostly dominating in nature, without being able to apply Ubuntu practices.

Colonialism effected fundamental changes by establishing an extra category of leadership based upon external, dominating systems, vested defacto outside of Ubuntu. Coloniality erodes the utilisation of the mechanisms to regulate peace through indigenous means and practices.

Ubuntu, paradigm and components

Summarising various authors and texts on Ubuntu, the following working-description emerges:

> Ubuntu is an epistemology emerging from an African paradigm. It is a metaphor, embodying the significance of group solidarity. It encapsulates a key to African values, involving collective personhood and collective morality. Ubuntu spells out the principle of caring for each others' well-being in a spirit of mutual support. Ubuntu shows how people are people through other people, recognising that an individual's humanity is expressed through that person's relationship with others and theirs in turn through a recognition of an individual's humanity. Ubuntu provides for the acknowledgement of the rights and the responsibilities of every citizen in promoting societal and individual well-being.

In short, Ubuntu captures the African essence of what it means to be human.

Ubuntu activated

Khoza (2005) tabulates a whole range of concepts that are part of Ubuntu. The common denominator is the way these concepts aim for unity. The concepts involve words like "interconnection", "integration" and "continuation". Other words incorporate moral overtones like "respect", "dignity" and "reconciliation". "Trust", "sharing", and "participation" feature too. Among the tangible outcomes of Ubuntu is "communal enterprise", where ownership of opportunities, responsibility and challenges are shared as in an extended family system. It prescribes "participatory decision-making" and "consultation" as a value orientation. In all endeavours, Ubuntu prioritises people and relationships over things and views interdependence as superior value to independence.

In Ubuntu, a human being finds genuine human expression in human relationships with other humans. Therefore, apart from the concepts, Ubuntu instils behaviour that is open and available to others. It affirms the other in his/her wholeness of being. Therefore, the collective is glad when others are able and good. Self-assurance is derived from recognising a belonging in a greater whole.

Important for peace, Ubuntu instils an understanding that an individual diminishes when others are humiliated, tortured or oppressed.

Ubuntu and law

In the South African Equality Court, in the case of "Afri-Forum and Another v Malema and Others", Judge Lamont in his assessment recognised the strength of Ubuntu as being "an important source of law within the context of strained or broken relationships amongst individuals or communities and as an aid for providing remedies which contribute towards more mutually acceptable remedies for the parties in such cases" (Lamont, 2011). In his assessment, leading to designating a certain utterance as hate speech, Lamont deduces from jurisprudence that Ubuntu opposes vengeance. It dictates that a high value be placed on life of a human being and a premium on dignity, compassion, humaneness and respect for the humanity of another. Within Ubuntu, a shift takes place from confrontation to mediation and conciliation, in an environment fuelled by good attitudes and shared concern.

Lamont understands Ubuntu to favour the re-establishment of harmony in the relationship between parties, aiming at the restoration of the dignity of the plaintiff without ruining the defendant, in a restorative rather than retributive justice. Therefore, Ubuntu operates in a direction favouring reconciliation rather than estrangement. This involves sensitising a disputant or a defendant in litigation to the hurtful impact of his actions to the other party and towards changing such conduct, rather than merely punishing the disputant. The outcome of such framing of the guidance from law is: mutual understanding rather than punishment, face-to-face encounters of disputants to facilitate resolving of differences rather than conflict and victory for the most powerful; and civilised dialogue premised on mutual tolerance.

Previously, the Constitutional Court of South Africa noted "It is values like (Ubuntu) that (the Constitution) requires to be promoted. They give meaning and texture to the principles of a society based on freedom and equality" (South Africa: Constitutional Court, 1995, §307).

Women, peace and reconciliation

Within Ubuntu, no gender segregation is made, in the sense that everyone exists by the grace of the other. Therefore, a de-construction of Ubuntu and gender in Western sociological or individualistic terms may not provide an effective frame of analysis. I found that a typical response to my questioning about Ubuntu and gender is:

> There is a way in which women are supposed to behave at different stages in their lives. And men as well. There are no questions about analysing gender,

as everybody assumes it. Elders deal with the details of everything.[5]

When approaching the subject of Ubuntu and women from the imagination of masculinity and femininity, then different meanings surface. Such meaning gives instruction on the different roles of women and men in protecting the harmony in society. Feminine and masculine attributes to peacekeeping are defined and revealed in stories, songs and expressions. In those narratives, the power of women as peace-builders is often celebrated, as shown in this example of a myth of the Yoruba in Nigeria on the creation of the earth:

> When they were coming to the Earth
> Women had no powers from Olodumare
> Women asked themselves as to what powers they had
> To do all they wanted to do on earth
> Men were maltreating the women
> Men enslaved them and treated them harshly
> Women returned to Olodumare and reported the case
> Olodumare was moved with compassion
> Olodumare promised them a power greater than that of men
> Olodumare gave women power over men
> Women were instructed not to use the power indiscriminately
> Olodumare endowed women with the power of aje[6]

Within Ubuntu, peace exists in situations where harmony is characterised by the presence of virtuous interpersonal relationships in the presence of dignity and order that serves the interest of all. Peace allows for diversity and the local expression of values. It allows the local culture to flourish.

An Ubuntu-based peace process is one of reconciliation. The South African Truth and Reconciliation Commission is a prime example of how reconciliatory processes defused a potentially explosive situation (Mamdani, 2001), although this process failed to deal with the needs for reconciliation in communities and especially the situation that had evolved for women after the conflict. Most transitional processes have focused on the state, but have forgotten to address the reconciliation within the communities which have been torn apart by conflict. The traditional processes of reconciliation at community level may enhance the participation of women in transition, if they adequately address the issues of justice, reparation and forgiveness. This

---

5   Interaction in Harare, Zimbabwe, July 2014
6   According to Oyeronke Olajubu, this part of Yoruba mythology explains the origin of how Olodumare created the Earth, the unintended gender bias that arose, and how eventually the power returned to women (Aderibigbe, 2013, 692)

is especially so where conflict has targeted women and the women's body, and when many of the perpetrators are men, even originating from the local communities themselves, leaving women without a place to return to, unless these crimes are addressed and reconciliation has allowed communities to heal. Van Reisen and Mekonnen (2011), in their study concerning transitional justice in Eritrea and Zimbabwe, explored how traditional justice systems may be instrumental in truth-finding, conflict resolution, reparation, and reconciliation. They substantiate the need for contextual societal specifics to be taken into account.

Murithi (2006) shows that the peace-making process found among Ubuntu societies goes through distinctive phases. These stages encompass an acknowledgement of guilt, showing remorse and repentance, asking for and giving forgiveness, and paying compensation or reparation, as a prelude to reconciliation. These steps are all focused on restoration of relationships as the ultimate target, and "being together" as the aim of Ubuntu, recognising the wrongdoing and need for reparation. Within Ubuntu, it is understood that the perpetrator is also a victim, and that reconciliation must involve perpetrator as well as the victim.

Women who are still rooted in traditional settings potentially have a lot to gain from reconciliation processes that focus on the communities. They can also provide more leadership if the rooting of peace in communities is recognized and institutionalized through locally rooted practices. During a meeting in Harare with a small group of women, the role of women in peace building was discussed. From the transcript printed here below, one can read how much women can feel excluded from peace building. They discuss in this citation the aftermath of the pre-election violence in 2008 in Zimbabwe and refer to the UN resolution 1325 being introduced in Zimbabwe:

> After the violence, there was that resolution saying: Let's look at the traditional model that exists, and see how we could incorporate it in peace building. Women, being placed in homes and having that domestic role to look after the family, there was that realisation why don't we involve the women? They are at home, they are responsible for raising the families, why don't we involve them and ensure that they can mould the young men to become peaceful people. They can involve their husbands to influence them not to take part in tensions. That is the model that is being used now. It seems to be very very effective, women are now at the centre of running the family, they are responsible for the upbringing, the socialisation of the children and the family.
>
> It has been thought: let's adopt that model where we women restructure societal thinking. That is the model that is currently being used. Elevate women from that position that they were previously disadvantaged and take

it to something positive that can bring some societal change.[7]

The arsenal of women in peace-building centres around Ubuntu's guidance in the area of giving and receiving forgiveness, however hard and difficult this may seem. The Ubuntu value is efficacious in attaining peaceful homes. In this fashion, women have power within Ubuntu to bringing about harmony and healing as well as transcending the deeply ingrained angers felt by victims of conflict at all levels. Aberibigbe (2013) calls for a reorientation of understanding these roles that give women agency in society, by recognising the rooting society must have in communities and in families:

> Thus, the status of the woman to Africans as portrayed in African traditional religion is not dependent on what has developed as male generosity as owner and dispenser of social roles and functions, which place him over and above women. My strong submission is that, ultimately, the status of women should not be viewed as something to be struggled for as a "call out" from oppression and subjugation. It is an innate right, divinely bestowed, and is to be enjoyed by women for the physical and spiritual wellbeing of everyone – the family, the community and the entire society.
>
> Finally, the claimed subjugation of women usually ascribed to African traditional societies cannot be said to have been derived from traditional religion. Any claim that places such subjugation within the dynamics of religion portrays at best an unfortunate misunderstanding and misrepresentation of the position of African religion on the role and status of women. Indeed the subjugation of women can be regarded as a violation of the central principles and values of African religion in its unique worldview on the origin, multiplication and sustenance of the human race. (Aderibigbe, 2013, 699)

Homes, families and communities are the backbone of peaceful societies. Ubuntu is practical. The African saying, "The home belongs to the women. If that woman is not there, there is no home" indicates the existence of a pivotal role of women as the mothers of communities in Ubuntu society. Women have power as guardians of peace, as mediators, negotiators and as strategists, as educators, as communicators and as economists, providers of food and providers of care. If women want peace, they have the power to build homes of peace, communities of peace and societies of peace.

Conclusions

Ubuntu says that we are all guardians of peace. Ubuntu facilitates indigenous processes for conflict resolution and maintenance of peace. Ubuntu

---

7 Interaction in Harare, Zimbabwe, July 2014

components do not separate nor reduce each other, and there is no separation of the process from the goal. Ubuntu is dynamic, is exercised through embodiment of its virtues within the lived environment. The interconnectedness of African life lived out through Ubuntu, focuses all interactions on inclusion of the other.

Ubuntu facilitates the authority of women in their capacity to create harmony in communities and societies by emphasising the importance of home and of care taking of each other. This gives her authority to speak out on behalf of families, communities and societies, especially when harmony is undermined.

The restorative processes of transitional justice focus on the state, but lack focus on communities and have mostly failed to properly integrate women. The traditional practices rooted in Ubuntu-epistemology, in creating peace through truth-finding, reparation, asking for forgiveness and reconciliation include the perpetrator and the victim. This may help women especially. These old traditions may help overcome the pain and the subjugation and exclusion experienced as a result of violence. It may above all help women regain confidence and authority that Ubuntu instils the idea of motherhood as the guardian of peace in societies who are expected to care for everyone but so often fail to do so and end up in conflict.

"The home belongs to the woman. If that woman is not there, there is no home" is a statement of the authority women have in making homes. That is the basic understanding of Ubuntu. Everyone belongs, everyone has a home. A peaceful society is a home, a home in which everyone belongs.

References

Adebajo, A. (2011) *UN Peacekeeping in Africa. From the Suez Crisis to the Sudan Conflicts*. Fanele, Auckland Park.

Aderibigbe, I. (2013) Womanhood in African Worldview and Religion. In: T Falola & B Teboh (Eds.), *The power of gender, the gender of power: Women's labor, rights and responsibility in africa*. Africa World Press, Trenton, NJ.

Anzaldua, G. (1987) *Borderlands/La Frontera: The New Mestiza*. Spinsters/Aunt Lute, San Francisco, CA.

April, K. and Ephraim, N. (2006) Implementing African Leadership: An Empirical Basis to Move Beyond Theory. In *1st international conference on values-based leadership*. Stellenbosch University, South Africa.

Bets, J., Stam, van, G. and Voorhoeve, A. (2012) Modeling and Practise of Integral Development in rural Zambia. Case Macha. In K. Jonas, I. Rai, & M. Tchuente (Eds.), *Fourth international IEEE EAI conference on e-infrastructure and e-services for developing countries* (Africomm 2012). Springer, Yaounde.

Chimakonam, J. (2012) *Introducing African Science Systematic and Philosphical Approach*. AuthorHouse, Calabar.

Colff, van der, L. (2003) Leadership lessons from the African tree. *Management Decision*, 41(3), pp. 257–261.

Collins, P. (2000) *Black Feminist Thought: Knowledge, Consciousness, and the Politics of Empowerment*, 2nd ed. Routledge, New York, NY

Colson, E. (2006) *Tonga Religious Life in the Twentieth Century*. Bookworld Publishers, Lusaka.

Cortright, D. (2008) *Peace: A History of Movements and Ideas*. Cambridge University Press, Cambridge.

Davies, C., Gadsby, M., Peterson, C. and Williams, H. (Eds.). (2003) *Decolonizing the Academy: African Diaspora Studies*. Africa World Press, Trenton, NJ.

Du Bois, W. (1994) *The Souls of Black Folk*. Gramercy Books, Avenel, NJ.

Fanon, F. (1963) *The Wretched of the Earth*. Grove Press, New York, NY.

Fanon, F. (1967) *Black Skin, White Masks*. Grove Press, New York, NY.

Gade, C. (2012) What is Ubuntu? Different Interpretations among South Africans of African Descent. *South African Journal of Philosophy*, 31(3), pp. 484–503.

Galtung, J. (1971) A Structural Theory of Imperialism. *Journal of Peace Research*, 8(2), pp. 81–117.

Garcia, E. (Ed.), (1994) *Pilgrim Voices: Citizens as Peacemakers*. International Alert, London.

Government of Republic of South Africa (1993) *Constitution of the Republic of South Africa Act 200 of 1993*. UCDP, Pretoria.

Grosfoguel, R. (2011) Decolonizing Post-Colonial Studies and Paradigms of Political Economy: Transmodernity, Decolonial Thinking, and Global Coloniality. *Journal of Peripheral Cultural Production of the Luso-Hispanic World*, 1(1).

Haraway, D. (1988) Situated Knowledges: The Science Question in Feminism and the Privilege of Partial Perspective. *Feminist Studies*, 14(3), pp. 575–599.

Hountondji, P. (1996) *African Philosophy: Myth and Reality*, Second Edition. Indiana University Press, Bloomington and Indianapolis.

Janheinz, J. (1961). *Muntu: An Outline of the New African Culture*. Grove Press, New York, NY.

Kaoma, K. (2010) *Ubuntu, Jesus, and Earth: Integrating African Religion and Christianity in Ecological Ethics*. Boston University, Boston, MA.

Khoza, R. (2005) *Let Africa Lead: African Transformational Leadership for 21st century Business*. VezuBuntu, Sunninghill.

Lamont, J. (2011) *Afri-Forum and Another v Malema and Others*. Southern African Legal Information Institute (SAFLII).

Louw, D. (1998) Ubuntu: An African Assessment of the Religious Other. In *Proceedings of the 20th world congress of philosophy*. Boston, Massachusetts.

Louw, D. (2002) *Ubuntu and the Challenges of Multiculturalism in post-apartheid South Africa*. Expertisecentrum Zuidelijk Afrika, Sovenga.

Mamdani, M. (2001) *When Victims Become Killers: Colonialism, Nativism, and the Genocide in Rwanda*. Princeton University Press, Princeton, NJ.

Mangaliso, C. and Mzamo, P. (2001) *Building competitive advantage from Ubuntu: Management lessons from South Africa*. Academy of Management Executives, 15(3), pp. 23–33.

Mazrui, A. (2003) Towards Re-Africanizing African Universities: Who Killed Intellectualism in the Post Colonial Era? *Turkish Journal of International Relations*, 2(3), pp. 135–163.

Mbigi, L. (1997) *Ubuntu: The African Dream in Management*. Knowledge Resources, Randburg.

Mbigi, L. and Maree, J. (2005) *Ubuntu: The Spirit of African Transformation Management*. Knowres Publishing, Randburg.

Mignolo, W. (2000) Local Histories/Global Designs: Coloniality, Subaltern Knowledges, and Border Thinking. In S. Ortner, N. Dirks, & G. Eley (Eds.), *Local histories/global designs*. Princeton University Press, Princeton, NJ.

Moraga, C. and Anzaldua, G. (Eds.), (1983) *This Bridge Called My Back. Writing by Radical Women of Color*, 2nd ed. Kitchen Table. Women of Color Press, Latham, NY

Murithi, T. (2006) Practical Peacemaking Wisdom from Africa: Reflections on Ubuntu. *The Journal of Pan African Studies*, 1(4), pp. 25–35.

Mwanzi, H. (2010) Reflections on Orality and Cultural Expression: Orality as a Peace Culture. *Journal des Africanistes*, 80(1-2), pp. 63–74.

Ndaba, W. (1994) *Ubuntu in comparison to Western philosophies*. Ubuntu School of Philosophy, Pretoria.

Ndlovu-Gatsheni, S. (2013a) *Coloniality of Power in Postcolonial Africa: Myths of Decolonization*. Codesria, Dakar.

Ndlovu-Gatsheni, S. (2013b). Decolonising the University in Africa. *The Thinker*, 51, pp. 46–51.

Reisen, van, M. and Mekonnen, D. (2011) Exploring New Spaces for Women in Transitional Justice in Eritrea and Zimbabwe In *2nd international symposium of the international research centre for intercultural studies*. Brussels, Belgium.

Sheneberger, K. and Stam, van, G. (2011) Relatio: An Examination of the Relational Dimension of Resource Allocation. *Economics and Finance Review*, 1(4), pp. 26–33.

South Africa: Constitutional Court (1995) S v Makwanyane and Another.

Stam, van, G. (2012) Towards an Africanised Expression of ICT. In K. Jonas, I. Rai, and M. Tchuente (Eds.), *Fourth international IEEE*

EAI conference on e-infrastructure and e-services for developing countries (Africomm 2012). Springer, Yaounde.

Stam, van, G. (2013a) *A Strategy to make ICT accessible in rural Zambia: A case study of Macha*. NMMU, Port Elizabeth.

Stam, van, G. (2013b) Information and Knowledge Transfer in the rural community of Macha, Zambia. *The Journal of Community Informatics*, 9(1).

CHAPTER 4. WOMEN HAVE ALWAYS HAD THEIR SPECIAL PLACE IN HISTORY AS PEACE-MAKERS: WOMEN AND PEACE BUILDING IN THE GREAT LAKES REGION

Pamela K. Mbabazi

Introduction

The region of the Great Lakes of Africa (GLR) is undoubtedly conflict prone, but it also harbours countries like Uganda and Rwanda, which have reached quite a high level of resilience to conflict. Although both countries have a long history of internal conflict, they are currently also islands of relative peace, stability and development in a volatile region. Women have always had their special place in history as peacemakers. There are clearly things that have worked in both countries from which we can draw lessons to further promote our societies. It is important that we always take stock of what has worked in our societies and the different sectors and spheres and critically understand what explains relative success in one area, where as there is total failure in the other... so as to ensure sustainable progress. But what exactly have been the real experiences of Women in Peace-Building in Rwanda and Uganda and in all the other countries in the Great Lakes Region? What lessons can we draw from each of these countries? This paper tries to highlight the contributions and experiences of women in both

Uganda and Rwanda with regard to peace building.

Overcoming gender inequality

It is a fact that men have always overlooked women and "put them in their place" in many societies throughout history, although of late this trend is undoubtedly changing and perhaps even more so in today's Rwanda. The bias against women, or rather the lesser stature of women, permeates legends and social traditions the world over. However there are moments in history that depict women as strong pillars in society with examples of women who have led nations into war, propelled societies into social and economic progress hitherto unknown, and presided over remarkable social transformations. Joan of Arc, nicknamed "The Maid of Orleans" provided leadership of the French army in the 15th Century and went on to win many battles during the hundred (100) years war that paved the way for the coronation of King Charles the VII. More closer to home, we have such examples as Prof. Wangare Mathai, the first African Woman to receive a Nobel Peace Prize. She was followed immediately by two more African women in Liberia, Ellen Johnson Sirleaf, The Liberian President, and Lymah Gbowee, a woman social worker in Liberia who led Liberian women to rise up against oppression and dictatorship by men at a time when it was not so easy to do so. To share the Nobel Prize with the two African women was Tawakkul Karman from Yemen who has been a leading figure in the protests against President Ali Abdullah Saleh for some time now. The Nobel committee said the three women had been chosen "for their non-violent struggle for the safety of women and for women's rights to full participation in peace-building work" (Norwegian Nobel Committee, 2011). We obviously cannot achieve democracy and lasting peace in this region and the world at large, unless women obtain the same opportunities as men to influence developments at all levels of society.

Measuring how far women have come to achieve equality with men in East Africa by the numbers that have been elected to parliament in Uganda, Rwanda, Kenya, Tanzania and Burundi is well known. However, in Rwanda, a small country in the region, the outcome of the 2013 parliamentary elections beat her own world record of 59% women representation in parliament set after the 2008 parliamentary elections. Today female representation in Rwanda's parliament stands at 64%, arguably the highest number in any legislature anywhere in the world.

Interestingly, Uganda, another post-conflict country and a pioneer of gender equality insights that promotes women's central role in society in the region, still stands at 34%, some 28 years since the coming to power of the National Resistance Movement (NRM) in 1986 and the introduction of the politics of women's empowerment. Initially in Rwanda, politics were based on ethnicity, while in Uganda it was based on tribal differences. Arguably, the effects of genocide in Rwanda has given a platform for women to participate in politics. In the case of Uganda however, a woman usually stands for politics on the basis of her marriage. If the marriage breaks, that is often the end of her participation on the political scene. The case of our former Vice-President, Dr. Specioza Wandera Kazibwe, is a case in point.

The underrepresentation and presence of women in national legislatures in high numbers has been studied and explained (Matland & Montgomery, 2003; Lovenduski & Norris, 1993; Norris & Lovenduski 1995; Goetz & Hassim, 2003; Ahikire, 2006; Powley, 2004; Longman, 2006; Burnet, 2008) largely using socio-economic, institutional and cultural variables or affirmative action. In the economically affluent West, there is a high number of women in legislature and the reverse is true with the less affluent polities of Africa. Due to a focus on quotas (i.e. the legal constitutional quota in most countries of 30% representation), there are few women aspiring to be members of parliament which makes the understanding of the phenomenon of the impacts of either high or low presence in parliament partial and insufficient.

Equal participation by both men and women in political decision-making provides a balance that more accurately reflects the composition of society and it enhances the legitimacy of political processes by making them more democratic and responsive to the concerns and perspectives of all segments of society.

Violent conflict situations in Africa and particularly in Rwanda, Uganda and the larger Great Lakes Region have raised women's awareness of the necessity to take strong positions in ending conflicts. However, as women seek to engage in peace building processes such as bridging reconciliation across conflict divided communities, leading community peace campaigns or community dialogues, they are often frustrated by the structures that deny them equal opportunities shared by their male counterparts.

In the case of Uganda, since the liberation war of 1986 and the coming to power of President Museveni's ruling NRM Government, Ugandan women have fought side by side with men and have proved that they are capable of enduring tough situations, demonstrating great courage and dying for a cause. In recognition of the vital role women have played in the success of the liberation war in Uganda, a woman was appointed Vice President (Dr. Wandira Kazibwe) and women ministers have been appointed in key positions like Hon. Jessica Alupo (Uganda's current minister for Education and a retired Major General August 2014). Hon. Rebecca Kadaga also holds the top position of Speaker of Parliament of Uganda and there are several more decision-making positions held by women. The current Uganda government policy on women aims at raising the status of women and fostering their emancipation from socio-economic, political and cultural bondages. This has largely been through programmes to review and reformulate sectoral policies to ensure that gender aware implementation strategies are put in place.

It is clear that the GLR faces many challenges ranging from poverty and epidemics to conflicts. The conflicts have cost the region immensely in terms of development, resources and human resource. In Rwanda, the effects of the Genocide are still fresh in many people's minds. There are still cases of trauma among genocide survivors while some families of genocide survivors are yet to get shelter over their heads. What is more critical however, is the fact that while violent conflicts affect both women and men, women in Rwanda probably bore the brunt of the genocide more than their male counterparts. This is common wherever there is a violent conflict, largely because of the women's biological make up - as most war crimes target women. As noted earlier, they are subjected to rape, defilement, and forced marriages, all of which expose them to HIV.

Rwandan women have stood up against the many conflicts that have plagued that country in order to foster peace. Their success in this noble cause, underscores the fact that women can take charge of the situation, not only for their own security, but also to protect their male compatriots. Most recently, the joint military operation of Rwanda-Congo against FDLR rebels, negotiated by among others the Foreign Affairs Minister, Rosemary Museminali, is a clear manifestation of the Rwandan women's determination to make peace prevail in the country by tackling threats to current peace. In addition, the role of Fatuma Ndangiza, as the Executive Secretary of the National Unity and Reconciliation Commission (NURC) further testifies to women's readiness to contribute to peace building in Rwanda. Ndangiza has played a pivitol role in uniting a society that had been deeply divided along ethnic lines. Other women like Rose Kabuye, the Director of State Protocol, and Senator Aloise are examples of women in high positions of decision making which has a positive impact.

Despite the many efforts in both countries to promote women, however, critical issues such as access to power and resources, as well as women's participation in decision-making, still need to be addressed to enable women to participate as effective pillars and stakeholders in the well-intended peace building initiatives of these two post conflict nations. Women have been portrayed as the main bearers of the consequences of the violence, as widows, as victims of rape, as heads of disrupted families in many post war settings. At the same time, extreme violence has been identified as a potential opportunity to redefine or reconstruct gender relationships, as it can be argued has been the case in Rwanda and indeed Uganda. Women have now become actors as well as benficiaries of reconstruction, reconciliation and peace building in Rwandan society following the period of genocide.

It is important to recognise that while violent conflicts, including genocide, are unfortunate, certain wars and types of violence create opportunities for formally marginalized groups, like women, to access sites of power that have been formally closed to them. Understanding how political power is organized and legitimized is critical to understanding why certain societies have managed to promote the advancement of women in politics while other have failed. The role of the dominant elite discourse in constructing and justifying the presence (or absence) of sites of power is also crucial.

Women's roles in the liberation movements across Africa has been at the centre of peace and security in different countries, such as during Namibia's struggle for independence, during the struggle against apartheid in South Africa, in Rwanda during the genocide, and in Uganda during the Kony war. Although many societies are male dominated, the liberation struggles in many African countries provided avenues for women to participate alongside men. Women's involvement in the liberation struggles has contributed to peace, enhanced education, strengthened the provision of women's rights and contributed to the development of their countries.

While women have demonstrated a willingness to participate, cultural constraints and traditional beliefs remained continued to constrain women from participating effectively. Women do not automatically have adequate tools in the form of skills, exposure, access to resources and freedom to participate and the only way to enhance their participation is by changing people's perceptions on the role of women and by breaking down the cultural barriers that demean women. If countries of Africa, and in particular those in the GLR, are to realize peace and security, women must be put at the centre of conflict resolutions and post conflict reconstruction.

Prof. Anyang noted in his recent lecture in Makerere on 'Ending the Servitude of Life Givers': "The reality is that we have not done as much as we should through our declarations and intentions." (Anyang' Nyong'o, 2011) There is still so much more we can do to point society in the right direction as far as women's roles and positions are concerned. It is appropriate that Rwanda as a small country within the East African sub-region that has done much better than most, to host the international conference on "Women's Participation in Peace-Building in the GLR", because others need to learn from the experiences and understand critically what it takes to put women in the fore, and what this means for societal transformation. Undoubtedly, Rwanda has done better, especially when we look at women's roles in decision making and in public offices and to some extent in business. Arguably, this could be explained by the existence of a much more progressive political leadership that values and respects the role of women in society and upholds the universal principles of equality for all.

In East Africa's history, it was President Julius Nyerere who first led this drive to raise the level of consciousness in society about Women's central role and pointed out the dangers of patriarchy and social bigotry as enemies of social progress. He raised alarm bells for female emancipation at independence when he said:

> If women want to take their rightful places in the community and if they do not want to be looked down upon, they have to prove this by leaving behind old practices and prejudices which push them back into the kitchen…..They have to prove that the confidence placed in them is justified since the party and the government have given full support for women. (Anyang' Nyong'o, 2011: 3)

This support from Government at that time was not simply given in form, through formal equality enshrined in law; it was also expressed in concrete programmes and projects that the independence government initiated to empower women, such as the adult education programme. In 1962 for example, 75% of those enrolled for adult education in the then Tanganyika were women from the countryside. This ultimately enabled women to compete with men on a more equal footing in the political, social and economic market. Undoubtedly, increased access to education has seen more women elected to parliament and local government institutions throughout the GLR, and to occupy top positions in the civil service, academia and leading professions.

While all these measures are important and indeed paint a clear picture of the extent to which equality of opportunity exists in our societies, it must be understand that it is equally important to start with the cultural revolution to demystify the old-age dominance over women and their relegation to beings of a lesser kind. As one scholar has noted: *"The Revolution Begins at Home by inculcating the confidence of self"*. (Anyang' Nyong'o, 2011: 5) It all begins with such simple acts like fathers (and mothers) recognizing and appreciating their daughters as individuals who can be and can achieve all that is great, and form the ethos of their society. No doubt we have many girls and women in East Africa who are great achievers, some whom we have celebrated but many we have simply wished away and appreciated only in passing.

Women are key in peace building in the GLR as they take a central part in socialization, which normally starts within the home right from child-birth up to adulthood. That is arguably why one's first language is referred to as the mother tongue. On the Economic development front, associations and cooperatives that involve women have promoted peace building through sharing of experiences, education, bargaining power, extending assistance to the vulnerable and sustainable peace. Women should be actively involved at all levels as nothing can be successful without women. The elite women are the ones that often take the lead in most women associations and all communication is done in English leaving non-educated women behind.

We cannot forget to applaud the majority of women in rural areas and in the slums of our cities who have given birth to many of us and have fed and looked after the workers and peasants that sustain our economies. As long as we do not question why the male side of the equation performs better than the female side under similar circumstances, then we shall continue to consign the majority of women to indignities, slave labour and human suffering, despite any progress made in woman's emancipation.

There is a need for the modification of our culture so as to eliminate prejudicial practices that block women's involvement in peace building. The crucial role played by social actors after conflict demonstrates the strong link between women and nation reconstruction, as clearly seen in Rwanda after the genocide. In Nyamirambo, for example, a women's group helped genocide survivors gain skills such as in computer applications, hand crafts and the use of sewing machines to develop themselves and their families. This created a means of livelihoods for many families that were previously desperate. Women are arguably more tolerant, give life and think of others as being more like their family than men.

While women's difficulties in times of armed struggle have recently featured more prominently on the international agenda for war-to-peace transitions, women's positive contributions to peace-building and post-war reconstruction remain largely unrecognized and undervalued. There is a need to overcome the obstacles that hinder women from participating more in peace building and post-conflict resolution and reconstruction processes. Women need to take advantage of the transformative experiences of war and the resulting weakened patriarchal order to build up a strong women's movement before it is too late -- before traditions that oppress women return to take over the space that has opened momentarily. Women need to build a strong movement before conflict starts and to sustain it through the war that may follow, as well as after the ceasefire. The movement should help to build bridges between different groups in civil society, thus bolstering the continued struggle for respect for women's rights without waiting for the end of the hostility to be achieved.

Furthermore, in order to make progress towards gender equality, we have to empower women by eliminating gender disparities in the enrollment in primary and secondary education and in access to higher education and learning in all professions. In the reproductive cycle of society in which women play the central role and bear the most burdens, maternal and child mortality must be reduced to near zero and access to reproductive health services made accessible to all women of child bearing age. However social change cannot really happen without profound ideological and cultural change at the level of ideas, beliefs and social norms. As Tadesse noted in the title of her presentation of the 2002 meeting of African Scholars in Ethiopia, we must all be in the "search of gender justice" (Tadesse 2002: 1).

References

Ahikire, J. (2006) *Localised or Localising Democracy Gender and the Politics of Decentralisation in Contemporary Uganda*. Fountain Publishers, Kampala.

Anyang' Nyong'o, P. (2011) Ending the Servitude of Life Givers: The Liberation of East African Women since Nyerere's Equality Call, *Makerere Africa Celebrations re-launching Makerere Africa Lecture Series*, (2 December 2011), Makerere.

Bop, C. (2001) Women in Conflicts: Their Gains and Their Losses, In: S. Meintjes, A. Pillay & M. Turshen (eds.), *The Aftermath. Women in Post-Conflict Transformation,* pp. 19-34. Zed Books London.

Brett, A. (1996) Testimonies of War Trauma in Uganda, In: T. Allen, (ed.) *In Search of Cool Ground: War, Women and Health in Eritrea*, pp. 278-92. Africa World Press, Trenton NJ, 278-92.

Burnet, J. (2008) Gender balance and the meanings of women in governance in post-genocide Rwanda. *African Affairs*, 107(428), pp. 361–386.

El-Bushra, J. (2000) Transformation conflict: Some thoughts on a gendered understanding of conflict processes. In S. Jacobs, R. Jacobson & J. Marchbank (Eds.), *States of Conflicts: Gender Violence and Resistance,* pp. 66-83. Zed Press, London

Goetz, A. and Hassim, S. (eds.) (2003) *No shortcuts to power: African women in politics and policy-making*. Zed Books, Cape Town – Available at: http://www.hsrc.ac.za/en/research-outputs/view/82#sthash.PjKq9Fko.dpuf (accessed 2 August 2014).

Longman, T. (2006) Rwanda: Achieving equality or serving and authoritarian state? In G. Bauer, & H. Britton (Eds.), *Women in African parliament,* pp. 133–150. Lynne Rienner, Boulder.

Lovenduski, J. and Norris, P. (1993) *Gender and Party Politics*. Sage, London.

Kagame P. (2002) The Great Lakes conflict: Factors, actors. And challenges. *Inaugural lecture at the Nigeria War College, Abuja, Nigeria*. (6 September 16, 2002). University for Peace, Geneva.

Matland, R. and Montgomery, K. (eds.), (2003) *Women's Access to Political Power in Post-Communist Europe*, Oxford University Press, Oxford.

Miall, H., Ramsbotham, O. and Woodhouse, T. (1999) *Contemporary conflict resolution: The prevention, management and transformation of deadly conflicts*. Polity Press, Cambridge.

Miller, C. and King, M. (2003) *A glossary of terms and concepts in peace and conflict studies*. University for Peace Africa Programme, Addis Abba.

Mwansasu, B. & Bugoya, W. (1999) *Overview of the Burundi Peace Process*. Mwalimu Nyerere Foundation Dar es Salaam.

Norris, P. and Lovenduski, J. (1995) *Political Recruitment: Gender, Race and Class in the British Parliament*. Cambridge University Press, Cambridge.

Norwegian Nobel Committee (2011) *The Nobel Peace Prize for 2011.* Nobelprize.org [online] Available at: http://www.nobelprize.org/nobel_prizes/peace/laureates/2011/press.html (accessed 5 September 2014).

Powley, T. (2004) *Strengthening Governance: The Role of Women in Rwanda's Transition. A Summary.* OSAGI, United Nations, New York.

Tadesse, Z. (2002) In Search of Gender Justice: Lessons from the Past and unveiling the 'new' NEPAD, *Presentation at African Scholars meeting 26-28 April 2002*, pp. 275-284.

Wallace, T. (Ed.), (1996) *Changing Perceptions: Writings on Gender and Development*, pp. 210-19. OXFAM, Oxford.

CHAPTER 5. THE POLITICS OF THE BODY IN CONFLICT: FOLLOWING WOMEN'S FOOTSTEPS: A HOLISTIC RESPONSE TO END SEXUAL VIOLENCE

Ruth Ojiambo Ochieng and Sandra Tumwesigye

Introduction

Our bodies are our primary means of participating socially, economically, politically, spiritually and creatively in society. They are the beginning point of the practical application of rights; the place in which rights are exercised, and for women in particular, the place where rights are most often violated. Without knowledge of and control over our bodies, including our sexuality, women's rights can neither be fully exercised nor enjoyed. (Isis-WICCE, 2013)

Devota Mbabazi an ex-combatant in Uganda and her experience of armed conflict bares a strong likeness to the stories of women in armed conflict-affected communities as far-flung as the Democratic Republic of the Congo (DRC), South Sudan, Liberia, Nepal, Kashmir, and many more others who have experienced sexual violence and the effects it played out on their bodies, minds and spirits. The experiences of these women and girls, demonstrate the multifaceted effects of armed conflict on the female gender and the need for a holistic response to end sexual violence against women in armed conflict if sustained peace is to be achieved.

Isis-WICCE has witnessed the value of a holistic approach to post conflict recovery programmes since meeting Devota, a survivor of rape by 21 soldiers. Despite existing 'peace', she was living in a remote village in central Uganda, unable to resume normal life or be integrated into the army due to her lack of a formal education. She had contracted HIV and AIDS as well as a glut of sexual and reproductive health compilations including fistula. Owing to her failed reintegration, she was unable to access social services to deal with her psychological trauma as well as her gynaecological health needs, which worsened her experience of stigma and inability to productively participate in recovery of her community. As a result, Isis-WICCE was impelled to adopt a model that enables women war survivors to fully and meaningfully participate, by striking a balance between restoring the dignity of women, and advocating for redress through equitable redistribution of resources in post-conflict settings.

The personal is political

Following over two decades of documenting and responding to the effects of conflict on women in armed conflict and post-conflict setting, Isis-WICCE has become well acquainted with the struggle for national sovereignty at the expense of women's bodily integrity. These experiences, which are reproduced at household, community, national and international levels, have made it increasingly clear that for women, the personal is indeed political. This politics is played out when the bodies of women and girls, are turned into battlegrounds through multiple experiences of abuse, particularly sexual violence. The same politics continues when conflicts are resolved and the damaged bodies are deemed ineligible in contributing to peace as peace processes and post-conflict recovery exclude them and their specific needs.

Ultimately, women's bodies continue to experience this very same politics through post-conflict decisions about national priorities, resource allocation, capacity development, and women's effective participation that do not prioritise gender responsiveness specifically addressing their meaningful participation, psychological, sexual and reproductive health needs. As such, even after the guns fall silent, women who have borne the brunt of the conflict are unable to participate in peace building or post-conflict recovery because their bodies, minds and spirits have not been restored.

The impact of sexual violence

Isis-WICCE has observed first-hand the markedly different way that women and girls experience the impact of sexual violence on their bodies, minds, spirits as well as their overall existence. Women in different settings experience rape, sexual mutilation, sexual humiliation, burning and mutilation of their body parts, forced prostitution, forced pregnancy or sexual slavery. Each case varies with the profile of the survivor, the motive of the perpetrator, the level of impunity and culture of militarism. As a result of their disadvantaged position in all societies, each woman or girl disproportionately suffers the effects.

In Liberia, Isis-WICCE found that 62.5% of women and girls in four counties of Banga Lofa Maryland and Grand Kru had experienced sexual violence. 73.9% had been raped and anecdotal evidence revealed forced prostitution in exchange for food from soldiers (Isis-WICCE, 2008). Women and girls in Sierra Leone experienced sex trafficking and in Central African Republic they were raped in front of their husbands or fathers (Isis-WICCE, 2011). In Jonglei, South Sudan, abducted girls are used as bargaining chips into sexual slavery and forced marriages, while women in Abyei and Northern Bahr-el-Gazal report rape by occupied forces (Isis-WICCE, 2013). Women in the Democratic Republic of Congo (DRC) reported high incidences of rape and sexual slavery by armed groups, the army/police and civilians in Rutshuru, Walikali, Lubero and other conflict affected territories of North and South Kivu. (Isis-WICCE, 2013)

In all these cases, the vulnerability of these women and girls to further injustice is heightened, and Isis-WICCE through its research and healing interventions has discovered that if unaddressed, women continue to suffer the impact of sexual violence on their minds, bodies and spirits.

The Body

Survivors experience grave damage to their reproductive systems and gynaecological issues such as infertility, abnormal vaginal discharge, chronic pelvic pain, sexually transmitted infections, vaginal tears, prolapsed uteruses and traumatic gynaecologic fistulae [1] which affects their sexual and reproductive health as well as their capacity for their daily living or social integration. In the case of Sierra Leone, of the 44.9% female survivors of the conflict, a great majority suffered a range of serious reproductive and gynecological health consequences. The most severe of them was vaginal destruction from violent sexual assault and gang rapes resulting in vesico vaginal fistula (VVF) and rectal vaginal fistula (RVF). During the healing intervention camps in Kitgum district, northern Uganda, Isis-WICCE found

---

1   Traumatic gynaecologic fistula—an injury that can result from violent sexual assault, often in conflict settings. Brutal rape (by one or more assailants or by the use of gun barrels, beer bottles, or sticks) can result in a tear, or fistula, between a woman's vagina and her bladder or rectum, or both. Women with traumatic fistula are unable to control the flow of their urine and/or faeces, and they find it impossible to keep themselves clean. (Traumatic Gynaecologic Fistula: A Consequence of Sexual Violence in Conflict Settings, ACQUIRE Project 2006).

that of the reproductive health complications exhibited by women, vesico vaginal fistula was experience among 6% of the survivors of sexual violence. In the Democratic Republic of Congo, a growing number of women dealing with fistula reported it as the result of gang rape, forced penetration with foreign objects or rape-induced spontaneous abortion. In certain cases, women who had been raped while pregnant suffered fistula as a result of unsuccessful attempts to extract the stillborn babies in remote health units.

Women with fistula and other ailments are unable to participate in society or support their families economically, due to fear of publicly bleeding or leaking urine and from overall weakness. They lack access to special health services that addresses these specific conditions. For example sexually transmitted infections (STIs) acquired following rape result in tubal blockage and thus infertility. This gynaecological condition leads to social stigma and affects the family stability worsening the effects of the experience on their bodied minds and spirit. In these settings some of the survivors are also faced with unwanted pregnancies and sexually transmitted infections such as HIV/AIDS, which put them at risk of carrying babies with no identity thus causing further stigma to the mother and later, the child. Some of the survivors have even attempted suicide and others have committed suicide even after delivering the children.

The Mind

While sexual violence is primarily administered on the body, the minds of survivors suffer grave and potentially long-term effects. Isis-WICCE research has revealed the severe psychological trauma among survivors of sexual violence. For instance, in Northern Uganda, women survivors had psychiatric disorders including post-traumatic stress disorder, depression, alcohol abuse disorder, panic anxiety disorder, agoraphobia, social phobia, somatoform disorder and suicidal thoughts. The findings also show that 6% of such women had homicidal thoughts just as a result of sexual violence. These psychological effects had impaired their ability to function normally or participate within their societies.

The Spirit

The power behind these survivors is destroyed and suffers social stigma, rejection and elimination, which inhibit their social reintegration. For instance women and girls with children resulting from rape and sexual slavery during conflict are doubly marginalised due to their children's questioned cultural identity and their association with rape. They suffer low esteem and hence have limited ability to effectively participate in socioeconomic opportunities. Such survivors are often ostracised by their husbands and families, thus driving them to leave their communities and discontinue their education. As a result they cannot access information about the government programmes as they have no fixed aboard, and their homes are the streets in townships.

Ultimately, Isis-WICCE has ascertained that without addressing the immediate impact of sexual violence on women's bodies, minds and spirits, survivors are not only unable to enjoy their rights or benefit from development, but the vicious cycle of sexual violence remains unbroken. This is well illustrated in the case of the approximately 300 ex-combatants and women formerly associated with armed groups in Uganda. These women with the average age of 27 years are survivors of sexual slavery. Some 62% of them were single mothers, 63% were ostracised by their families and communities, and 87% were unable to access land. They were all unable to successfully reintegrate or provide for their families. As a result, they are displaced and unable to engage in more productive activities, and instead survive on the meagre resources they get though commercial sex work in exchange for food items. The have sex with 2 to 6 clients a night to earn 72,000 ($30) a month. 67% of them would like to be able to earn an income without resorting to sex work. Despite purportedly living in peace or post-conflict, they are exposed to deeper levels of vulnerability and further sexual violence (IOM, 2010) that continue to make them insecure and thus not at peace. In these circumstances their communities and the nation at large can be at peace.

Consensus exists on the fact that while sexual violence is highest during armed conflict, it continues at alarming rates in post-conflict settings if the specific causes and associated dynamics are not addressed. As such, notwithstanding the existence of international and national laws criminalising sexual violence, such as the Rome Statute or local laws against rape and defilement. A holistic gender responsive approach is necessary in order to promote gender equality, challenge social constructs of violent masculinities and society's attitudes to women's bodies, dismantle cultures of militarism and build communities' capacities for conflict transformation. This will ultimately cause post-conflict recovery action that responds to women's specific judicial and bodily needs resulting from their experiences of conflict.

Impunity and liability for damage to women's bodies, minds and spirits

Over the years, Isis-WICCE has witnessed great strides taken on the part of governments and the international community in expressing their commitments to gender equality and more particularly to prevent sexual violence, impunity, and respond to the needs of survivors of violence. For instance, in the DRC as in Liberia, the governments have put in place national protocols on medical assistance, psychosocial support, legal referral and socioeconomic reintegration for survivors. Liberia's Ministry of Gender and Development, was a pioneer in developing a comprehensive National Gender-Based Violence Plan of Action, with the goal of reducing sexual violence and responding with appropriate services to survivors. A growing number of States like South Sudan are currently developing National Action Plans for UNSCR 1325 (2000), geared to providing women's rights, opening doors for women to participate in the post conflict development plans, preventing sexual violence, ending impunity and responding to the needs of survivors of abuse.

The leadership of Burundi, Uganda and DRC (among others), for example ratified the International Conference of the Great Lakes Region Protocol on the Prevention and Suppression of Sexual Violence Against Women and Children (2006) as well as the Goma Declaration on Eradication of Sexual Violence and Ending Impunity (2008). They also signed the December 2012 International Conference of the Great Lakes Region (ICGLR) Kampala Declaration, and launched the Zero Tolerance campaign to improve the effectiveness of judicial responses for sexual violence, as well as to ensure a one-stop centre where survivors can get medical and legal support. This year a regional Sexual and Gender-Based Violence (SGBV) centre has been established and has a major aim of building the capacity of the police and judiciary to effectively address the scourge of SGBV. Even more Heads of States signed and ratified the Maputo Protocol (2003), the protocol to the African Charter on Human and Peoples' Rights on the Rights of Women in Africa, as well as the Convention on the Elimination of All Forms of Discrimination against Women. These represent a sample of policy and legal frameworks that have been put in place to the same vein.

Nonetheless, despite the strong expressions of commitment in these policies, their corresponding impact on the bodies, minds and souls of women affected by armed conflict has yet to be registered. The problem of sexual violence in armed conflict persists and the needs of survivors in post-conflict settings largely remain unaddressed. In cases such as Burundi, Uganda, Liberia, South Sudan and DRC, women human rights defenders continue to advocate for the efficient implementation of these expressed commitments. The distinctive message underlying this is the need to walk the talk by prioritizing women's needs and addressing the impact of sexual violence in conflict on their bodies, minds and spirits.

An illustration can be seen in the case of sexual violence survivors in north and northeastern Uganda, where, in 2002, Isis-WICCE held a healing intervention camp in Soroti district in eastern Uganda. Survivors reported having unsuccessfully sought medical attention for their gynecological problems from the national health centres a decade later, and 2 years into the implementation of the post-conflict peace and reconstruction plan (PRDP). This is because the PRDP has prioritized physical structures, with limited focus being given to human security which is embedded in the body of individuals and thus the need for quality health services to repair women's minds and bodies.(Isis-WICCE; 2011).

Armed conflict inevitably destroys infrastructure and affects the provision of public services all of which calls for the post-conflict reconstruction of these institutions and facilities, and this takes time to be achieved. However, the same armed conflict damages the humaneness (IOM 2007).

This ultimately begs the question of who is liable for the damage to women's bodies that results from abuse in conflict? It can be argued that denying liability or disregarding the psychosocial, sexual and reproductive health needs of survivors of sexual violence represents a form of impunity for the perpetrators. In armed conflict and post-conflict settings where governments do not prioritise the needs of survivors there is an implicit message being sent that even though women's bodies are turned into battlegrounds, the repair of the infrastructural battlegrounds is of greater value. Consequently, in order to address the impact of sexual violence, women call for governments to express their commitment with plans and programmes backed with sufficient allotment of resources and capacities to address survivors' central needs so that they can reclaim their dignity, self-esteem and adjust the world so as to be accountable to these survivors. Ultimately, these responses should place women as prime agents able to significantly participate in processes of social transformation, peace building and post-conflict development.

Weaving women's power into peace

Since 1996, Isis-WICCE has been following the footsteps of women in different armed conflict and post-conflict settings of Africa and Asia. Over the years, through this practice of amplifying women's voices, documenting their experiences, exposing the underlying violent structures and conditions, as well as effecting positive change with their participation, a specific approach to feminist peace building has been honed.

This has been encapsulated in what is now referred to as the Isis-WICCE model of 'Weaving Women's Power into Peace'. This holistic model looks at a woman during her life span and works with five major ingredients. 'Illumination' focusing on research and documentation of the situation of women in armed conflict and post conflict, while 'Healing' repairs their body, mind and spirit. Under 'Synergy', women's skills are built to address critical issues and challenge the political status quo, while 'Advocacy' puts in place innovative strategies to influence androcentric post-conflict reconstruction policies and programmes. Finally through 'Radiation' Isis-WICCE mentors community based women's groups to implement activities that contribute to total peace building and gender responsive post-conflict rehabilitation; an aspect that builds a sustainable peace.

As a result, various shifts have been witnessed in women's ability to participate and contribute to peace building and development, in their respective communities and countries. Viewing women holistically and reaffirming their agency and personhood, while challenging the structures that oppress and perpetuate violence against women has brought about some positive results.

Illumination: Documenting violence against women in armed conflict

> "If the president will be able to watch this on television and become aware of my experiences as an ex-soldier and survivor of armed conflict, then I want every detail to be made known for my sake and for the sake of other women in a situation similar to mine." Devota Mbabazi

Centering women's bodies, minds and spirits

At the heart of the Isis-WICCE technique is the view of sexual violence survivors not simply as data sources but as 'knowers' and prospective change agents. As such, while the documentation process seeks information on their experience of sexual violence, it also seeks their views on the appropriate responses to prevention and protection from sexual violence in their contexts. These women are therefore not viewed as victims of a sexual crime but also as valued actors with a right to contribute to decision-making and any plans or programmes concerning their plight such as possible reparation or post-conflict recovery plans (Isis-WICCE Model; 2013). This fits within Isis-WICCE's view that all action on behalf of women should result from a bottom-up process that captures their views and priorities and is ultimately implemented with their participation.

Isis-WICCE also adopts a method that puts women's bodies, minds and spirits at the centre. To this end, storytelling is used as a distinctive tool to gather information while promoting the survivors' psychosocial wellbeing. It has been discovered in different contexts that by allowing women to tell their own personal stories, they experience healing because it allows them to challenge the shame and conspiracy of silence surrounding their bodily attack. Their bodies are put at the centre by facilitating emergency interventions to their sexual and reproductive health needs. Over the years, Isis-WICCE has applied this action-oriented approach by setting up healing camps and mobilizing health professionals to respond with treatment and surgery for the different sexual and reproductive health and psychological ailments in Uganda, Liberia and South Sudan.

In some cases some of the stories have become tools of advocacy and have supported calls to leaders to address the needs of survivors. As such the documentation process contributes to long-term processes such as gender responsive transitional justice or post-conflict recovery and reconstruction processes.

Collaboration and capacity development

This same principle of contributing to local processes is reflected in Isis-WICCE's practice of building a self-sustaining mechanism for timely data collection and respond to issues associated with women's situation in armed conflict and post-conflict. Through its international capacity building programme, Isis-WICCE has developed the capacity of a vanguard of women leaders and human rights defenders, at local level to document and respond to women's issues. These women activists regularly document their own realities and women's experiences of SGBV for further action. For instance, following the documentation of women's experience of armed conflict, an institute alumna from northeastern Uganda responded by forming a Community Based Organisation, The Teso Women's Peace Activists (TEWPA), which has been instrumental in peace building, and engendering post-conflict recovery efforts in the region.

Through equipping a movement of documenters and working with local women leaders, Isis-WICCE has been able to address issues posed by the International Protocol process such as the question of sensitivity. Local women and women's organisations are knowledgeable of their contexts and are also well able to gather evidence from other women while maintaining sensitivity and providing support to the survivors. Through this approach, Isis-WICCE has been able to receive information from various armed conflict areas it would otherwise be unable to reach. An example is the documentation of rape and sexual humiliation in rural Zimbabwe (by Alumna), in areas that purported to supported the political opposition during the 2008 elections when NGOs were denied access and mobility was restricted (Isis-WICCE; 2012).

In a similar vein, several documenting and investigating processes of sexual violence in conflict have been curtailed due to female survivors' low willingness to report. This was the case in Rwanda where the local culture frowns upon discussing sexual violence, thus the low precedence for justice for sexual crimes of this nature. Another case is the truth and reconciliation processes in Sierra Leone and Liberia where many women and girls did not approach the commission to share their experiences due to the associated stigma, as well as gender insensitivity in data collection and presentation. Trust and local credibility is required in order for survivors to willingly share their experiences. Isis-WICCE has been able to overcome these hurdles by consistently working in collaboration with active local women and women's groups in their communities for a long time. Involving government departments is critical for continuity, responsibility and accountability.

As such, since the International Protocol seeks to promote practices that nurture mutual support, it would be profitable to collaborate with local women's groups and organisations already concerned with providing support to survivors. Ultimately, the process of documentation and investigation of cases should contribute to a more long-term impact and social transformation. Consequently, in the absence of strong institutions, it is recommended that women's capacity and the capacity of women's organisations is developed to take charge of the documentation and investigation of violation of women's rights in their settings.

Radiation: Women's meaningful participation for peace and post-conflict rehabilitation

The value of women's participation extends beyond their ability to effectively gather information of evidentiary value on sexual violence against women. Women's roles as proactive change agents in addressing peace and human security in various countries is widely recognized and well documented. It is common knowledge that the women of what is now the Republic of South Sudan are largely responsible for the outcome of the 2011 referendum, which relied on their full participation and saw women's groups and Member sof Parliament mobilizing women from door to door, providing water, food and in some cases transportation for women to participate in the referendum. The significant contribution of women's participation to peace and security in Burundi is also widely known. It is acknowledged that without the existence of local women's groups, there would be no structures to reach widespread communities to participate in peace and reconciliation, and close gaps in development across gender and ethnic lines.

Women peace activists in Sierra Leone were at the forefront of the movement for peace. The various creative initiatives used by the women's movement in Uganda, Liberia and Nepal, agitating for the peaceful resolution of the respective armed conflicts. The roles of women in bringing conflicting parties, as well as their spirited agitation for the criminalization of sexual violence in conflict-affected DRC, fall in this same category. Despite these demonstrations of women's capacities, women are consistently excluded from formal peace processes whose peace agreements and post-conflict reconstructions plans also exclude women's needs. An assessment of 24 major peace processes reflects this same dynamic with only 3% women signatories, 8% participation in negotiations and women visibly underrepresented when making vital decisions about post conflict recovery (UNIFEM 2010). As a result, the same script is played out in post-conflict settings with women agitating for inclusion in post-conflict settlements and for their needs resulting from sexual violence in conflict to be addressed in the programmes developed.

Reframing women's participation

Women's experience in formal peace and reconciliation processes has proven the insufficiency of participation without concrete influence. While different governments expressed their commitment to address sexual violence and women's associated needs at the peace tables, actual implementation of the post-conflict recovery plans do not reflect this. In many countries, such as Liberia, Burundi and Uganda among others, these commitments are not fully implemented and government machineries often lack sufficient funds and capacities to do so, (Isis-WICCE 2012). As such, it is inadequate to solely view and promote women's participation as women's representation in these formal structures and processes. Over time women have become discontent with solely seeking a seat at the table and continuously agitating for a slice of the pie even when all decision makers acknowledge the fact that women bore the brunt of the conflict.

Women are therefore taking the same proactive approach to address issues of violence against women in armed conflict setting and beyond. Women are advocating and applying pressure for governments to directly address the psychosocial and reproductive health and rights needs of survivors of sexual violence, as an expression of their commitment and accountability to post-conflict recovery and ending sexual violence. At the same time women and women's organizations are seeking partnerships with governments and other actors to break the cycle of sexual violence by taking direct action to prevent, mitigate and respond to the conflict that is played out on women's bodies, as is the case with Isis-WICCE's healing camps. This two-pronged method enables women to effectively **participate** in, and contribute to a genuine peace and reconstruction that prioritizes the bodies, minds and spirits of conflict-affected women and girls.

Additionally, instead of purely taking a reactive stance by ensuring that a representative number of women is included in formal peace and recovery processes, women's organizations such as Isis-WICCE now promote a proactive approach that develops the capacity of larger constituencies of women over a period of time, to prevent violent conflict, to transform household and community conflicts, to make decisions that protect women and girls from sexual violence and ultimately to participate in determining and influencing interventions planned on their behalf. Consequently support for interventions of this nature that do not always fit neatly into the more popular quick impact project frameworks, goes a long way in improving women's participation in sustainable peace, security and prevention of sexual violence.

Advocacy: women's innovative strategies for peace, human security and post-conflict rehabilitation.

In harmony with Isis-WICCE's survivor-centric approach that puts women's bodies, minds and spirits at the centre of rebuilding the shattered nations, it goes without saying that efforts to prevent sexual violence against women and girls in conflict must include and be driven by women and women's armed groups/organizations. In this regard, UN Security Council Resolution 1366 supplements UNSCR 1325, in emphasising the importance of women's vital role in conflict prevention. In addition, Isis-WICCE's experience over the years has highlighted the value of their participation in early warning and conflict mitigation, as well as the risks associated with excluding women's knowledge and participation.

This is well illustrated in the case of Uganda where in Karamoja (in north eastern Uganda), women were privy to valuable early warning information concerning planned armed raids, routes to be used and storage of firearms (Isis-WICCE 2009, Stites & Akabwai 2009) but this was never used to mitigate conflict or their experience of sexual violence. In Luwero, women who also experienced sexual violence spoke of having been lured to support the civil war with promises of quick delivery out of poverty (Isis-WICCE 1998). These women did not understand their vulnerability in a context of conflict. In 1989, when no one had the courage, a group of women wore rags and sang funeral songs as they walked through Gulu town, in northern Uganda, demanding an end to violence (Isis-WICCE 2000). These women understood their power to spark change for peace. These cases demonstrate the need to build women's capacity to participate at their different levels in making valuable decisions before, during and after armed conflict, to understand the nature of violent conflict and ultimately appreciate their role in preventing sexual violence in conflict.

Early warning for prevention of violence against women

In taking emergency action with the goal of prevention, humanitarian agencies only stand to benefit from close collaboration with local civil society actors and particularly women's groups or organizations already working with communities on issues of sexual violence. By engaging women and community members, these efforts benefit from a deeper understanding of the context, which is particularly important in appreciating and interpreting issues of gender, which differ depending on the society and in relation to sexual violence. In addition, they often fill a capacity gap by providing the financial and institutional support needed to set up sustainable mechanisms to support long-term efforts to prevent sexual violence during periods of unrest.

Isis-WICCE received reports of women in South Sudan who were aware of the impending armed violence. However because these women did not have a mechanism or the resources to reach a large number of women quickly, they walked from house to house and several women and girls did benefit from this early warning information. Moreover, several women and girls who were aware of the imminent threat did not have the benefit of a protection mechanism.

Consequently, according to the UNMISS human rights report, large numbers of women and girls were raped by soldiers in Juba and opposition forces in Bor and Malakal. Among those that did managed to flee their homes, more women and girls were raped by civilians seeking refuge at the UN Mission (UNMISS 2014). Cases of this nature emphasize the need to prioritise, popularise and apply early warning frameworks and mechanisms for sexual violence along with self-defence or personal protection mechanisms for women and girls. This could be embedded in the structures of women's organisations and groups. In 2011 UN Action against Sexual Violence in Conflict, UN Women and the Department of Peacekeeping Operations developed a framework of early warning indicators focused on conflict related sexual violence. However knowledge and use of this framework appears limited and not broadly shared.

This calls for collaboration between humanitarian agencies and women's groups and organizations that have long-term relationships with women and already operate in these areas, but lack sufficient financial and human capacity for extensive impact. Solid early warning and protection mechanisms for sexual violence are also needed and would benefit from strategic linkages due to numerous dynamics.

Analysis of different cases in DRC and South Sudan promote the value of collaborating with local women's organizations. They connect a relationship between a profound understanding of various elements of a specific context to the ability to foretell increased levels of sexual violence. This includes a strong knowledge of the actors including leadership, sources of funding, and methods of conscription, ethnic composition, and the past history of abuses. This can then be assessed together with information on the specific conditions on the ground so as to increase prevention. At the same tile this can improve the efficient protection by security actors and self-defence by affected communities (UNWOMEN 2012). This role is best executed by local actors already taking action on sexual violence, such as women's organisations. A midterm review of the implementation of Uganda's post-conflict peace and reconstruction programme confirms the value of women's organizations in mitigating conflict as they were ranked highest (56%) for their work to this end (Isis-WICCE; 2011).

Funding for women's bodies

In the case of Burundi, women were consulted while the priorities for the countries post-conflict reconstruction were being determined. However final decisions were influenced by the Bretton Woods institutions and major funders who did not prioritise women's reproductive health needs (Isis-WICCE; 2012). In South Sudan, the allocation of resources over a six-year post-conflict period revealed the government's priorities with 29% being allocated to security, 12% to roads, 7% to basic education and 3% to health. It therefore comes as no surprise that the meagre financing for health did not emphasize women's health needs, which includes addressing increasing rates of HIV/AIDS in armed conflict and post-conflict sections of the country, (USIP; 2009). This lack of a focus in prioritization or funding on women's specific needs has resulted in post-conflict recovery programmes that do not adequately promote gender equality and women's total health, which are a prerequisite to sustainable peace.

In all these contexts, women decry the absence of health service delivery mechanisms that respond to their needs and situations, particularly those transiting out of armed conflict. Survivors face challenges of drug shortages, lack of medical equipment, scarcity of skilled medical personnel and quality gynecological services as well as inadequate health infrastructure to address their special sexual and reproductive health needs. In the DRC, there has been some level of free treatment for post rape survivors. However, most of these centres are urban based, with no mechanisms to facilitate moving traumatised survivors to the centres given that most of the rapes are committed in remote areas, Their remote locations and the long distance to health units therefore renders these services inaccessible to most of the survivors. While in Uganda, the health budget in the post-conflict Peace, Recovery and Development Plan (PRDP) prioritises construction of health centres and purchase of transport equipment (ambulances), but it has not allotted sufficient resources to reproductive health care or the repair of survivors' bodies. As such, gynecologists are only located at referral hospitals and women have to travel long distances for these services and in some cases even pay 60,000 shillings ($24), to use the government ambulance due to corruption. Health centres in hard-to-reach areas lack skilled health workers and women have complained of a lack of HIV testing kits for pregnant women in some units. (Isis-WICCE; 2011).

Across the board, women sexual violence survivors are calling for governments to put their money where their mouth is. The commitment expressed in policies to respond to the needs of sexual violence survivors should be translated into funding to heal women's bodies, minds and spirits. Funding for post-conflict recovery programmes such as the PRDP in Uganda should prioritize psychosocial support for sexual violence survivors.

These resources should also focus on recruiting and training health workers to identify and treat psychosomatic, sexual and reproductive health conditions. Funding should also address the shortages of medical officers, midwives and gynecologists as well as women's challenges to accessing health centres.

For more sustained and holistic support, there should be coordination between women's organisation, which play a first call post with government institutions responsible for the peace and recovery programs. Due to the limited number of staff within national health systems, these local organisations should be trained to provide complimentary support in trauma management. Funding should also be directed to organisations providing these much needed services.

Other civil society organisations such as AYINET[2] and Isis-WICCE have partnered with governments (such as Uganda's Ministry of Health and Ministry of Local Government), to directly respond with treatment and surgery for survivors' sexual and reproductive health problems. In Liberia, Isis-WICCE worked with the Ministry of Health and Social Welfare, the Ministry of Gender and WANEP/WIPNET, to provide specialised health care to women survivors, build the capacity of local health workers in the management of reproductive and surgical complications of war, trained primary care health workers to provide psychological support to survivors and resourced reproductive health kits to rural health units. The team reached twelve health centres and two hospitals in two counties, in a period of one month. About 1200 survivors received counselling and treatment for fistulae, genital prolapses and fertility problems. The power of networking among the Isis-WICCE team of doctors influenced them to sell the idea of providing mental health clinics to these war ravaged areas. The Peter Alderman Foundation in the USA, supported the establishment of a trauma centre in one of the affected communities in Uganda; and in Banga, in Liberia, and contracted a Ugandan psychologists to support the hospital.

This medical intervention has been replicated in different conflict-affected parts of Uganda such as Luweero, Gulu, Soroti, Kitgum, Kasese, Lira and Kotido districts, as well as South Sudan, where Isis-WICCE partnered with the Ministry of Health and Totto Chan Trauma Centre. In order to contribute to the healing of women's bodies, minds and spirits, it is important that these partnerships with government are promoted and funding is also allocated to civil society organisations that have demonstrated transformative impact in directly addressing survivors' psychosocial as well as sexual and reproductive health needs. Presently a team of feminists Across

---

2. The African Youth Initiative Network (AYINET). It is committed to making peace and justice a reality for victims and survivors of war.

Africa have established a model with support from the Stephen Lewis Foundation, named the Africa Integrated Response for survivors of crisis to support the coordination of women's interventions and provision of appropriate skilled personnel for appropriate action.

Looking to the future: The post-2015 development agenda

Based on the level of progress achieved in promoting gender equality, ending sexual violence in armed conflict and post-conflict settings or responding to survivors' sexual and reproductive health needs, it is safe to say that governments and global actors cannot rest on their laurels. In line with the transformative shifts currently underpinning the post-2015 development agenda, it is clear that gender inequality must be addressed in order to leave no one behind, building peace and putting sustainable development at the centre.

The post-2015 framework echoes the sentiments of this paper in its recognition of vulnerability, the importance of protection, inclusiveness and participation. As such in order to build on this and the existing commitments in the millennium development goals (MDGs), the post-2015 framework should be framed to prioritise a specific focus on gender inequality as an expression of true commitment to sustainable development.

By specifically focusing on addressing gender inequality, national and international actors will have an implementation and accountability mechanism to address women's marginalisation and the structural inequalities that make women and girls vulnerable to sexual violence in armed conflict and susceptible to gender discrimination in the allocation of post-conflict recovery resources.

The framework should also include specific sub-goals and targets concerned with addressing the specific sexual and reproductive health needs of women associated with conflict and their experience of sexual violence. This includes explicitly prioritising sexual and reproductive health and rights responses, as well as adequate and quality health service delivery for survivors in order to improve past national and global performance in this area, which has been characterised by a lot of lip service. To consolidate and build on progress made under goal 3 of the MDGs, the post-2015 framework should prioritise these gender equality issues by strengthening the gender and peace pillars without which there can be no guarantee of global development, peace and security.

The opportunities to address this lie within the existing goals of the framework, for instance under goal 4. Women's mental, sexual and reproductive health needs should be specifically addressed as their health is the starting point for their meaningful participation in development, which is hit hardest in armed conflict and post-conflict countries. Goal 10 must centre on women's meaningful participation and acknowledge their role as transformational actors in order to be able to boast of truly good governance and effective institutions. Without prioritising gender responsive post-conflict reconstruction that addresses women's bodily integrity, and their specific needs, goal 11 cannot expect to effectively ensure stable and peaceful societies. Ultimately, in creating a global enabling environment and ensuring long-term finance, the post 2015 development framework should ensure equitable resource allocation for women's concerns as well as funding women engagement in peace building and development.

Conclusion

It is important to bring back into focus the mind, body and spirit of women affected by armed conflict, which must be restored in order for women to be able to contribute to the social, economic, political, spiritual wellbeing of societies, and be at peace with self and others.

References

International Organisation for Migration (2010) *Land Or Else: Land-based Conflict, Vulnerability and Disintegration in Northern Uganda.* IOM, Kampala.

Isis-WICCE (1998) Women's Experiences of Armed Conflict in Uganda, Luweero District 1980-1986, Uganda. *Paper.* Isis-WICCE, Kampala.

Isis-WICCE (2000) Women's Experiences of Armed Conflict in Uganda, Gulu District 1986-1999, Uganda. *Paper.* Isis-WICCE, Kampala.

Isis-WICCE (2008) Touching the Unreached: A Medical Intervention in Liberia. *Paper.* Isis-WICCE, Kampala.

Isis-WICCE (2009) Baseline Study of Women's Leadership for Peace and Security in Uganda. *Paper.* Isis-WICCE, Kampala.

Isis-WICCE (2012) Women's Leadership in Peace Building in South Sudan. *Paper.* Isis-WICCE, Kampala.

Isis-WICCE (2012) Mid-term Review Report of the Peace, Recovery and Development Plan for Northern Uganda. *Paper.* Isis-WICCE, Kampala.

UN WOMEN (2012) *Women's Participation in Peace Negotiations: Connections Between Presence and Influence.* UN WOMEN, New York.

UN WOMEN (2012) *Gender Responsive Early Warning: An Overview and How-To Guide.* UN WOMEN, New York.

Isis-WICCE (2013) Who we are [online] Available at: http://www.isis.or.ug/who-we-are/who-we-are/ (accessed 14 September 2014).

Isis-WICCE (2013) *Pushed to the Periphery: The Necessity of Women's Innovation in Activating Post-Conflict Reconstruction*. Isis-WICCE, Kampala.

UN Mission in the Republic of South Sudan (2014) *Conflict in South Sudan: A Human Rights Report*. United Nations, Juba.

United States Institute for Peace (2009) *Post-Conflict Health Reconstruction, New Foundations for US Policy*. USIP, Washington, DC.

CHAPTER 6. AGEING AND CHANGING COMMUNITY DYNAMICS IN AFRICA

Antony Ong'ayo Otieno

Introduction

African is a continent that constantly draws global attention for all kinds of human and natural disasters. In recent years however Africa has been undergoing significant societal transformation partly due to increased interconnectedness of global dynamics with local realities. The dynamism within the continent has led to significant leaps from the impact of colonialism and the decades of dictatorship and political instability. The continent has shown enormous resilience to the impact of the global economic crisis with a number of countries currently experiencing impressive economic growth rates of 5% and above. A growing middle class accompanies the observed growth, though with varying degrees in different countries. The noted economic growth is also linked to a change in population structure in terms of the number of youth and elderly, health status and level of education.

Demographically, life expectancy in Africa has seen a jump from 50 years in 2000, to 57 in 2012, compared to the global average of 70 (WHO, 2012). Mortality rates in Africa have not gone down but the local dynamics in Africa are further driven by population growth with studies showing a more youthful population (Young, 2005). While previous studies largely focused on the factors influencing demographic changes in Africa namely: poverty, lack of basic necessities, disease, drought, famine, floods and conflicts, another strand of literature started to also give attention to ageing (Bigala & Ayiga, 2014; Apt, 2012; Golaz & Rutaremwa, 2011; Oppong, 2006; Adamchak, 1989). Elderly care however has only received limited focus. The impressive economic growth and increasing life expectancy currently witnessed in many stable African countries need not overshadow the challenges of ageing as an important demographic feature in contemporary Africa. The family unit has been an important safety net in Africa, but currently faces enormous pressures from tendencies linked to modernization and urbanization. Urbanization in rural areas and rural-urban migration (Remi et al., 2014) have brought new challenges with regards to the care for the elderly in the context of marginalization, the increasing gap between rich and poor and between different localities in the same polity.

Part of this process started much earlier with the commodification of labour and the colonial labour legacy, which forced many young persons to leave rural areas for settler farms (Ong'ayo et al. 2013). Current mobility patterns are influenced by both push and pull factors (Remi et al. 2014) like economic decline and poverty in rural areas. In attempts to escape from poverty, and find means to support their families, large numbers of young people in Africa are leaving the rural areas in search of better opportunities in cities and other countries. This has also been dubbed the intergenerational 'migration contract' between a migrant and his or her parents, in which the (usually male) migrant moves and sends remittances in expectation of a subsequent inheritance (Black et al. 2006 p45). Migration studies also point to the socio-cultural and economic development implications of migration (Riccio, 2008; Adepoju, 2002), in relation to rural depopulation and reduced manpower for agricultural production.

In recent times rural-urban migration has led to the abandonment of elderly parents without safety nets that cushion them from the impact of globalization. The family structure which has been a bedrock of care and support in the African context is fast disintegrating as many communities experience enormous pressures to cope with threatened livelihoods linked to unemployment, climate change and food insecurity. Those that have left rural areas for cities increasingly adopt new cultures in what has been described as globalization of cultures (Nederveen, 2004). Challenges with blind aping or adoption of new cultures without reflection has since put many African urbanites at a cross roads due to their inability to completely de-Africanize and westernize at the same time. The social-cultural crises in Africa is further exacerbates by a failure to adapt valuable practices from both worlds. These dynamics have implications of how traditional values and family systems on care for the elderly are viewed in Africa.

In this paper we seek to provide an overview of the ageing situation in Africa. The paper further examines the challenges and opportunities for addressing current and future needs in elderly care in the continent. It uses the legacy of Marga Klompé (van Reisen & Borgman, 2012) on ethical approaches to Health Care as its philosophical underpinning in order to derive complementary values and practices of care from other cultures in the context of globalisation. This perspective brings to the fore the questions of gender and masculinity in the area of ageing and care within specific national and cultural contexts. Part of the data used in this paper is derived from a study that examined the health sector activities of Dutch-based diaspora organisations (Ong'ayo, 2014). This is augmented by excerpts of two interviews conducted with a Dutch-based Ghanaian diaspora who has taken a number of elderly care initiatives in Ghana and an elderly person in Kenya who has been dealing with challenges of care in the absence of family and institutionalized forms of care in a rural setting.

This paper is structured as follows: Part one presents a critical assessment of ageing and changing family structures and community dynamics in Africa. This is important for understanding the kind of social changes currently taking place in Africa and how they impact on traditional care and safety nets for the elderly. Part two examines issues at stake in ageing and elderly care in Africa in terms of cultural and socio-economic conditions and the political, institutional and policy response to ageing and care. Part three discusses how challenges in ageing and care in Africa can be addressed through innovations that are contextually and culturally relevant, economically viable, sustainable and humane. The final part presents a set of reflection points with implications for policy and intervention

Critical assessment of ageing and changing family structure in Africa

In 2013, the population in Africa topped 1 billion people with the expectation of an annual average increase of 2%. A large proportion of this population consist of young persons at 46.2% (table1). Life expectancy has also changed significantly from a low 52 years in 1990 to 57 in 2010. By 2030 it is projected to reach 63 years (UNDESA, 2012). Female life expectancy in the same period stood at 53 and 57 respectively. The elderly population in Africa was estimated at 36 million in 2010. It is projected to increase by 10% in 2015 (UNDESA, 2012). As table 1 shows, the population in the 65+ brackets constituted 3.6% of the total continental population. North Africa and Southern Africa recorded the highest old age at 5.1% and 4.9% respectively. East and West Africa both had 3.2%. Central Africa had the lowest number of elderly persons at 2.9%. In 2015, the total African population above 65 years of age will be about 102,000. Current old age dependency is about 6.2% and it is expected to reach 7.0% in 2030. Urbanisation in Africa has also rapidly increased from 14.7 in 1950 to 36.2% in 2000 (UNDESA, 2012). These demographic changes generate new challenges in terms of care for the elderly. This is more so in the context of a lack of data on the actual situation in rural areas, and inadequate institutional and policy preparedness.

Table 1. Population by age groups - continents and sub regions as at July 2013

Age	0-14	15-44	45-64	65+	Total
World	1,864,072,480	3,292,837,689	1,406,651,977	566,451,615	7,130,013,761
Africa	435,599,165	494,601,127	124,903,796	39,632,587	1,094,736,675
Eastern Africa	149,220,753	156,019,657	34,071,329	11,074,205	350,385,944
Middle Africa	60,212,613	59,378,390	13,173,239	3,947,057	136,711,299
Northern Africa	67,985,151	106,110,669	34,728,479	11,191,548	220,015,847
Southern Africa	17,786,005	29,193,003	9,076,738	2,881,720	58,937,466
Western Africa	140,394,643	143,899,408	33,854,011	10,538,057	328,686,119

Source: UNDESA (2012)

These challenges are further exacerbated by the social changes currently taking place in Africa especially at the family level. From a livelihoods perspective (Chambers & Conway, 1992) the family unit in Africa has been central in providing for all needs. These directly relate to the capabilities, assets and activities that enable them to secure livelihoods, health, and means of living through participation in the economic sphere. Through these activities, the family is guaranteed security in terms food, nutrition, health, water, shelter and education. Struggles by many families to address these factors thus become one major cause of the disintegration of the family unit. Consequently, the struggles are reshaping at the same time being reshaped by new roles that family members have to play including children and the elderly.

Changes in the way the contemporary African family functions have implications for care practices that are embedded in values and practices that have sustained communities for years. Values have been a critical component of traditional care safety nets in case of illness and disability. Historically, the role of the elderly in African society has been that of a mentor, counsellor, mediators in conflict situations and a safety net of support to grandchildren. In recent years the elderly, especially grandmothers, have become the primary carers for grandchildren in the context of AIDS related deaths of their own children. This situation raises the question about who takes care of the care of the elderly caregivers (Beilsma & Asio, 2013). In situations where there are surviving children, the elderly have traditionally been cared for within the family unit. It is for this reason that many African countries still lacking institutionalised forms of elderly care. However, as the family unit is disintegrating under the pressures of globalisation, as well as local social and economic transformation, new or alternative forms of care become necessary.

As a result of the noted transformations and disintegration of the family unit, many elderly people in Africa are experiencing different kinds of abuse. Firstly because the role of the elderly is losing value compared to previous times when old age was revered and treated with respect. Secondly, the loss of these values has also informed the emerging abusive treatment of the elderly in African today. An example is the unorthodox interpretation of culture in ways that perceive the aging conditions such as dementia as witchcraft (Boatemah, 2012). Such perceptions and ignorance have led to physical abuse of the elderly including, ostracism and physical removal from the vicinity of the community. Other forms of elderly abuse include sexual, emotional and financial abuse (Bigala, & Ayiga, 2014). Observations in Ghana suggest that even in cases where children are highly educated and have means, elderly parents still encounter neglect (physical and emotional) as a result of claimed modern influence and perceptions about dementia as sign of witchcraft. Many middle classes in urban areas are less inclined to have their elderly parents living with them in their modern house in the cities. These conditions have given the impetus for alternative forms of care including home services by professionals even though these services are still under developed.

The family unit in the majority of African communities plays an important role in the economic sphere. This relates to production, which has a collective dimension. This entails collective participation in productive activities and in care of members of the family. Changes in mode of production has a significant impact on the socio-economic aspects of community life. This is more so in the context of agrarian and land reforms that have disrupted land ownership and production but also the conflicts that have emerged as a result of competition for scarce resources. Adding more complexity to the function of the family unit and its struggles with care is climate change, which has affected agricultural production, especially in rural areas where households rely on subsistence farming. Low agricultural productivity also impacts on a major source of livelihood as well as from a nutrition and health point of view.

The failure of many countries to facilitate the integration of all parts of the polity into the national, and consequently global economy continues to marginalise large populations from sources of livelihoods. A shift to a more market oriented economic system has left many households in vulnerable situations since a majority cannot participate in the modern economy due to lack of education and the necessary skills. For families that have managed to send children to school, employment opportunities are scares hence the safety net role of children in most African communities is in jeopardy.

Socio-economic conditions at the family level thus have a significant impact on families and by extension the elderly who rely on the safety nets for survival in the absence of state provided institutionalised care.

Issues at stake in aging and elderly care in Africa

As the demographic structure changes in Africa there is still limited understanding of the demographics of aging in terms of well-documented patterns and trends influencing factors and implications (box 1). This includes the social welfare, health status and conditions of disability of older people and patterns of change and care that the elderly require.

Box 1. Issues on aging and care
- Social welfare
- Health care
- Housing an environment
- Food and Nutrition
- Support services
- Culture, value and practices
- Technological input
- Education and training

The first critical issue relates to the limited comprehension of traditional care and social support mechanisms that can still serve as models to be upgraded and up-scaled in order to reach poor segments. Such models could be fused with modern approaches in order to tap into values and practices that informed care. This is more imperative in an era of high costs of giving care. State provided care might not be the long-term solution, but coming with a middle way is likely to be confronted by the fading away of the valuable traditional care practises as many people aspire to adopt modern lifestyles including western models of care.

A second critical issue relates to the socio-economic conditions that underpin living, health and care in Africa. The patterns of demographic change in Africa further requires an in-depth understanding of influencing factors as the precondition for developing appropriate responses. The socio-economic conditions influence the overall social welfare of the elderly. This includes such aspects as secure livelihoods, healthy living, environment and capacities for mitigating the challenges that come with aging in contemporary times. A third important issue is the political condition in the local context. Many African countries have experienced conflicts of different kinds and a significant number continue to undergo reconstruction, reconciliation and putting in place essential services. The political angle to aging and care also relates to the question of inclusivity or exclusivity in resource distribution. This is important in terms of resource allocation for the establishment of the necessary infrastructure for elderly care as well as the necessary space for collaboration between government and non-state actors (civil society and private sector). The political system is also critical for addressing such concerns as rights of the most vulnerable such as women, children and the elderly through appropriate institutional, policy and legislative frameworks. Political stability also plays an important enabling role for addressing societal challenges.

The forth issue relates to the approach and interventions that seek to address aging and care in Africa in ways that takes into account the numerous challenges and opportunities in the continent. This concerns the questions of addressing elderly care in a context where there is increased interconnections to developments elsewhere without being fully integrated into the global systems. The increasing use of ICT in Africa, rapid flow of information and images, expose local populations to a broad spectrum of products and a consumerism mentality that require a certain level of socio-economic foundation. These influences include the use of products and technology for solutions to local problems. This situation gives the impetus for exploring new developments and knowledge that could address contemporary and future aging challenges in Africa

Addressing challenges in aging and care in Africa

In terms of political, institutional and policy response to aging and care, demographic shifts have implications for the development trajectory in any polity depending on how its various dimensions are managed. The main concerns are pressures on health and education systems, infrastructure and the conflicts that are likely to arise due to resource scarcity. However the health of a population is most important since it determines participation in all spheres of life, and consequently the productivity of individuals and society. In the context of the observed challenges caused by demographics changes in Africa the main concern is to what extent are the political, institutional and policy frameworks responsive to these transformations. The centrality of political will in shaping policy outcomes gives the impetus for interrogating the political establishment in Africa with regards to aging and care for the elderly. The policy and institutional response thus concerns issues such as facilities, service delivery and the continuous search for solutions that meet constantly shifting care needs.

Community-based care (Moetlo et al., 2011; Kangethe, 2010; Kidman et al., 2007) is not new to Africa. The approach is often presented as an alternative form of care but such practices have existed in Africa from time immemorial. The problem lies with its prescription without linking them to the values and practices that underpinned such approaches. These challenges thus call for rethinking hybridity (Gunaratnam, 2014) in approaching care in different cultures and contexts that are undergoing dramatic societal transformation. These dynamics further call for redefining the family unity, community values, gender roles and the traditional care practices that provided safety nets for members of the family including the elderly, women and children. Additionally a redefinition of gender roles is critical since family situations are changing in Africa to the extent that roles are increasingly switching. More females are performing tasks that have been traditionally in male domains. At the same time men are also increasingly performing roles previously left for females. An example is a situation where a male is a widower or the only caregiver in a family environment that is predominantly female.

In the face of an increasing deteriorating state of the social safety nets in Africa what lessons can we learn from Marga Klompe's visionary approach to these issues in her time? What kind of inspiration can we derive from the temporality of her vision and pragmatism in the area of social security and elderly care? Looking at Marga Klompe's legacy as represented by the Social Security Bill, Elderly Homes Bill, Caravan Bill and her work in education, politics and religion is a stark reminder of the timelessness, unbounded and transcendent character of the values she stood for. Her legacy and the value she stood for are very relevant to both past and present Africa in which vulnerability is pervading every area of human dignity. This is more so in cases of persons that continue to experience conditions of socio-economic and political marginalisation.

Challenges facing Africa today are reminiscent of Marga's own time, hence it gives an impetus for rethinking the issues for which Marga Klompe stood. This ought to be approached from the perspective of reclaiming the values that have been lost or being lost in the process of modernisation, and increased consumerism and individualism; retaining the values and practices that are still relevant, adapting new practices of care bases on a principle of cross-cultural exchange, reciprocity and win-win scenarios. This imperative is informed by the increasing interconnectedness of people and places through basic human needs and de-territorialised forms of interdependency. The new challenges posed by aging in the context of contemporary transitions (aging and care in Europe and Aging, young population and care in Africa) are thus intertwined with global and local processes, hence responses need to tap into values and practices from both contexts while at the same time protecting human dignity through care that is humane.

Conclusion

In the context of globalisation and dominance of neo-liberal economic policies addressing aging and elderly care challenges in African will not be immune to external influences. The main concern is how the externally led interventions will pay attention to local context perspectives and knowledge and needs in the prescribed solutions. This concern calls for interrogating new ideas being proposed as part of on-going and future social and technological innovations. The on-going social and economic transformations in Africa will be accompanied by technological challenges and opportunities as part of new solutions, especially in the health and care sector. The main players in the health sector from industry, to knowledge institutes and civil society will have to rethink their entry strategy but also how to develop products in line with local needs and capacities. Such an approach thus calls for innovations that are context and culturally relevant.

In addition, costs are always inherent in new innovations and the extent to which new innovations can be rolled out through mass production and use has to take into account the question of affordability. While this is a normal calculation within the entrepreneurial logical there is evidence that disregard for affordability of life saving products has ended up excluding the most vulnerable and needy segments of society. Innovative undertaking in the health sector are capital intensive and the framework for their product in and application vary significantly between developing and highly industrialised countries. Hence new ways of ensuring cost returns and affordability, and sustainability need to be factored into any initiative that seeks to address the aging and care challenges in Africa. From an ethical perspective, and drawing on Marga Klompe's philosophy on humane care, innovations that target developing countries should align their concerns over costs and profit motives with humane dimensions of the end use of their products. At the same time users in the targeted contexts need to be made aware of the interests and costs that underpin innovations and interventions. Users of products and services could be included in measures that target the sustainability of systems, products and services if their needs are the focus.

The observed dynamics in Africa might present a bleak picture, but given a different angle, they also present opportunities, which can complement the on-going social and economic transformations. First, these challenges present an opportunity for rethinking care in Africa and the significance of combining approaches that borrow from valuable sides of global interconnectedness. Secondly the challenges present opportunities for reviving creativity and innovation in Africa and to up-scaling successful models. Combining models that include social enterprise inherently address the concerns about returns on investment, and sustainable interventions through local input. Such a framework taps into the added value of multi-stakeholder approaches in care, leading to reciprocity and win-win outcomes.

Marga's ideals of humanity, justice, and emancipation of women further serves as a reminder to the fundamental issues that need to underpin all kinds of intervention. Political systems, institutional, policy and legislative frameworks that address aging and care need to be underpinned by certain values that orient interventions towards more humane forms of care. This touches on the rights of the elderly, caregivers and more so the position of women as caregivers and persons that deserve care on equal measure. Science and technology also stands to serve humanity if innovations are informed by humane values. In the case of aging and elderly care in Africa, innovations based on actual needs and input from the targeted groups need to pay attention to resilience in Africa. Solutions informed by local perspectives and experiences have the potentials to provide a framework for sustainability of innovations and interventions and return on investments. The design of interventions if informed by values will inherently address ethical and moral concerns and consequently the realisation of humane care. Such practices will require models of exchange and multi-stakeholder collaborations that facilitate reciprocity, and win-win outcomes

Interviews

Interview with Dorothy Boatemah,[1] Delft the Netherlands

Based on your family and professional experience with aging and care in Ghana what do you see as the major challenges for elderly care in Africa?

I became aware of elderly care challenges from my own family experience. My father was very ill and when taken to a hospital the substandard treatment he received compelled me to do something...It was a problem of lack of knowledge on the complications of old age and unpreparedness of health workers to handle palliative care.

What did you do then?

Upon returning to the Netherlands, I went back to study geriatrics and palliative care next to my regular work in a care home. With these tools I decided to organize skills training and awareness creation activities mainly targeting poor communities.

What kind of gaps have you observed in the last 6 years that you have been going back to share your skills and experiences from the Netherlands?

In the course of my involvement, which included participation in IOM's MIDA health programme, I experienced first hand the many gaps in the health care system...what I see as major challenges are absence of Government national health policies, inadequacy of essential medical policies; inappropriate education policy, poor public awareness and understanding on elderly care. I also noticed that people in need of palliative care have no rights yet many are in very vulnerable situations.

To what extent are current interventions addressing the needs you have observed over the years?

---

1. Ms Boatemah is a health worker in elderly care in the Netherlands. She is originally from Ghana where she has been involved in skills transfer in the area do elderly care and awareness creation on dementia. Ms Boatemah is also involved in lobbying the Ghanaian parliament to include elderly care in the health policy and service delivery

One important thing to note is that even though the concept of palliative care within Africa has its roots in the western models, we believe it must be adapted to African traditions, beliefs and cultures – all of which vary between communities and countries. Care should be provided, where possible by a multidisciplinary team, which includes community workers and traditional healers, as well as nurses, doctors and other health care professionals. Provision varies according to context, but Africa currently faces extremely restricted access to the multidisciplinary teams needed to deliver holistic palliative care tailored to each patient. Most health facilities have no palliative care teams, or health care providers working with different colleagues at different times. The reality is often simply a nurse and community volunteers, working with family members – an arrangement which is overwhelming for hard-pressed health care workers and inadequate for meeting patients' needs.

What are your views on the role of women in relation to the aging and elderly care needs in Africa?

I believe we are all equal when it comes to our roles from the level of our families to our communities and the nation. In terms of community development African woman represent a potent force for change as custodians of family and community values and norms. The African woman is good in helping each other, building peace and harmony, and pushing for stable communities and neighbourhoods.

What are the challenges for women as caregivers and people who also need care in old age?

For us African migrant women what is important is to see ourselves as one group facing challenges of discrimination, abuse, marginalization, unemployment, deprivation, and many obstacles which block us from using our full potential and exercising our rights.

Interview with Mama Matilda Ong'ayo[2], Asembo, Kenya

How are you coping in your current conditions?

---

2. Mama Matilda Ong'ayo is 87 years old widow living in East Asembo, Siaya County in Kenya. Three children out of ten and thirteen grandchildren survive her. Due to her advanced age, her care has become complex in the context of changing family circumstances. Her care is currently being arranged through a close network of her children and those of her twin sister who lives in close vicinity to her home.

I cannot complain much. For me it is even a dream that I am alive today. We grew up as orphans, and with my twin sister, we almost died because we lacked the necessary care after the death of our mother. But now I am 87 years I look back with disbelief...My twin sister is 87, my elder sister died at 92 and recently my only brother died at 93 years. I see this as a miracle because we came from a poor family. We could not finish primary school and got married so early. Life has been a struggle all through....but each one of us has brought up their children under difficult circumstance. Education was important for us even though we only managed class 4. That some children have gone to university is a miracle but also a dream to us.

What role has the family played in care and support for its members in the past?

When I was young, after the death of our mother, we had to live with some relatives but not everyone treated us well. A sister to our mother took us in and provided the care we needed till we started school. The family has always been important especially when children loose a parent. Grandparents or uncles or aunts will always take care. I have been close to my twin sister, and we have always supported each other. We also had friends in the village and took care of each other including children. Today many of you young people are living far away not like in the past. But you have to maintain contact, with people close to you.

Who provides you with every day care in areas that you cannot do yourself?

I have my children and not all of them are around every time. They have arranged for someone to help because not everyone in the village can help as before...people in the village are also struggling...besides my own children, my sister's children have been looking after me. They bring me to hospital; they pass by from time to time. You know that I cannot travel anymore, but the little miracle, the little telephone is enabling me to reach the children.... now you see why education is important... I can call the children, or ask for help... I can also read my medicine... those who are employed to help me are also not very efficient. Today people are not keen on things they do... we used to work from the heart, helping was not forced, it can form the heart and because of that we gave our best.

If there were a home for old people in the village or nearby city would you live there?

No... I have a home and a house here, I am getting too old....I don't want to be away too long. Even when the children send me for treatment in the city, I prefer to come back home to recover from here. You know these days everything is very expensive.... here `I don't pay anything.... except food we eat.... I still have friends, my network is here and from time to time I get help from those close to me...in our tradition it is not possible for someone old like me to leave her home and stay in another home.

References

Adamchak, D (1989) 'Population aging in Sub-Saharan Africa: The effects of development on the elderly.' *Population and Environment,* 10(3): 162-176.

Adepoju, A. (2002) 'Fostering Free Movement of Persons in West Africa: Achievements, Constraints, and Prospects for Intra-regional Migration.' *International Migration Quarterly Review,* 40(2): pp. 3-28.

Apt, N. (2012) 'Aging in Africa: Past Experiences and Strategic Directions.' *Aging International,* 37: pp. 93-103.

Beilsma, C. and Asio, P. (2013) *Who take care of Whom? Orientation of the care-giving role of Grannies in Uganda and The Netherlands.* World Granny, Amsterdam.

Bigala, P. and Ayiga, N. (2014) 'Prevalence and Predictors of elder abuse in Mafikeng Local Municipality in South Africa.' *African Population and Health,* 28(1): 463-474.

Black, R., Crush, J., Peberdy, S., Ammassari, S., McLean H., Mouillesseux, S., Pooley, C. and Rajkotia, R. (2006) *Migration and Development in Africa: An Overview,* Migration and Development Series, Southern African Migration Project, Cape Town, South Africa, and Kingston, Ontario.

Boatemah, D. (2012) *Report on Basic Training on Palliative Care/Treatment, Volta River Authority (VRA) Hospital,* Akosombo – Ghana, Vosaw Healthcare System, and IOM Ghana Mida III Health Project.

Chambers, R. and Conway, G. (1992) Sustainable rural livelihoods: Practical concepts for the 21st century. *IDS Discussion Paper 296,* (pp.7-8). Institute for Development Studies, Brighton

Golaz, V. and Rutaremwa, G. (2011) 'The vulnerability of older adults: what do census data say? An application to Uganda.' *Journal of African Population Studies,* 25(2): pp. 605–620.

Gunaratnam, Y. (2014) 'Rethinking hybridity: Interrogating mixedness.' *Subjectivity,* 7(1): 1-17.

Kangethe, S (2010) 'Occupational care giving conditions and human rights: A study of elderly caregivers in Botswana.' *Indian J Palliat Care,* 16: pp. 79–82.

Kidman, R., Petrow, S. and Heymann, S. (2007) 'Africa's orphan crisis: two community-based models of care.' *Special Issue: Community Responses to HIV and AIDS,* 19(3): pp. 326-9.

Moetlo, G., Pengpid, S. and Peltzer, K. (2011) 'Evaluation of the Implementation of Integrated Community Home-Based Care Services in Vhembe District, South Africa.' *Indian J Palliat Care,* 17(2): pp. 137–142.

Nederveen, P. (2004) *Globalization and Culture*, Rowman and Littlefield, Lanham Maryland.

Ong'ayo, A., Oucho, J. and Oucho, L. (2013) *The Biggest Fish in the Sea? Dynamic Kenyan labour migration in the East African Community*, Brussels: ACP Observatory on Migration and International Organization for Migration (IOM) ACPOBS/2013/PUB02.

Oppong, C. (2006) 'Familial Roles and Social Transformations: Older men and Women in Sub-Sahara Africa.' *Research on Ageing*, 28: (6) pp. 654-668.

Remi, J., Christiaensen, L. and Gindelsky, M. (2014) "*Rural Push, Urban Pull and... Urban Push? New Historical Evidence from Developing Countries*" Working Papers 2014-04, George Washington University, Institute for International Economic Policy

Riccio, B. (2008) 'West African Transnationalisms Compared: Ghanaians and Senegalese in Italy.' *Journal of Ethnic and Migration Studies*, 34(2): pp. 217-234.

United Nations Department of Economic and Social Affairs (2012) *World Population Prospects: The 2012 Revision Volume II: Demographic Profiles*, United Nations, New York.

Reisen, van, M. and Borgman, E. (2012) *De verbeelding van Marga Klompe. Perspectieven op de toekomst*, Klemant, Zoetermeer.

World Health Organisation (2012) *Life Expectancy Global Health Observatory*, United Nations, New York.

Young, A. (2005) 'The Gift of the Dying: The Tragedy of Aids and the Welfare of Future African Generations.' *The Quarterly Journal of Economics*, 120(2): pp. 423–466.

PART II – WOMEN'S POLITICAL LEADERSHIP

CHAPTER 7. THE STRUGGLE OF THE SOUTH SUDANESE WOMEN

Betty Achan Ogwaro

Introduction and Background

South Sudan is characterised by years of war, underdevelopment, famine, drought and flood that have produced a crisis of enormous proportions across the country. The overall demand for food production, security, basic health and social services, infrastructure, income generation and capacity building is overwhelming. In addition to the tragedy caused by the war, there is continued loss of many lives, lost opportunities, destruction of infrastructure, devastation of livestock and crops, and displacement of many families.

Before its independence on 9 July 2011, South Sudan was under the Sudan, then Africa's largest nation. Sudan was divided into northern (predominantly Muslim) and southern (predominantly Christian) administrative zones under British colonial rule. In 1955, before the declaration of the independence of the Sudan, South Sudanese chiefs requested to have a separate administrative section from that of the North, preferably under a Federal system of governance. This however did not happen and resulted into the 1955 Torit mutiny in then Southern Sudan. During this period women concentrated on caring for families and had little public life.

After independence (1956), the Sudanese government from the North took control over the South, leading to tensions and the emergence of the Southern Sudan Liberation Movement (SSLM). The First Sudanese civil war (1955-1972) between the SSLM led by Lt General Joseph Lagu and the government resulted in the suffering and many deaths of women and children, as well as mass displacement as refugees into neighbouring countries, especially Uganda, Kenya and the Democratic Republic of Congo. The 17 years of war ended with the signing of the Addis Ababa Peace Agreement in 1972. The agreement gave the then Southern Sudan relative political autonomy and control over land and resources.

In 1980, the government of the Sudan redrew the north-south administrative borders, including the oilfields in the north. In September 1983, the government implemented Sharia Law throughout Sudan. The introduction of Sharia Law affected women of the Sudan negatively. Many women, who were bread winners for their families through cottage industries and as roadside vendors, lost their businesses as women were not to be seen serving in public places. It took a mass campaign by women of both the South and North Sudan to bring women back into small trades, and to achieve amendments in the regulations. The introduction of Sharia law also provoked the emergence of the Sudan People's Liberation Army (SPLA) under Col. John Garang, and led to the second civil war (1983-2005). An estimated 1.5 to 2 million people died as a result of the war and approximately 4.9 million were internally displaced or became refugees. The war ended with the signing of the Comprehensive Peace Agreement (CPA) in 2005, which included a clause about self-determination for the South (The Government of the Republic of South Sudan, 2005).

Women, politics and nation building

The participation of women in political and public affairs of South Sudan is a fairly recent phenomenon. This is partly due to the fact that, involvement in politics was, not seen as a woman's prerogative, a perspective that continues today. Traditionally South Sudanese women and men occupy different and unequal positions and power relations both within the family and society. Women are largely regarded as a source of wealth to the family (bringing in the bride price). They were denied education in favour of their brothers or male cousins. They were not allowed to speak in public as it was seen as disobedience to do so. They remained at home to help their mothers in doing the household chores, while mothers taught them the art of being a woman from cooking food to milking cows. However, as the war progressed the position of women soon began to change. Since the second half of the twentieth century, women in South Sudan have been able to venture into the political arena, business, and other occupations that were previously considered solely reserved for men.

Women's visibility in politics, however, though limited was evident in the Southern Sudan Regional Government established after the signing of the Addis Ababa Agreement in 1972. For instance, some women from South Sudan joined the Women Socialist Union created during the Nimieri regime

(1969-1985) and some became members of Parliament. One woman (Hon Agnes Lokudu) became a governor of Central Equatoria State (1993-1995).

For the women of South Sudan, the most notable achievement was the acceptance by both the SPLM/A and the Government of Sudan of the inclusion in the CPA that, all levels of government of Southern Sudan shall: "promote women's participation in public life and their representation at all levels of governance by at least twenty five percent as an affirmative action to redress imbalances created by history, customs and traditions [in accordance with Article 20, Sub article 4 paragraph (a)". The item is further clarified in Article 58 (1) b and Article 112 (30) of the Interim Constitution of Southern Sudan (2005) and the Transitional Constitution of South Sudan (2011).

The women who worked hard for this article to be included in the Comprehensive Peace Agreement and the Interim and Transitional Constitutions of Southern/South Sudan had a vision anchored in the values of gender equity and equality, social justice and fair representation. Women of South Sudan believe that a just and fair Sudan requires that all members of society (women and men, rich and poor, able and disable, advantaged and disadvantaged) are able to develop their full potential and contribute to, participate in and benefit from the political, social and economic life of the country. This provision is helpful as it assures women of the transformation of political structures and spaces, which are necessary for the viability of implementing equality-focused principles. Today, several women are playing parts in the Government of South Sudan in a variety of positions and roles. Such a small but important step is a big achievement for women to enter Parliament and Executive positions. Women in the Legislative Assembly have embraced affirmative actions for women being at least 25% of the total membership of the Legislative Assembly. Through their determination, today the women in South Sudan Legislative Assembly represent 31% of the total numbers of members

In 1986, women in the SPLM-controlled areas demanded a special unit in order to address women affairs. As a result, the position of Director for Women's Affairs was created in 1989, later to be known as the Commission for Gender, Youth and Social Welfare. Out of this the Commission developed into being the Ministry of Gender and Social Welfare. However, it became challenging to keep women's issues as a core and part of the public debate and action after the CPA was signed, and even more so after Independence (July 2011). Women seem to have lost the zeal they had during the war and have slipped back from being centre-stage, which they enjoyed during the war.

Although over the period of the war periods, 1955-1972 and 1983-2005, women were concerned about human rights abuses in the Sudan. After the signing of the CPA, women shifted their campaign to look at women's priorities and where they would position themselves in the Interim Southern Sudan post-CPA era in nation building. In 2005, Sudanese women met in Oslo, Norway and identified their priorities and presented these to the Donors Round Table (Sudanese Women's Priorities, 2005). Women realised that the affirmative action promised in the CPA was not reflected in resource flows or in the results of peace building and development. Women were not included in the meeting but worked their accreditation through Dr. John Garang. This gave them the opportunity to read the women's statement to the Donors and demanded that in the next round of the Donors Conference, women should be included in the official delegation.

In 2008 women met again in Oslo and identified the gap in financing for gender equality in the reconstruction period of the Sudan and South Sudan. Again they presented a paper to the Donors Conference requesting a part of the donation to be specifically allocated for financing for gender equality. Women of South Sudan struggled to occupy top ranks, especially in the fields of politics. Women are no longer physically unfit for military and police departments. We have women Police officers. Eastern Equatoria has shown us that women can excel in local government. Chief Magdalena Ihisa has been the head of chiefs in Eastern Equatoria State and has shown development in the traditional leadership. Yet, this inclusion of women in the peacekeeping institutions was not reflected in their political representation. This in turn led to inadequate funding allocations to areas to promote gender equality.

During the post-CPA period (2005-2011), women were optimistic that the priorities they presented to the Donors' conferences in Oslo (2005 and 2008) would make the critical stakeholders pay attention to the voices of women so as to ensure an improvement in the lives of the women of South Sudan but little was attained. Taking ownership and consolidating the gains; ensuring that the promises are met; allowing women to be part and parcel of the democratic space and governance processes of the government of South Sudan; and keeping women's issues core and part of the public debate and action were increasingly confronted by competing government and donors priorities, providing real dilemmas to the women's movement of South Sudan.

As female literacy on the whole is on the rise, women in South Sudan have now become more aware of their rights as individuals and they are now opting for higher positions at work at the same time aiming to be perfect housewifes at home. There are now many examples of women making major contributions to the national life of their states. Women managed to rise to the position of a Governor (Gemma Nunu 2007-2010; Nyandeng Malek Deleich was elected in 2010 in Warrap State and has remained in office to date); and Parliamentary Speaker (Hon Sabina Dario was elected in Eastern Equatoria 2007-2010). However these women met with resistance from men and also so often from fellow women too.

Continued pressure by women on the Presidency has seen women heading foreign missions. On 7 March 2012, South Sudan's President, Salva Kiir, issued four decrees announcing 90 ambassadors to be deployed throughout the world in various diplomatic and foreign services posts. Presidential Decree No. 18/2012, No. 19/2012, No. 20/2012, and No. 21/2012 appointed 10 Grade (1), 43 Grade (2) and 37 Grade (3) ambassadors. Out of the total of 90 ambassadors, nine were women: three from Grade (2) and six from Grade (3). This only represents 10% of ambassadors being women, most of whom are Grade (3). (Sudan Tribune, 2012)

Similarly, women also progressed and became Chairpersons of Commissions, Under Secretaries and heads of political Parties. These are positions normally accorded to men. Women continued to work hard to gain places in Parliament, the Executive, Judiciary, as administrators, officers, entrepreneurs, doctors, engineers, and almost in all spheres of activity contributing to social transformation and nation building. Although gender equality in its real sense is still far from being achieved.

During the interim period (2010-2011) there was an increase in the number of women in decision-making positions of the former Government of Southern Sudan. But this did not come easily. Women groups and civil societies played a big role in campaigning for the fulfilment of the Constitution's article 16 mentioned above. The women's critical mass campaign for the implementation of the minimum 25% quota representation, which was gladly joined by some men, resulted into the "Women Only" seats known in the Parliament as the Women List. This accorded 25% of the Parliamentary seats for women. Having achieved representation in Parliament, women were then faced with the challenge of taking leadership positions at all levels. For example, in 2009, women in the Legislative Assembly in Juba moved a motion for the Executive to implement the 25% minimum representation. This move saw men displaced from the National Assembly and the 25% quota implemented in the 10 State government Executives. Furthermore, after the elections of 2010, women attained 33% representation in the Parliament (25% came from the Women List, 3% from the Party List and 5% from the geographical List). However, women were initially appointed to only 24% of the positions of Chairpersons of the Specialised Committees. They were assigned to 26% of the positions as Deputies to the chairpersons.

After a tough negotiation with the Speaker of the House, Rt Hon James Wani Igga, a breakthrough was achieved and women were accorded more seats in the leadership of the Assembly, which then brought their representation to 29%. This consistency in demand set a precedent and now women enjoy 25 % of seats in the executive at all levels of governments.

There is still a great imbalance in the appointment of leaders such as Ministers, Ambassadors and Head of Commissions. The current constitution is very clear about the representation of women but the problem is in its implementation and the political will to implement the provisions.

Another of the achievements of women is the outcome of the Referendum for self-determination that counted on the numeric superiority of women (52% of voters were women) and the roles that they played to ensure that communities came out to vote peacefully. South Sudanese women withstood the consequences of armed conflict and continued to be the social glue keeping a community together at times where its leaders differ fiercely and sometimes brutally.

Women's participation in War and Peace-building

Women in the armed forces

The women of South Sudan played an instrumental role in the country's liberation struggle and will continue to make sure their voices ring loud and clear. Women participated in many fronts, besides taking care of families: nursing wounded soldiers, and preparing food for soldiers, even serving in the front line. During the 1st armed conflict (1955-1972), which ended with the Addis Ababa Agreement in 1972, women's participation in war and other types of violent conflict was quite invisible. During the SPLM war, the then Southern Sudanese women became the backbone of the liberation struggle in the Sudan. They fought alongside men at the war front during the 21 years of struggle for equality, democracy and peace in the Sudan. Since 1984 women became actively involved in the SPLM and created the Girls' battalions (Katiba banat). Today many women are officers in the Army.

Women at the Peace Negotiation Tables and Peace building

Women of South Sudan have a varied and long history of working towards peace and the betterment of women's position in society. Women used their lobbying skills to make their voices on peace heard in several forums. For years Sudanese women's groups and civil society have been involved in community peace building and advocacy among the communities. They also lobbied for inclusion in the formal peace negotiations.

In 1995 Sudanese women made their voices heard at the UN World Women's Conference in Beijing and at the UNIFEM-Carter Peace dialogue in Nairobi. The Joint Assessment Mission for Sudan (JAM) offered the opportunity for greater participation as it sought to identify those structures, policies and practices, which would help perpetuate patterns of disadvantages and inequalities for women and men. UNIFEM provided the lead in mainstreaming gender issues into the JAM process. Gender analysis, as a methodology for the JAM, began at the level of the household by considering ways in which women and men participate differently in the household economy and in society. It also sought to identify structures (institutional, political and social), policies and practices, which act to perpetuate patterns of women's and men's disadvantages and inequalities. In articulating the primary responsibilities of the government, the obligation of "ensuring the protection of the rights and interests of the people in Southern Sudan" is important for women.

In 2000, a coalition of Sudanese and international human rights and women's groups created a shared vision for a future transitional government in the Sudan expressed as the Second Declaration on Human Rights, Democracy and Development in the Transitional Sudan.

Despite the involvement of women's groups in peace activism, women were not included in the negotiations of the CPA, which were completely controlled by military forces. Consequently, the agreement does not contemplate gender concerns and, instead, specifically protects customary law, which is often detrimental to women's rights. To address this, women held several meetings and workshops that were convened to identify gaps and women's priorities. These meetings included the Yei Women's Conference in March 2005; Nairobi Women's Consultation meeting in March 2005; Oslo Women Symposium in May 2005 pre-Donors Conference; Sudanese Women Consultative meeting in Kampala July 2005; Oslo Women's Symposium in May 2008 pre-Donors Conference and many other consultative meetings.

Although the CPA did not adequately address gender equality, it was more inclusive of women than previous peace negotiations. The recognition of the ability of women in Mediation was achieved first in 2006, when the Government of Southern Sudan appointed two women (Hon Betty Achan Ogwaro and Hon Mary Nyaolang) out of five in the peace Mediation Team negotiating a peace settlement between the Government of Uganda and the Lord's Resistance Army (LRA).

Internal Conflict of December 2013

Ever since the conflict broke out in South Sudan on 15 December 2013, women's organisations have tirelessly been advocating for peace. This has led to both sides actually having women representatives at the peace talks. The women campaigned towards the government quoting the UN Security Council Resolution 1325 which explicitly called for all parties in the conflict to respect women's rights, and to support their participation in peace negotiations and post conflict reconstruction, as well as on South Sudan

Constitution's provision of 25% minimum representation of women at all levels. South Sudan has made steps towards the development of a 1325 National Action Plan (NAP) and the Parliament has passed ratification of CEDAW.

As early as 20 December 2013, just 5 days after the recent crisis broke out, women leaders and other women civil society actors called for peace in South Sudan. They made a press statement condemning the crisis. They called upon President Salva Kirr to restore peace and stability in the country, and they called on the SPLM in opposition to lay down their arms. Women met in the capital Juba and later in Kampala, Nairobi and in New Yolk, U.S, to mobilize for an end to the conflict and for women's participation in peace negotiations. When the African (AU) summit took place in Addis Ababa 21-31 January, the women also gathered there, releasing a statement that addressed these issues as well as the need for the protection of women and children. In the US, women lobbied the Troika – Norway, UK and U.S – and the seven-member East African regional bloc Intergovernmental Authority on Development (IGAD). A ceasefire was brokered on 23 January 2014. Peace talks then resumed in Addis Ababa on 11 February. Women went further to meet the IGAD Chief Negotiator, Seyoum Mesfin, Norway's Minister of Foreign Affairs, Borge Brende, the delegation of the government of South Sudan and other important actors in the peace process.

The government initially thought it was not important to include women on the team. According to Makuei Lueth, the government spokesperson, said, "What is important is not the gender representation but what is important is the achievement of the objective" (Marthe van der Wolf, VOA 16 January 2014). Governor Clement Wani said, in a meeting of the three Equatoria States, it was not yet time to include women because the situation was still too harsh for women. However, women strongly objected to this statement. As a result of the advocacy by South Sudanese women and international pressure there are now three women on the government side. Despite all these changes, women's role as negotiators, mediators, signatories or even witnesses remained notably low.

Internally Displaced and Refugee Women

The majority of refugees and displaced are women, children and older people. Women refugees and displaced persons encounter gender-specific constraints. Women face difficulties in accessing their homes, land and property rights in South Sudan. South Sudanese women like many women in war situations suffer gruesome journeys as they flee from the war zone. Sometimes they struggle with sickness and diseases on the way. Children die and they have no alternative but to bury and leave their children in shallow graves and move on. On arrival in a new destination they struggle with homelessness in their new locations or host countries. Often women refugees or IDPs have to develop coping mechanisms to survive. They struggle with learning new languages and culture. Lack of access to routine care puts pregnant women and their babies at risk. Women at the camp struggle to survive, including in fetching water and looking for firewood. They often walk long distances even while pregnant, which increases the risk of complications. They are vulnerable to sexual assault while in the bush collecting firewood, with it risk of unwanted children and diseases such HIV/AIDS.

Obstacles to women's participation in political and public life

South Sudanese women's involvement in politics and public life face numerous challenges which include socio-cultural, low educational status, class, family background, ethnic and regional variations, economic, etc. Women themselves become obstacle to their cause. In fact women became more confused and started working as small groups instead of working together. Disparity became clearer when the crisis of December 2013 occurred. There is a gap between the women at the negotiating table and the rest of the women back home. Women have voiced their concern about the lack of communication between themselves and women at the negotiation tables.

Funding for gender activities

One of the difficulties South Sudanese women face is funding their struggle, thus South Sudanese women have voiced the need for opportunities, empowerment, participation and inclusion of women in the establishment of legislative and constitutional systems. The gender symposium held on the eve of the Oslo Donors Conference in 2008 produced a common set of priorities and recommendations for funding for gender activities (The Sudan Consortium, 2008), but so far women still struggle to fund their activities.

Low educational status of women

The low educational status of women in South Sudan has often been used as an excuse not to appoint women to high positions, thus reducing the chances for women competing for leadership positions. 53% of women have had no formal education and only 37% have attained primary/junior level education. Several factors contribute to such a high illiteracy rate among women, including the consequences of over 50 years of civil war (1955-2005) as well as cultural perceptions that undervalue girls and women's education. With poor social services the gaps in health provision are also high. The war impacted greatly on the physical and psychological wellbeing of over 60% of women and girls (Southern Sudan Centre for Census, 2010).

Lack of knowledge of the negotiation and mediation peace talks

One of the excuses that men have used to keep women away from the negotiation table is their low educational status and lack of knowledge of negotiation and mediation peace talks. Arguably, men face the same problem but this is normally not considered. Women of South Sudan have organised to attend negotiation and mediation training sessions but such capacity building is far from sufficient to equip women to stand up to the challenges posed by men.

Lack of coordination of various women's initiatives

During this current crisis, which started in December 2013 in South Sudan, it became evident that despite the gains made during the SPLM/A war, women have slipped back into their heterogeneous groups. Differences based on educational achievement, financial situation, age, marital status, political party affiliation, ethnic and regional affiliation, religion, and other forms of social difference started to emerge. These social differences in turn shape and influence women's decisions, their chances, and the choices they make regarding their participation in political activities and public life at large. Currently, there is a lack of proper coordination of the various initiatives for women. This hinders their ability to consolidate their efforts so as to reach a consensus through a dialogue that would enable alternative messages to be developed, which may be critical for sustainable peace.

Cultural Practices and Perceptions

Cultural practices and perceptions in South Sudan view women as suited only for domestic responsibilities, while involvement in politics is seen as the domain of men. A Sudanese rural woman, for example, gets up at five o'clock in the morning to walk up to five kilometres, just to bring 20 litres of water. After the long walk she would spend another five hours working on the family farm, and would then come home to make the family meal.

This represents a major obstacle to women's participation in politics and other public affairs. In addition, a number of communities in South Sudan encourage early, forced, and/or arranged marriages. Such practices limit women's chances to continue education, which would allow them to pursue careers in politics and other professions.

When requesting the 30% minimum participation of women in decision-making, Dr. John Garang commented that "women are the marginalized of the marginalized whose suffering goes beyond description", according to minutes of a meeting of the SPLM Secretariat of Information (1994). Customary laws in the South also have influenced the role of women in public life, in particular political participation. The existing customary laws make it harder for women to escape the bondage of domestic roles, which relegated them to the status of second-class citizens. It is true that under customary law women are valued and respected as mothers. They are also valued and cherished as daughters because they are expected to bring wealth to the family upon marriage. Women are also seen as guardians of culture and traditions and are charged with imparting cultural values to the younger generation. However, this accord of respect is not usually complemented by many other parts of customary law as they pertain to women's lives. Aspects of the law are sometimes used to marginalize women's voices and rights, as well as to justify women's exclusion from political participation and decision-making processes.

Women themselves

South Sudanese women themselves have lost the zeal for fighting for their rights. Many times the progress women activists make is derailed by attitudes of other women who begin to dislike and/or feel reluctant to get involved in politics, having to get permission or approval from their husbands, or men from their communities, to do so. This is also seen in parliamentary discussions over contentious issues, even if the issue affects women. Women openly criticise their fellow women colleagues. Politically active women are sometimes labelled as "unfeminine," "irresponsible wives," "loose women," "spoilers", "ring leaders" or other derogatory terms.

South Sudanese women's priorities

During the war women were particularly concerned with human rights abuses in South Sudan. However, after the CPA insufficient attention has been given to critical issues affecting women by both the government and development partners. A compilation of Sudanese women's priorities taken from all the meetings held by the women from 2005 to 2010 found that every year women emphasized the same issues (ISIS-WICCE, 2013). The priorities in this booklet were developed to identify the key areas of concern for women of South Sudan including across age, livelihood, and political ideology.

The priorities of South Sudanese women are important because:

A new nation has its new diverse issues. Despite women's achievements during the war, new challenges impacting on their advancement continue to arise. Politics changes for the better when women are able to play their full part. There can be no real development without women;

> Insufficient attention is given to critical issues affecting women;
> It is important to remember the past in order to shape the future.

The key areas needing to be addressed are:

> Peace and Security;
> The elimination of gender based violence;
> Basic social services;
> Governance and the rule of law;
> Economic empowerment and poverty reduction;
> Institutional building.

The meetings included from which these concerns and priorities were collated include:

> Yei women's Conference (March 2005),
> Nairobi Consultation (March 2005);
> OSLO Women's Symposium (pre-Donor's Conference); May 2005
> Kampala consultative meeting reflecting on Oslo Donor Conference; July 2005
> OSLO Women's Symposium (pre-Donor's Conference) May 2008
> Thereafter, several Juba Consultative workshops and Conferences (2006-2010)
> Juba review of priorities April 2011

Participants included women leaders from the government, state administrations, women Parliamentarians, women groups and women actors from civil society.

Summary and Conclusion

South Sudanese women played a significant role in the war, fighting and supporting the multiple armed movements. Women also suffered sexual violence throughout the struggle. The trauma suffered as a consequence has remained largely unaddressed.

South Sudanese women play a central role in Sudanese society, in physical and psychological welfare as well as in conflict prevention, resolution and peace building. South Sudanese women play a role in shaping community life, assisting with fundraising when a member is in need, nurturing healthy families, raising future generations and providing for family needs. The efforts that Sudanese women put into building strong, vibrant and healthy communities should be recognised.

Despite the importance of women in communities, their post-conflict status is among the lowest of all groups in South Sudan, regardless of ethnic background. The recent crisis in South Sudan has shifted the focus of donors and humanitarian actors to emergency response. It will be important not to lose sight of the importance of gender equality in this context too, as women become refugees or internally displaced persons.

There is still a long way to go for women throughout South Sudan to realize their rights, including for housing, land and property rights and to achieve durable solutions. Attention is needed to address the low literacy rate among women and girls, harmful traditions, customs, male domination and gender insensitivity of men, all of which act as barriers to women's active participation and being leaders in decision making.

In conclusion, so long as women are not uplifted and granted equal status with men in all walks of life – in political, social, economic, domestic and educational areas, progress in South Sudan will be slow. Despite the evident progress and opportunity for securing peace, development and women's empowerment, it is crucial to recognise that the struggles of South Sudanese women are not over and that the challenges ahead are immense and numerous.

References

Government of the Republic of South Sudan (2005) *Comprehensive Peace Agreement (CPA) between the Government of the Republic of the Sudan and the Sudan People's Liberation Movement/Sudan People's Liberation Army*. [online]. Available at: http://unmis.unmissions.org/Portals/UNMIS/Documents/General/cpa-en.pdf (accessed 7 August 2014).

Government of Republic of South Sudan (2011) *The Transitional Constitution of the Republic of South Sudan 2011*. [online]. Available at: http://www.sudantribune.com/IMG/pdf/The_Draft_Transitional_Constitution_of_the_ROSS2-2.pdf (accessed 2 August 2014).

Government of Southern Sudan (2005) *The Interim Constitution of Southern Sudan*. [online]. Available at: http://www.refworld.org/pdfid/4ba74c4a2.pdf (accessed 2 August 2014).

Government of Southern Sudan (2011) *Statistical Yearbook for Southern Sudan 2010,* Southern Sudan Centre for Census, Statistics and Evaluation. [online]. Available at: http://ssnbs.org/storage/Statistical%20Year%202010.pdf (accessed 7 August 2014).

ISIS-WICCE (2013) Invest in Women Develop South Sudan: South Sudanese Women's Priorities. *Paper.* Isis-WICCE, Kampala.

John Garang (1994) Speech of the Chairman and Commander-In-Chief to the First SPLM/SPLA National Convention. *In Report of First SPLM/SPLA National Convention.* Secretariat of Information and Culture, Sudan People's Liberation Movement, Nairobi, p. 43.

Southern Sudan Centre for Census (2010) *Key Indicators for Southern Sudan.* Southern Sudan Centre for Census, Statistics and Evaluation, Juba.

Sudan Consortium, The (2008) *Conclusions Women's Preparatory Conference*, 5-7 May 2008. [online]. Available at: http://www.inclusivesecurity.org/wp-content/uploads/2012/09/Oslo-2008-Womens-Preparatory-Conference-Conclusions.pdf (accessed 7 August 2014).

Sudan Tribune (2012) 'Kiir appoints 78 ambassadors, directs immediate transfers.' (10 March 2012) *Sudan Tribune* [online]. Available at: http://www.sudantribune.com/spip.php?article41859 (accessed 7 August 2014).

Sudan Tribune (2012) *The Transitional Constitution of the Republic of South Sudan*, 2011. *Sunday Tribune* [online]. Available at: http://www.sudantribune.com/IMG/pdf/The_Draft_Transitional_Constitution_of_the_ROSS2-2.pdf (accessed 7 August 2014).

Sudan Tribune (2008) 'South Sudan's women warriors suffer in peace.' *Sudan Tribune*, [online]. Available at: http://www.sudantribune.com/spip.php?article29415 [accessed on 7 August 2014).

Sudanese Women's Priorities and Recommendations to the Oslo Donors' Conference on Sudan (2005) in *Towards Achieving the MDGs in Sudan: Centrality of Women's Leadership and Gender Equality*, UNIFEM, Norwegian MFA and NIIA, pp. 47-52.

Wolf, van der, M. (2014) Interview with Betty Ogwaro. Interview on Voice of America. [radio] *Voice of America*, 16 January 2014.

Zambakari, C. (2012) South Sudan: institutional legacy of colonialism and the making of a new state. *The Journal of North African Studies*, 17(3), pp. 515-532.

CHAPTER 8. REVOLVING REVOLUTIONS: THE INCLUSION OF WOMEN IN PEACE BUILDING IN NEPAL AFTER THE WAR

Susan Sellars-Shrestha and Leena Rikkila Tamang

The story of Yogmaya

Any story about women and peace building in Nepal must start with the story of Yogmaya Neupane, whose integrity and courage is still inspiring women today. Born in the 1860s, Yogmaya Neupane was widowed soon after becoming a child bride. She remarried – three times – breaking all kinds of social taboos.

In the early 1900s, she became an ascetic and a religious leader, meditating in a cave and following strict austerity practices. Her teachings were against corruption and injustice and, in the dark days of the Rana regime, she championed the powerless and exploited, including women and Dalits (so-called 'untouchables'). She fought against practices such as child marriage, dowry and sati. She condemned caste discrimination and demanded education for girls. Her's was the first serious attack on social traditions. She attracted thousands of followers who called her *Shakti Maya* (Power Love).

In the early 1900s, Yogmaya submitted a list of demands for equality for the downtrodden and oppressed, including women, to the Rana Prime Minister, Chandra Shamsher Jung Bahadur Rana. This led to the abolition of the practice of sati in 1920 (Neupane, 2001).

In 1936, not long after the death of Chandra Shamsher, Yogmaya travelled to the capital to meet with his successor Juddha Shumsher Rana, who came to the holy temple of Pashupatinath in Kathmandu to seek her blessing. Juddha Shumsher gave Yogmaya a plate of gold coins, which she refused asking only for the creation of a humane state. He agreed, but after she returned home to Bhojpur in the east of Nepal, Juddha Shumsher sentenced her and four others to death.

In 1940, Juddha Shumsher arrested Yogmaya and four other activists, whom he labelled revolutionaries. Yogmaya was jailed, but released a few months later. The four others were executed.

On 14 July 1941, Yogmaya waded into the Arun River in defiance of the repression of what she saw as an inalienable truth – that we are all equal. Sixty-seven of her followers waded in after her and were washed away. Their deaths lifted their truth up high, above politics, and gave it immortality, so it could no longer be denied (Republica, 2007; International IDEA et al., 2011; Aziz, 2001).

Revolving revolutions

Since the time of Yogmaya Neupane, Nepal has seen many revolutions – all promising inclusion and with the stated aim of ending oppression. In the 1950s, the people of Nepal lived under the autocratic Rana regime. The Ranas came to power after a coup and ruled as Prime Ministers, keeping the Shah Kings as powerless figureheads. The Rana regime banned education for anyone other than the ruling classes and reinforced a feudal system that kept the people poor and the elites rich. The regime was brutal and the people were oppressed mercilessly.

This regime was toppled in 1951 by revolutionaries who trained across the border in India, under the auspices of the 'Nepali National Congress', the precursor to the Nepali Congress party, Nepal's first political party and the largest mainstream party to this day. Most of the soldiers in this army were Gorkhas who had returned from World War II – some of them educated in India (Darjeeling and Sikkim) and even Myanmar. The revolutionary army took the major Terai towns one by one, toppling each feudal lord and eventually marching on the capital. The Ranas yielded before the army reached Kathmandu (Edingo, 2010).

The mood of the time was pro-change. There was a new world order after World War II; colonial powers and oppressive regimes were being replaced by democratic governments on every continent. Hence, the revolutionaries of the Nepali Congress were labelled 'freedom fighters' and their cause considered just.

A new constitution was promulgated and democracy was trialled in 1951, but the new regime was reluctant to give women the right to vote. Nepali women who had actively participated in the movement against the Rana regime were being cut out of participating in the new government – or even voting for the new government (International IDEA et al., 2011). But the women who had watched the revolution from their houses and kitchens, and many who had participated in it, would not be silenced. The seed had been planted by Yogmaya Neupane and others and women were aware that there could be a different life for them. They staged a demonstration and sent a delegation to meet with the Prime Minister, who was compelled to grant them voting rights. In the first municipal elections in 1951, the Nepali people voted for the first time – and women proudly cast their vote and ran as candidates (International IDEA et al., 2011).

Political women of Nepal

Mangala Devi Singh: Early leader of the women's movement

Mangala Devi Singh (1925–1996) was one of the women who went to Prime Minister Padma Shamsher demanding equal voting rights for women. She led the democratic faction of Nepal Mahila Sangh, an organisation established to work for women's rights. The women of Nepal Mahila Sangh united against the Rana regime, visited political activists who had been jailed, carried letters to and from the jail, and educated women on politics. However, after democracy was established in 1950, these women were fragmented into different parties and lost their single platform. During her political career, Mangala Devi was imprisoned and tortured. She participated in Jana Andolan I (People's Movement) in 1990 and contested in the first parliamentary election after the restoration of democracy in Nepal.
Source: International IDEA et al. 2011; Pradhan 1996

Kamakshya Devi: Uniting women in one platform

Kamakshya Devi (1924–1987) believed that the tradition to limit women to domestic chores should be broken down. On meeting a fellow politician who was sentenced to death, she said, "Brother, I will not chew betel nut leaf until the work you have initiated for the country and the people is completed." With this oath she entered into politics. She believed that women should not be divided on the issues of women and accommodated women of disparate views. She established Nepal Mahila Sangh to unite all women for equality in the one platform.
Source: International IDEA et al. 2011

Unfortunately, the first exercise in democracy was brief and King Mahendra instituted the feudal Panchayat system of local government in 1962, in which women had little space or political voice. Inevitably, another revolution took place a short time later in the form of the 1990s People's Movement (Jana Andolan I). This movement, which included many strong women, culminated in a march to the palace gates, where the people demanded democracy. King Birendra readily agreed and became a constitutional monarch. But what did this democracy bring? The same political families and the same Brahmin and Chhetri men divided up the power and the spoils. True equality and a functional democracy seemed far away and many looked back on the party-less Panchayat system with nostalgia citing that at least it was a functional form of decentralised local government.

A short 6 years later the Maoists started what would become a 10-year civil war in the Far West of Nepal. Their rally cry was again freedom from oppression and equal rights for women and the downtrodden. The people of the Far West of Nepal had suffered much due to poverty and had historically been neglected by the state. Much of the arable land in the Far West was owned by feudal lords, many of whom did not even live in the area, and farmed by local residents. When the land reforms promised during the 1990 revolution did not materialise, the people undertook their own reforms, declaring fields that they had farmed for generations to be their own. The army and police responded brutally with Operation Romeo in 1995 and Operation Kilo Sera II in 1998 (Bisht 2008). These operations played into the hands of the Maoist by radicalising the people of the Far West, the most forgotten region of Nepal, who readily took up arms, as much to defend themselves against the army and police as to fight for freedom. But the global mood had changed after 9/11 and these revolutionaries were labelled 'terrorists' by the government in Kathmandu and some western governments, including the United States of America. Indeed these new revolutionaries were fighting against a democratically elected government, not an autocratic regime, but these are labels that had little meaning for the farmers who found themselves still without access to the means of production and still without a voice in this new 'democracy'.

Women as Maoist combatants: Equality on the battlefield

In the 10-year civil war (1996–2006) by the Communist Party of Nepal (Maoist) against the state, women fought beside male combatants on the battlefield for a 'new Nepal' that was to include women and people from disadvantaged and oppressed groups in political and social processes. The Maoist revolt was basically a revolt against oppression by the ruling classes and the Maoists rose to power on the promise of equality. You may get the feeling in reading this that history is about to repeat itself. You would not be far wrong; more than four decades after the Rana regime was toppled, little had changed in rural Nepal. Although some argue that development indexes had started to improve in the 1990s and that the Maoist war interrupted this (Dixit 2011; Dixit and Ramachandran 2002), these pockets of development were mainly among the emerging middle class – precious little had changed at the bottom of the hierarchy. Early experiments in democracy in Nepal had proved to be simply new ways of justifying the use of power by the same power elites. Leaders in the capital wrestled with each other to lead the government; people in the Far West starved; people in the Terai produced, only to have their wealth exploited by those in the capital; people in the mountains of the North lived in isolation – nothing much changed.

Women's political space in Nepal

After the 1990 revolution

Before the civil war between the Maoists and the state, although the women's movement was strong, women had virtually no role as elected representatives. Sahana Pradhan was the only female minister in the 11-member interim coalition government formed after democracy was established in 1990 and there were no women in the 9-member Constitution Recommendation Commission. As a result, there was no space for women to participate in the making of the 1990 Constitution (Pathak and Pyakurel, 2008 cited in International IDEA et al., 2011). Women were once again deprived of their political rights – despite having fully participated in the revolution that established democracy in 1990. Accordingly, after the Constitution of the Kingdom of Nepal 1990 was promulgated, nearly 100 laws that discriminated against women continued in force (International IDEA et al., 2011). Women's participation in the House of Representatives between 1991 and 1999 ranged from 3 to 6%, a dismal reward for their efforts in the fight for democracy (Didi Bahini, 2008, cited in International IDEA et al., 2011).

Besides central level politics, women have also been active at the local level. In 1997, the laws governing local bodies/elections (The Decentralization Act 1982, Village Development Committee Act 1992 and District Development Committee Act 1992) were amended (Government of Nepal 1997) to ensure women's participation in local government. As a result, 44,120 women were elected to local bodies (municipalities and VDCs) in 1997, an increase from a mere 217 in 1992 (National Women's Commission 2008, cited in International IDEA et al., 2011). The fact that this number of women (although less than 10% overall) gained political experience is significant in the political landscape of Nepal. It is also important to note that this 'win' for the women's movement was possible only because of a legislative framework for the political inclusion of women.

Sahana Pradhan: Leader of the 1990 revolution and government minister

Sahana Pradhan (born 1941) fought against the Rana regime for the right to education for women. In the 1951 revolution she played a key role in mobilising women against the regime. She was detained in the army barracks in 1961 for participating in the democratic movement and expelled as a teacher during the Panchayat era for staging a protest against the party-less Panchayat system. Sahana Pradhan then led the United Left Front during the historic People's Movement of 1990 and went on to hold the portfolio of Minister for Industry and Commerce in the interim government. She went on to serve in the Ministry of Industry and Commerce, Ministry of Forest and Soil Conservation, and Ministry of Women and Social Welfare. After Nepal was declared a republic, she served as Minister of Foreign Affairs.

Source: Prabhat 1996, cited in International IDEA et al. 2011; Republica 2014

Women in the Maoist movement: A paradigm shift

Women's liberation was one of the key agendas of the Communist Party of Nepal (Maoist) and women were given positions in the party and as combatants in the People's Liberation Army. Rural women, many of whom were facing extreme forms of discrimination and violence, left the villages and joined the Maoist movement by the thousands. The armed conflict redefined women in Nepal. Many young women realised for the first time that they could hold a gun, live in the camps with the men and fight on the battlefields. With 15% women in its political wing, 35% in the military wing, and 40% in the state and militia (Chand 2010, cited in International IDEA et al., 2011), women formed a critical mass in the Maoist movement. Despite this, women were glaringly absent "in peace dialogues and negotiation committees that brought the war to an end", which "reflects the patriarchal mindset and disapproval of women as leaders" (International IDEA et al., 2011, p 22). As explained by International IDEA in its publication 'Women members of the Constituent Assembly: A study on the contribution of women in constitution making in Nepal':

> The significant participation of women and their important role in the Maoist war helped overcome traditional images and roles associated with Nepali women, and changed Nepali society's perception of women. To a certain extent, this has helped to overcome social and religious norms and values that view women's core responsibility as to engage in household chores, give birth and raise children. Values that segregated certain work for men were also torn down. (International IDEA et al., 2011, p 44)

Hemanti Syanda's story: Life as a woman in the People's Liberation Army

Hemanti was 16-years old when she joined the women's wing of the People's Liberation Army in 2002. She had heard about Maoist ideas from a Maoist woman who had come to her village and spoken about gender and caste-based discrimination. "I immediately understood her as we witnessed the same problems every day around us. Then I decided I wanted to be a part of that movement", says Hemanti.

Hemanti became an Area Committee Member. Instead of fighting, she visited communities and talked about women and Dalits' rights and about the change that the Maoists wanted to bring about. She led a double life: during the day she lived in the traditional way, but at night she visited the surrounding villages. This posed a great danger to her family and the other villagers: "When the people in my village and my family found out that I was a Maoist they became very angry." Eventually, the police came to her village and burned down her family's house.

Hemanti was regularly trained for two or three days in a row. The topics included mostly political orientation and sometimes the use of weapons. It was a hard way of life: "We had to mistrust everybody because there were many army informants around. We did not know whether people were on our side or not. I carried a rifle and a hand grenade to defend myself, but I never had to fire a shot, even though I witnessed two battles." After three years in the movement, Hemanti was appointed vice president of the district's Maoist women's wing.

At one point, she realised she was pregnant. She had married when she was 14-years old and her husband was also with the Maoists. She was still visiting villages during the late stages of her pregnancy. One night, while coming back from a political event, she went into labour. The people around her were afraid to be in contact with her, a Maoist, so she had to give birth outside the village. She brought a plastic sheet and a knife into the woods. A girl from the neighbouring village joined her to assist during childbirth, but the girl became so nervous that Hemanti had to comfort her – even while giving birth. "I cut the umbilical cord myself and washed my child. That was the moment when I realised that I can do everything if I am prepared for it."

Source: Extract reproduced with permission from Ministry of Peace and Reconstruction and GIZ (2013) 'From combatants to community members: Reintegration of ex-combatants.' Chapter in: *Improvement of Livelihoods in Rural Areas (ILRA)*. Kathmandu: Deutsche Gesellschaft für Internationale Zusammenarbeit (GIZ) GmbH, pp 94–96

Jana Andolan II

On 6 April 2006, to foil a demonstration in the capital called by the

Communist Party of Nepal (Maoist) and the seven party alliance (an alliance of the main political parties), King Gyanendra called a 'shoot on sight' curfew. The Maoists had trucked thousands into Kathmandu from the villages to demonstrate against the King, who had dissolved the elected parliament in 2004 and seized executive power in 2005. The demonstrators defied the curfew and the King sent the army into the fray. The demonstrators did not back down. The army showed great restraint – perhaps they saw the writing on the wall? The curfew was extended. The Internet was cut and the airport closed. The newspapers of the time carried photographs of sari-clad women sitting in between riot police and activist in the laneways of New Road, arms crossed, rocks littered around them (Nepali Times 2006 and 2007). Defiance is the word that springs to mind.

As well as these women, who were at the forefront of student groups, political parties and members of the Maoist movement, there were also other women – housewives, women who worked in hospitality, and legal professionals – who staged protests in this movement, which came to be known as Jana Andolan II, or People's Movement II (Nepali Times 2006). These women, and many other groups of non-politically active citizens – musicians, tourism entrepreneurs, traders – gathered in small groups at different points in the capital to oppose the curfew. Many were not politically aligned with any particular group. The mood was not so much pro-Maoist as it was pro-change. The people did not want to stay in their houses under another curfew called by another autocratic ruler who wanted to control them.

Towards the end of what stretched into a nearly three-week curfew, everyone seemed to come out onto the streets – either to march or watch; some played hand drums; some gave water to the protesters to drink as they circled the ring road. King Gyanendra had no choice but to step down. The seven mainstream political parties and the Communist Party of Nepal (Maoist) formed an Interim Government and promulgated an Interim Constitution, with the promise of elections for a constituent assembly to write a new constitution.

Interim Constitution: Legally defining the space for women

When the Maoists joined mainstream politics they brought with them the women who had participated in the revolution – but not in leadership positions. During Jana Andolan II, women demonstrators were arrested and killed: "Of the 26 people who lost their lives in course of the movement, 6 were women" (International IDEA et al., 2011, pp. 45–46). Initially, there were no women in the 16-member Interim Constitution Drafting Committee. Women protested and the committee was reorganised to include four women – but it felt like an afterthought.

The Interim Constitution of Nepal promulgated in 2007 was a victory for women and there were 17% women in the reinstated Interim Parliament. The reinstated Parliament passed a women's rights resolution requiring 33% participation by women in each and every organ of the state. This paved the way for women's participation in the Constituent Assembly.

Constituent Assembly Election 2008: Landmark women's representation

In what some would say is a surprising turn of events, the Electoral Commission of Nepal enforced the quota set for female candidates in the Interim Constitution through proportional representation (Nepal applies a mixed electoral system of first-past-the-post and proportionate representation). Political parties who submitted lists of candidates that did not meet the quota for women under proportional representation were sent back to the drawing board. As a result of this, and the fact that the Community Party of Nepal (Maoist) fielded a lot of female candidates in the first-past-the post system, women constituted 33% of the members of the first Constituent Assembly, elected in 2008.

However, their participation in constitution building as a part of peacebuilding was not assured by this landmark level of representation. Instead they were sidelined from decision-making processes, both formal and informal, and represented often by the press as token women, without the education or expertise to contribute.

Despite this, the Constituent Assembly stands as the greatest achievement of the women's movement in Nepal to date and has created a paradigm shift in terms of women's participation in politics (International IDEA et al., 2011). Women united in the new Constituent Assembly, across party lines, in the Women's Caucus. The Women's Caucus in the Constituent Assembly was able to ensure that important women's issues were included in the preliminary drafts of the Constituent Assembly's thematic committees. The right to inheritance, to proportionate inclusive representation based on population size, and to equality in citizenship regardless of gender were some of the issues successfully raised (International IDEA et al., 2011). However, the term of the Constituent Assembly, although extended several times, lapsed before a new constitution could be written.

Constituent Assembly Election 2013: Eroded space for women

Unfortunately, the gains of the 2008 election are being eroded. Part of the reason for the 33% representation of women in the first Constituent Assembly in 2008 was the strict enforcement of the quota (through proportional representation) by the Electoral Commission of Nepal. The other part of the reason is that so many Maoist women won under the first-past-the-post system; in other words, they were directly elected with the support of their parties and constituencies.

Unfortunately, this 'space' for women narrowed in the second Constituent Assembly election in 2013 with only 10 women elected through first-past-the-post, compared to 30 in 2008. One of the reasons for the low number of women elected through first-past-the-post is that only 10% of all of the first-past-the-post candidates were women (International IDEA, 2013), which is the minimum that the parties needed to meet the requirement in the Interim Constitution 2007. Also, whereas in 2008 strong women candidates were fielded with a fair amount of party support, in 2013 the candidates simply did not have 'winnable' tickets – either because they were fielded against strong male candidates or they did not have sufficient party support, including campaign funds (International IDEA, 2014 – forthcoming). The onus is on the political parties to improve this.

A recent Nepal Democracy Survey conducted by the State of Democracy in South Asia, Nepal Chapter and International IDEA, '*Citizen Survey 2013: Nepal in Transition*', indicates that people in Nepal are ready to vote for women; 45% of respondents said that they would prefer a female candidate in the Constituent Assembly elections, compared to only 25% who preferred a male candidate (International IDEA, 2013).

A strong legal framework for inclusion and a bona fide attitude towards the inclusion of women (and other marginalised groups) on the part of the political parties and the Electoral Commission is needed to consolidate the gains made by the first Constituent Assembly election (International IDEA, 2014 – forthcoming).

In the meantime, the second Constituent Assembly has started its work by going through the drafts prepared by the first Constituent Assembly and identifying resolved and unresolved issues. Issues that have been resolved are being forwarded to the constitution drafting committee for finalisation and inclusion in the new constitution; those that are unresolved are being put before the political dialogue committee. In terms of the women's agenda, it seems that most of the achievements on women's issues in the first Constituent Assembly are considered 'resolved' and now in the drafting process. The main outstanding contentious issue is that of citizenship by descent and by marriage (through the man or woman, or both).

In terms of positions held by women, again the vice chair – very much a ceremonial role – is a woman and two out of the five committee chairs are women. However, the two committees chaired by women are the ones considered 'less important' and were given to small parties within the Constituent Assembly, while the major political parties and men took the chair positions of the political dialogue committee, drafting committee and the committee reviewing the work of the first Constituent Assembly. It is yet to be seen whether the women Constituent Assembly members will come together across party lines to ensure a women-friendly constitution and to what extent the male Constituent Assembly members are ready to support the same.

Interviews: One Maoist woman and one Nepali Congress woman share their experiences of politics in Nepal

The following interviews were conducted with prominent women in Nepali politics (from the two main political parties) who have been through the people's war, were members of the Constituent Assembly in 2008 and who are still in politics today. Their interviews were conducted to ascertain their views on the 'space' for women in politics and peace building in Nepal after the civil war and what they think needs to be done to expand that space.

Hisila Yami

"It is also a leadership question; very few women were able to get positions in which to grow into the bigger responsibilities. […] After the war, men started to relegate women back to the private sphere."

Hisila Yami (born 1959) is one of the leaders of the Communist Party of Nepal (Maoist) party. During the People's War (1996–2006) she served as a central leader of the Maoist party, staying 'underground'. In 2006, when the Communist Party of Nepal (Maoist) party resurfaced as a mainstream political party, Hisila became Minister for Physical Planning and Works in the Interim Parliament. After winning her seat in the election of 2008, she became Minister of Tourism and Civil Aviation and a member of the Constituent Assembly tasked with writing the constitution (2008–2012). She has authored books including 'People's War, Women's Liberation in Nepal', and 'Marxism and Women's Liberation', which she co-authored with her husband, Dr Baburam Bhattarai. Hisila comes from a political family. Her mother and father both spent time in jail in the 1940s for their political activism. Her father, Dharma Ratna Yami, was a founding member of the Nepali Democratic Congress Party, which joined forces with the Nepali National Congress to overthrow the Rana regime in 1950. When asked why she joined the Maoist movement, she tells of her first trip to India in the 1970s where she saw the suffering of Nepali labour migrants firsthand. Not only was the work they did pitiful (mostly menial jobs such as watchmen, household servants, and dishwashers, as well as in the 'red light' areas), their sense of dignity was completely crushed. When she saw this, Hisila felt she had to do something for her country.

You were part of the People's War (1996–2006) and Jana Andolan II (April 2006) and have been in politics ever since, what is your view:

Did the revolution change the role of women in politics in Nepal? Were the promises of the revolution, in terms of gender equality, kept?

One of the reasons for us [women] not being able to seize the momentum after the revolution was that various oppressed and marginalised groups did not bring the issue of gender up as part of the overall struggle. Women are part of all these groups too. But it is also a leadership question; very few women were able to get positions in which to grow into the bigger responsibilities.

Secondly, when peace settled in, the 'heat' on issues like women's political participation went down, and issues like emancipation were pushed aside. To my mind, the reason for this is simple: we still live in a feudal patriarchy. After the war, men started to relegate women back to the private sphere. They started to think of their personal life and asked: where do they want women to be; at home, or in politics? During the war, children were taken care of by the community in our party. Who is taking care of the children now?

What do you think is the role of the law in creating an enabling environment for women to participate in politics?

In 2008, the law and the government were ahead of the political parties in terms of gender equality; without the electoral laws and the quotas there would not have been so many women in the first Constituent Assembly – or even in the second. It is the political parties that are lagging behind. I am also very critical of the fact that other parties, for example, the Unified Marxist-Leninist and Nepali Congress [the other two main parties in Nepal], are doing much better in terms of the internal inclusion of women in their party structures than the Communist Party of Nepal (Maoist).

The Maoist party was seen as the champion of women and other marginalised groups, but since we lost, or came third, in the November 2013 elections, naturally these questions also lost some prominence in the political discussions.

Where do you see yourself in 10 years' time, still in politics?

Yes, politics is my life. Both my parents were in politics and I was lucky to be able to pursue my own path. My father was very progressive. There have never been any *'ifs'* or *'buts'* from my husband either [Maoist party leader and former Prime Minister of Nepal, Dr Baburam Bhattarai]. I want to be part of transforming society – you need political power in order to change things.

What do you wish for your daughter?

We [my husband and I] have left her to choose her own path; but I am very proud that she is now doing her PhD at the Jawaharlal University in India, the place were both myself and my husband studied.

Pushpa Bhusal

"The political parties provided very little support to women candidates: no financial or campaign support and even moral support was precious little. Only strong constitutional provisions and laws will ensure women's political participation in the future."

Pushpa Bhusal (born 1961) is a lawyer by training and former elected member of the Constituent Assembly (2008–2012) for the Nepali Congress party. She was chair of the committee that drafted the Truth and Reconciliation Act. She was also a member of the drafting committee for the Interim Constitution (2007). Pushpa comes from a political family; her father was a Minister in the cabinet of Prime Minister BP Koirala in 1959. On 15 December 1959, when the then King Mahendra dissolved the cabinet and took over power, Pushpa's father went into self-exile in India, followed by his family, where they remained for 13 years. Following in her father's footsteps, Pushpa was attracted to the Nepali Congress since childhood. She feels that it was the Nepali Congress that led the movement for democracy in Nepal. Pushpa says that she is committed to making the Nepali Congress a democratic and even more effective political party in the future.

Do women in Nepal have more space in political decision-making forums now than before Jana Andolan II in 2006?

I do think that Jana Andolan II, the Peace Agreement in 2006 and the subsequent Interim Constitution 2007 changed a lot for women. Already earlier, at the beginning of the 1990s, Nepal had signed many important international treaties such as the Convention on the Elimination of all forms of Discrimination against Women (CEDAW) and agreements against racial discrimination etc., but our parliament, as well as the Supreme Court, only produced 'messages' for greater participation, but no binding action, no new laws or policies were produced.

I do give it to the Maoist movement – it was largely because of them that issues of inclusion, discrimination and gender equality were taken seriously by the state institutions. I think that the Maoists used these groups [women and marginalised groups] and themes [equality for all] strategically in order to get support for their movement and attract people to the war, but the results were also there. The Interim Constitution 2007 made radical changes to the provision for 'citizenship' [which was changed from by male descent to by both female and male descent], it also states that the human rights commission needs to include women. Furthermore, the parliament passed laws for social inclusion in all of the public services [organs of the state] and the election law is very progressive. All these were unthinkable before Jana Andolan II. To an extent, the People's Movement [Jana Andolan II] forced cultural changes in the party leadership, even if the inner circle of party decision-making remains male and Brahmin /Chettri (so called 'upper castes').

Nepali women seem to have achieved numbers in politics, but do they have power?

Women have played important roles in the peace committees at the village levels, but it is true that there were no women at the most important tables during the peace process. And yet many of the peace process issues affect mostly women; women suffered as victims and the disappearances and displacements affected women in multiple ways – as victims, mothers, wives, sisters and care givers. In the Constituent Assembly too, women do have the numbers, but they are not in the important positions; not as chairs of the important committees, or even of subcommittees, nor are they in sufficient numbers in the critical negotiation teams – formal or informal.

Why is this so and what can be done to change it?

Women should raise their voices themselves, that is true. Women should also propose each other to important positions. Men always expect that the few women leaders who are there are seeking positions for themselves. I am always suggesting: why don't we appoint Chitra Lekha Yadav or Meena Pandey [prominent Nepali Congress women] to such and such position.

The new constitution is the document in which women need to include a maximum amount of rights, and the proportionate representation [of women] cannot be left to the political parties. That is why it is so important to use this constitutional momentum for ensuring women's equal participation in politics. In the 2013 Constituent Assembly elections, the political parties provided only 10% of the first-past-the-post ticket to women, and even then only because the Interim Constitution forced them to do so. The political parties provided very little support to women candidates: no financial or campaign support and even moral support was precious little. Only strong constitutional provisions and laws will ensure women's political participation in the future.

Do you see any hope for the younger generation in political parties?

It is very difficult to get a position in a party in the short term; you need to be there with a long-term vision. I am afraid everyone gets opted by the system by the time they are in power. The Nepali Congress is a mass-based party and senior leaders make all the decisions. There is much interest among young women and men to participate, but very few platforms for them raise their voices. We need to start democratising our political parties.

Conclusion

The recent civil war in Nepal was fought for equality and the inclusion of previously excluded and marginalised groups, including women. However, as with the previous civil war (that over threw the Rana regime in the 1950s) and the first democratic movement (Jana Andolan I in 1990), the post-war landscape in Nepal is divided among the same players as always: Brahmin and Chhetri men and so-called 'high' caste political families. A simple fact of peacebuilding processes is that whoever participates in the process determines the outcome. So, if women are to have a say in the outcome of the peace process, they need to be able participate in the process – and not just in numbers, but in leadership positions.

Women's place in Nepali society is changing: Although it is hard to generalise, women are now being viewed differently. There has been a paradigm shift since the civil war. Many stereotypes about women (e.g., that their place is in the home and that public life is the work of men) were broken down by the Maoist movement. Before this war, women had participated in the revolutions, but not on the battlefield. Holding a gun and standing beside their male combatants changed how women were viewed and how they viewed themselves. However, as peace sets in, men are closing ranks to protect the status quo. Men in Nepal (and perhaps in most of the world) are simply not comfortable with women having real decision-making power – or submitting to the decision of a woman. However, while men in Nepal might initially succeed in putting logistical barriers in women's way in terms of their participation in politics (such as not allocating funds to women candidates for their political campaigns), the ideological war has been won: men have admitted that women have a right to be equal.

Although much ground has been won for women by the various revolutions in Nepal (including the right to education for girls after the Rana regime was toppled), revolutions in Nepal seem to succeed initially, only to fail in the long term as those in power are not willing to share the power with everyone, including women. Conflicts tend to be cyclical in nature: what remains not implemented from past peace agreements becomes the cause for the next conflict. Issues related to power sharing between the conflicting parties and political issues are generally more easily implemented, whereas providing for the wellbeing of those harmed by the conflict is more difficult to implement. The majority of Nepalis are still waiting for the dividends of peace in terms of improved economic situations and opportunities; almost 8 years since the peace agreement was signed, the promised truth and reconciliation process is yet to start.

Although the first Constituent Assembly was the most inclusive in the history of Nepal (in terms of women and other previously excluded groups), it appears that the dream of an inclusive state is fading as the power elites close ranks and divide up the spoils. If we do not learn the lessons from history, then history will repeat itself again and Nepal may find itself facing yet another revolution. How many revolutions do we need before we realise that everyone must have a say in governing their future – including and, especially, women?

Among other things, a strong legal framework is needed for equality for women in politics and the peace process more broadly – as those in power have never been known to share without compulsion. The women of the new Constituent Assembly have a vital role to play in this. Although the male leaders of Nepal seem to have closed ranks to protect the status quo, if organised properly, the more than a quarter women members of the Constituent Assembly can unite – and rise above party politics – to push the agenda for women home. The hour is upon us.

References

Aziz, B. (2001) *Heir to a silent song: Two rebel woman of Nepal*. Centre for Nepal and Asian Studies, Tribhuvan University, Kathmandu, p 50–51.

Bisht, R. (2008) *International Encyclopaedia of Himalayas*, Vol. 4. New Delhi: Mittal Publications.

Chand, N. (2010) *Women bulletin*, 12th Year, Vol 1. All Nepal Women's Association, Kathmandu, p 21.

Dixit, K. (2011) *Peace politics of Nepal. An opinion from within*. Himal Books, Lalitpur.

Dixit, K., Ramachandran, S. (2002) *State of Nepal*. Himal Books, Lalitpur

Didi Bahini (2008) *Rajnitima Mahila Sahabhagita*. (Third Revised Edition). Didi Bahini and UNIFEM, Kathmandu p 10. Cited in: International IDEA; Nepal Law Society; Women's Caucus, Constituent Assembly Secretariat (2011) *Women Members of the Constituent Assembly: A study on the contribution of women in constitution making in Nepal*. International IDEA, Kathmandu.

Edingo, D. (2010) *GB Yakthumba: A champion of democracy*. Indira Yakthumba, Kathmandu.

Government of Nepal (1997) *Nepal Gazette*, Section 2, Part 47, Additional Edition No. 23, 22 August 1997. Government of Nepal, Kathmandu.

International IDEA; Nepal Law Society; Women's Caucus, Constituent Assembly Secretariat (2011) *Women members of the Constituent Assembly: A study on the contribution of women in constitution making in Nepal*. International IDEA. Kathmandu.

International IDEA (2013) *Citizen Survey 2013: Nepal in Transition*. Nepal Democracy Survey Round III, a joint survey by State of Democracy in South Asia/Nepal Chapter and International IDEA. Available at: http://www.idea.int/asia_pacific/nepal/upload/Citizen-Survey-Report-2013.pdf (accessed 17 August 2014).

International IDEA (2014 – forthcoming) *The gender gap and gender-based violence in 2013 CA election, Nepal*. International IDEA, Kathmandu.

Ministry of Peace and Reconstruction, GIZ (2013) 'From combatants to community members: Reintegration of ex-combatants.' Chapter in: *Improvement of Livelihoods in Rural Areas (ILRA)*. Deutsche

Gesellschaft für Internationale Zusammenarbeit (GIZ) GmbH, Kathmandu, pp 94–96.

Nepali Times (2006) 'Protest in pictures.' *Nepali Times*, Issue 294, 14–20 April 2006. Available at: http://nepalitimes.com/news.php?id=11654 (accessed 17 August 2014).

Nepali Times (2007) 'Scenes from an uprising.' *Nepali Times*, Issue 345, 20 – 26 April 2007. Available at: http://nepalitimes.com/news.php?id=13451 (accessed 17 August 2014).

Neupane, G. (2001) *Upheavals in Nepal: Transforming the state and society*. Center for Development Studies, Nepal, Kathmandu.

Pradhan, S. (1996) *Direction of Nepali women movement*. Working Paper, Women Participation in Politics, Report of the National Women Gathering, 10–12 April 1996. Informal Service Sector Centre, Kathmandu.

Pathak, N., Pyakurel, B. (2008AD/2064BS) Nepal's Interim Constitution 2007 and Constitutional Records. (Second Edition) Kathmandu: Pairabi Publication. Cited in: International IDEA; Nepal Law Society; Women's Caucus, Constituent Assembly Secretariat (2011) *Women Members of the Constituent Assembly: A study on the contribution of women in constitution making in Nepal*. International IDEA, Kathmandu.

Republica (2011) 'Nepal: Yogmaya Neupane: Nepal's first female revolutionary.' Republica, 4 May 2011.

Republica (2014) 'Leader Sahana's health improves.' *Republica*, 21 July 2014. Available at: http://www.myrepublica.com/portal/index.php?action=news_details&news_id=79446 (accessed 17 August 2014).

National Women's Commission (2008) *Laingik aadhar ma vibhaajit tathyanka (2065 BS)*. Kathmandu: National Women's Commission.

CHAPTER 9. TOUGH CHOICES, LIMITED SPACES AND CONFLICTED LOYALTIES: WOMEN'S LEADERSHIP IN GOVERNANCE IN AFRICA TODAY: THE KENYAN EXPERIENCE

Stella Maranga

Under-representation of women in elective politics

Despite the major contribution women leaders in Kenya make towards governance processes and results, they face a dual struggle – ascending into leadership and governance positions and getting their voices and agenda to centre stage. This chapter looks at experiences of women leaders in Kenya during the period between the promulgation of the new constitution in 2010, and the first elections under the new dispensation in 2013. The chapter looks at the challenges that women faced in trying to realise the promise of the constitution, the experiences on the campaign trail and the subsequent experiences when women try to set the agenda. The central premise of this chapter is that for equality in leadership and governance to be realised fundamental inequalities in society, including gender inequalities, will need to be addressed. The chapter is based primarily on reports and documents written at this time and after, media reports during this period, and on the personal experiences of the author who worked as a gender and governance advisor during this period.

A key feature of women's participation in leadership in Kenya is the under-representation of women in elective politics. From Independence in 1963 to 2012 only fifty women had been elected to parliament. In the 10th parliament women comprised only 9.8% of members of parliament, the lowest in the East African region. The low numbers of women in leadership became the focus of feminist advocates, and a specific goal was to at least attain a critical minimum of 30% representation. Feminist advocates had realised that the political climate in Kenya was not ready for women to compete on an equal footing with men, and recognised the need for measures to address and redress the gender imbalance in leadership in Kenya; thus started a fifteen year journey to have a new constitutional dispensation that had gender equality at its core.

The Constitutional Review Process (1995 – 2010)

The Constitution of Kenya officially became law on 27 August 2010, after a historic referendum and a long journey to ensure that gender equity and human rights were entrenched. The Constitution had many gains for gender equality and human rights for men and women in Kenya. It delivered on many issues that had been at the heart of struggles for gender equality, democracy and fundamental human rights in Kenya. This constitution was a product of wide consultations with a wide range of stakeholders for whom this was the first time they had participated in a Constitutional review process. Women in particular had never been consulted and their under-representation inside parliament meant that their interests had not been well articulated. The constitution review journey, including the setting up of the review bodies such as the Constitution of Kenya Review Commission and the Committee of Experts, entailed a struggle to ensure gender equality and equity. Women lobbied to ensure that the review and harmonization processes included representation of women (Musembi et al, 2011). The process saw women learn how to engage with the centre, manage political machinations seeking to undermine women's meaningful participation, and how to get women's issues on the national agenda. Women negotiated under the umbrella of the Women Political Caucus, a loose umbrella organisation of women's organisation and groups.

The constitutional gains were far reaching and touched on many aspects that had previously been areas of contention for human rights advocates including: citizenship – women could now pass on citizenship to their children; family law – including women's rights to inheritance; and matrimonial property to name a few examples. The constitution also has a bill of rights that guarantees fundamental human rights for all Kenyans. On the political participation front, women made many gains including the provision to guarantee gender-balanced representation in elective public bodies. The constitution directs parliament to enact legislation for the special representation of certain groups of women, persons with disabilities, youth, ethnic and other minorities, and marginalized communities. With regard to women, in both the National Assembly and the Senate, a number of seats were reserved for women candidates - 47 in the National Assembly and 16 in the Senate. The 47 National Assembly seats are filled through elections in which only female candidates may participate. The 16 Senate seats for women are filled through party-based nomination, according to the proportion of each party's elected membership in the Senate. Further room for gender balance is provided in the seats set aside for youth, and for persons with disabilities. The two nominees representing each of these interests must consist of one man and one woman respectively.

On the development of party lists, the constitution requires that they alternate between male and female qualified candidates, opening greater possibilities for representation of women in the National Assembly. Kenya still retains the First Past the Post system, (FPTP), a system of voting favoured by former British colonies. This is a controversial system which has been criticised as one that distorts representivity:

> Voting takes place in single-member constituencies. Voters put a cross in a box next to their favoured candidate and the candidate with the most votes in the constituency wins. All other votes count for nothing. We believe FPTP is the very worst system for electing a representative government. (Electoral Reform Society, 2014)

The constitution chose to employ reservations rather than party-based quotas to boost women's political representation. Further gains for women were made within the provisions of the Political Parties and the Elections Parties Acts, both developed on the basis of Article 100 of the constitution that required political parties to respect the rights of all persons to participate, the inclusion of minority groups, and the requirement that parties "promote human rights and fundamental freedoms, and gender equality and equity".

Another notable gain for women in leadership and participation in governance was the provision for devolved government. The constitution provides for a devolved government structure (articles 174, 175 and 177), in order to promote democratic and accountable exercising of power, and to protect and promote the interests and rights of minorities and marginalised groups. Devolution had been at the centre of civic strife in Kenya and many Kenyans welcomed the provision they saw as eliminating the disenfranchisement they felt with the central government in Nairobi, and dominance at this level by some communities. Article 175 directs county governments to ensure that no more than two thirds of the members of representative bodies are of the same gender and article 177 established the County Assembly, which consists of elected members and special seats to ensure that the two-thirds requirement is met. So, where parliament was required to develop a formula for national level representation, the Constitution provided one for the county level.

Finally, to ensure that the constitution was implemented and that the spirit and letter of the law was respected, the Constitution established a number of commissions to oversee its implementation. A notable one for gender equality was the National Gender and Equality Commission (NGEC), whose role was to safeguard women's and gender equality provisions.

2010-2012: Getting the word out and finding a formula to implement the affirmative action provisions

Article 27 (8) of the Constitution states that "in addition to the measures contemplated in clause (6), the State shall take legislative and other measures to implement the principle that not more than two-thirds of the members of elective or appointive bodies shall be of the same gender." This left the onus on parliament to develop a formula to implement the provision. Women and gender advocates in Kenya realised very quickly that no matter how far reaching the articles were in the Constitution, the war was far from over for women's participation in leadership. Women advocates tried many times to get parliament to enact a law that would ensure that it was implemented, but each proposed draft had fundamental flaws and problems that would require the dismantling of some other fundamental legal provision or that would be impossible to realise. Apart from lacking an implementation formula the provision posed potential problems with the reserved seats already in place. Political parties and the electorate become even more hostile toward women seeking party nomination to compete in the elective politics. Any formula developed was increasing the number of legislators making parliament even bigger and more expensive. Since the article was air tight regarding the provisions on affirmative action, the winning party would not constitute a parliament without ensuring the one-third representation. Based on historical voting patterns, the chance of women being elected in enough numbers was nil. In the end parliament failed to pass a viable law and the matter was referred to the Supreme Court, which ruled that the provision was progressive and gave parliament until 2015 to find a formula (Supreme court of Kenya advisory opinion no. 2/2012). This gave parliament a lifeline to function without the 30% representation of women, to the great disappointment of women throughout Kenya. Women activists still maintain that with political will a formula can be found and that the absence of a formula right now is more an indication of the patriarchal nature of Kenyan politics, not a provision that is impossible to implement.

If the provision was complicated and confusing to the legislature and judiciary, it was much more confusing for civil society advocates trying to communicate to voters, most of who were sceptical of its viability and legitimacy. The messaging had to carry both the facts as provided for in the Constitution, and the rationale of feminist arguments for having affirmative action. This did not work as effectively as it could, due to time constraints. Civic educators had to quickly learn the new Constitution and the attendant acts to facilitate the first elections. They had to understand the new six elective positions compared to the previous three, the devolved structures and the new roles of the political parties. The constitution had been billed as a product of people's participation so there was a strong ownership of the document at the grassroots, and a high demand for public education. Unfortunately these demands were too much for civic education groups who were under time and other pressures, so any chance for addressing gender equality and the role of affirmative action was limited or lost.

2013: Women candidates get on the campaign trail

The first past the post system tends to favour already entrenched leaders and is harder to penetrate for new comers, marginalised groups and women. Civil society advocates were lobbying for a system of proportional representation, where candidates may not win the top position, but are still able to get in lower slots and, depending on a party's success, into the legislature. This was not adopted for the elections although some form of proportional representation was adopted for the reserved seat nominations.

For women to get elected they had first to get nominated as their party's candidate to vie against other candidates from other parties. This nomination process is perhaps more significant in Kenya than other countries because of the strongly entrenched identity politics. A candidate nominated by a party that was popular in a specific constituency was almost always assured of winning the seat. Party nominations were strongly contested and women had little chance of getting nominated by parties for these, particularly for safe seats. Affirmative action measures could have helped, but the Elections Act 2011 did not put in place any significant affirmative measures for candidates. Most seemed to have been minimal measures intended to ensure that the party qualified and, more importantly, accessed party funding which was contingent upon having a one-third representation of women. Very few women earned meaningful party nominations.

Those women who managed to get nominated faced a political campaign field that was highly masculinized. The campaign mode was overly aggressive, the perception of a leader was along very traditional male lines, and the concept of women as the weaker sex was often repeated on the campaign trail. Feminine leadership traits when displayed were used as evidence that women could not make good leaders. Any display of emotion was seen to confirm that women were too weak to lead. Because of the historical ethnic clashes that seemed to happen during elections, communities were looking for politicians who would protect their communities. Prominent politicians were given nicknames reminiscent of great warriors of past eras. Moreover, women wanting to join politics come with disparities in professional experience, minimal familial ties and obligations, and with the existing disadvantages in the labour market that meant limited access to finances and experience. Many women found this environment intimidating and did not present themselves as candidates or shied away from competitive seats, opting instead for the overcrowded women's seats.

One important fact to note here is that women did not gain seats as expected because fewer women were nominated to vie in the direct elections. Those who did get nominated performed fairly well compared to men according to the FIDA audit report: 14% of all men who vied for election won compared to 12% of women (Federation of Women Lawyers, 2013). It is at least a demonstration in that the sex of the candidate was in itself less of a barrier to getting elected than political parties assumed.

Election violence and violence against women

Since 1992 and probably earlier, Kenya has been prone to election and post-election violence and displacement. The violence has been largely ethnic and reached a tragic climax in the 2007 elections when over 1000 people were killed in ethnic clashes across the country. Tens of thousands were displaced. Some of who still remain displaced. Women experienced violence both as voters and as candidates and over 3,000 sexual violence cases were recorded.

> As reported by the Nairobi-based Centre for Rights Education and Awareness (CREAW), police data for 2007 indicated that there were approximately 3,000 cases of rape, defilement, indecent assault, and abduction reported. With hundreds of thousands of people displaced by the violence, women were sometimes forced to have sex in exchange for food and shelter, said Christina Siebert of the Heinrich Boll Foundation in Nairobi. (Simpson, 2012)

In 2013 the problem was not as widespread as 2007 but women still reported a number of cases of violence against women. One way in which things were different from 2007 was that there were better response mechanisms from civil society and democracy advocates to gender based electoral violence. UN Women for example provided support to both the peace building platforms to enable them to record, report and respond appropriately to incidences of violence against women. A UN Women observation mission recorded a number of incidents of harassment and violence.

> "I was confronted with a situation where I received threats on my life, while my supporters were physically intimidated" was reported directly to UN Women election observers.

The following incidents were reported by election observers, supported by UN Women, and contained in a report by Caroline Nyambura. Constituency names have been removed.

> In X constituency, there was a case of propaganda bordering on threats to a female candidate. The candidate's husband, who did not support her bid, fell sick and later passed on. She was accused of killing her husband and threatened with death, which intimidated her to the extent that she could not campaign despite being a competitive candidate.
> In another constituency, a male politician hired young men to circulate hateful and abusive leaflets about a strong woman candidate a day before the elections.
> In constituency Y, a female candidate vying for the county representatives position received threats from three male opponents, who were determined to frustrate her since she was the strongest candidate. Her vehicle's windscreen was shattered while on the way to a polling station. She subsequently received phone calls threatening her to not to leave her house for any polling station or she would be maimed. Another female candidate was threatened to the effect that she would pay heavily if she won, which was traumatizing because she did not know what her opponents anticipated to do to her or to those close to her. Another female candidate found her vehicle tyre deflated after leaving a polling station for another, which took her time to fix.
> There was a case of attempted rape of a female candidate during the campaigns in Z and reports of sexual harassment. (Nyambura, 2013,)

Another widely reported case in the Kenyan media involved a candidate from Central Region, Ms. Alice Wahome, who reported that on the eve of the party nominations her rivals distributed condoms to voters with the following inscription "A gift from Alice Wahome". The intention was to paint her as moving away from traditional values and encouraging promiscuity amongst the youth. She went on to win the election, but was to later share several examples of how gender based violence was used against women candidates.

❖ WOMEN'S LEADERSHIP IN PEACE BUILDING

Women in Kenyan Parliament – current situation

	Lower house	Senate
Total seats	350	68
Total women	67 (47 elected representatives, 16 elected members of parliament and 4 nominated women)	18 (all nominated)
% of women's representation	19%	26%
system	First Past the Post	

Source: Quotaproject,

Whether the elections were a success for women is a not that straightforward. This observation from FIDA's review sums up some of the perspectives of women activists.

> "The results disappointed backers of the new Constitution. In the National Assembly women won just 6% of directly elected constituency seats, down from 8% in 2007. Not a single woman was elected to the powerful position of governor or senator for the 47 newly created counties." (Migiro, 2013)

Despite the fact that the percentage of elected women was reduced compared to the 10th parliament, the reality is that there are more women in legislative assemblies than in any other period in Kenya's history. As shown in the table above, women form 19% and 26% respectively of the representation in the lower and upper houses of parliament.

The promise of devolution and bringing services closer to women

Devolution was intended to bring decision-making and services closer to the people. Not surprisingly with the devolution of power, many of the positions that had become available at that level now also attracted greater interest with male and seasoned politicians and women did not find the going any easier vying for such positions. The constitution provided for two seats that could be vied for at the devolved levels, the powerful county governor and his/deputy and the Ward representatives (Member of County Assembly - MCA). There was a lot of misinformation and propaganda applied to keep women away from being candidates for these seats. The most commonly applied tactic was that male politicians convinced the electorate that women already had their reserved seats and did not need to seek election for the competitive positions. Parties discouraged women from seeking the candidacy and promised women nominations instead. Eventually women only won 5% of the 1,450 MCA positions. Another 650 women were nominated to meet the constitutional threshold of one-third gender representation.

Analysis

Beyond numbers: some lessons emerging from 2013 elections

Despite a good track record for policy level advocacy and fairly decent domestic laws as far as gender equality is concerned, parliament has still not developed the legislative framework for realising the affirmative action provision. The timeline given by the Supreme Court is approaching but there is no formula developed yet. Indeed the constitutional provision is constantly under threat of being reviewed in a referendum. The numbers are vital for women to be effective in getting their voices heard, but numbers alone are not enough. For meaningful participation in governance, the focus will ultimately need to move beyond numbers. This section looks at some of the emerging issues that will be the focus of feminist advocacy in the next elections and beyond. Four key issues are identified as being important for women to participate effectively in politics.

Addressing underlying causes of inequality

Gender is an important factor in determining leadership styles, how people access or do not access leadership positions and how governance is structured. Gender is not the only factor that has an influence. Kenyan women's lives are complex. Pastoral women in northern Kenya experience inequality very differently from poor urban women in informal urban settlements, who in turn experience inequality very differently from middle class women in Nairobi. The different economic, social and cultural differences between and among women will need to inform the women's leadership discourse in Kenya. During previous elections one of the most frequently mentioned criticisms of this discourse was that most of the women nominated represented the middle class.

Recognising the inter-sectionality of women's representation need not be taken to mean women are divided along ethnic or class lines or even urban and rural lines. Rather it is a way of acknowledging how nuanced women's lives are, and the importance of getting all the voices heard. It means understanding how the ethnic and economic differences intersect with gender inequality to keep women unequal. It also means understanding other forms of marginalisation. In attempting to bring women's issues to the fore, it is important to start looking at the realities of the most marginalised women, as this is really where the historical, economic and other social injustices come into play.

Changing the perception and portrayal of women

The way that women are portrayed and perceived by the public and media is a major factor in keeping them from entering politics. Even after the campaign period women continue to face adverse and negative portrayal from both their male counterparts and from the media. A prominent politician was reported to have issued this threat to a female member of parliament in 2014. "If you are 35 and don't have a husband, there is something wrong… We will start demanding that you are married before you are elected". (BBC, 2014)

The MP was later to issue an apology after outrage from women's groups and other civil society organisations, but his view was far from an isolated case. The commonly held stereotype of women entering politics as single, frustrated or divorced women implicitly communicates that politics and leadership are a male domain and that a normal happy woman would not want to be part of the leadership. They should be at home with her family! Another woman candidate, Shakida Abdalla, who lost the elections but was nominated on a party ticket made this observation:

> Voters judge us by a different standard than they would a male candidate. For instance, a man's marital status hardly ever comes into consideration – we had a president (Daniel Arap Moi) who ruled Kenya for 24 years without taking a wife. But, in the case of women in electoral politics, whether they are single, divorced or widowed becomes an election issue. (Mushtak, 2008)

Tokenism

One of the major risks of having an affirmative action provision in an unwilling political climate will always be tokenism. This has been demonstrated in a number of ways: political parties nominated women to positions where their chance of influencing the agenda was limited. Tokenism is also demonstrated in other ways, by political parties nominating only those women whom they can control or who are affiliated to them in some way, while at the same time denying women who merit positions. By far the worst case of tokenism happened in the 2013 elections when women were edged out of competitive politics with the argument that they already had the reserved seats.

Agenda setting

Ultimately the aim of having women in leadership is so that they can set the agenda and influence governance for the benefit of all as a means to achieve equality. To do this, women need to take centre stage and to have their voices heard in national political discourse. Although it is too early to judge the performance of the current crop of women representatives, there are clearly some successes and some gaps. Women have taken centre stage and shown good leadership, for example, on issues of sexual offences and violence against women. There are certain issues where the capacities of women leaders are absent and where leadership has been absent. A good example was the debate on polygamy. In 2014, the President signed into law the Marriage Act (Marriage bill no 13 2013). When the bill was debated in parliament women were conspicuously absent.

This is what the Daily Nation reporter Ngirachu said about the law when it was passed:

> In amendments that appeared more designed to serve the marital needs and assuage the financial fears of male MPs, the House watered down the Marriage Bill, which had given wives the right to be consulted before their husbands brought home a second wife. (Ngirachu, 2014)

Women in county assemblies too have faced challenges in articulating women's issues and setting an agenda for gender equality in Kenya. This also is compounded by the fact the majority of women representatives are nominated and are yet to enjoy the full mandate of their positions. In the fullness of time it will be important for women's and gender issues to become not just an issue for women but national issues that inform our governance and development agenda. Currently women tend to be most vocal on issues that affect women or are seen as family issues. When they lead committees they are usually found in those committees that tend to reinforce their reproductive roles and their roles as mothers and carers.

Conclusions

For most Kenyan women working on these issues on a daily basis, it is easy to get absorbed in current challenges and to feel that not much has changed for women's participation. Of particular cause for concern is the on-going lack of political will to fully realise the constitutional provisions for women. This chapter attempted to show that there has been progress in women's representation and participation.

The progress has been primarily as a result of women organising and fighting for rights at every stage as demonstrated in the constitutional review process. Women's gains were also secured once women joined with other rights advocates and activists and identified the interconnectedness of their struggles. A progressive legal and policy framework is an important first step for women's participation, but more is needed to ensure that such participation is substantive. Women should not just be sitting at the table but also influencing decisions and making an impact on gender equality and the quality of life for all women. As demonstrated in the analysis above, this requires a look at the underlying causes of gender inequality, looking at other types of inequalities including ethnicity and economic status, and recognising the multifaceted nature of women's lives. The argument has been made that women are shying away from politics because of its highly masculinized nature of political discourse, and by the way women get into politics is portrayed. All of these will need to change to make space for women to engage.

In conclusion, the women who are actively engaged in leadership have made strong contributions to development and to gender equality in Kenya. They have shown tenacity and taught the Kenya nation that it is possible to be a leader despite the odds. What has been most impressive has been the way women have learnt how to negotiate the leadership terrain and find ways of being influential despite the limited space they currently hold. These gains can only improve as more women enter the fray.

References

BBC, 2014. (5 February 2014) 'Kenyan governor Kabogo apologises over single women slur.' *BBC*, [online]. Available at: http://www.bbc.com/news/world-africa-26049787 (Accessed 2 August 2014).

Bii, B. (2013) Female candidates claim discrimination in Kenyan elections. *Online Report*. Institute for War & Peace, [online]. Available at: http://www.iwpr.net/report-news/female-candidates-claim-discrimination-kenyan-elections (accessed 02 August 2014).

Electoral Reform Society UK (2014). 'First Past the Post.' *Online Report*. Available at: http://www.electoral-reform.org.uk/first-past-the-post/ (accessed 02 August 2014)

Federation of Women Lawyers, 2013. *Key Gains and Challenges: A Gender Audit of Kenya's 2013 Election Process*. FIDA, Nairobi.

Library of Congress (2014) 'Kenya: Parliament Passes Comprehensive Marriage Bill, Changes Process for Contracting Customary Marriages.' *Online Report*. Library of Congress [online]. Available at: http://www.loc.gov/lawweb/servlet/lloc_news?disp3_l205403910_text (accessed 2 August 2014).

Kamau, N. (2010) *Women and Political Leadership in Kenya: Ten Case Studies*. Heinrich Herbert Stiftung, Nairobi.

Kenya Law (2012) 'Advisory opinions application 2 of 2012.' *Online Report*. Available at: http://kenyalaw.org/caselaw/cases/view/85286 (accessed 18 September 2014).

Migiro, K. (2013) 'New Laws Ignored, So Women Trailed in Kenya 2013 Election.' *Allafrica.com*, Available at: http://allafrica.com/stories/201312091132.html (accessed 02 August 2014).

Morris, M and Bunjun, B. (2007) *Using intersectional feminist frameworks in research: A resource for embracing the complexities of women's lives*. Canadian Research Institute for Advancement of Women, Ottawa.

Mukabi, K., and Kimani, E. (2012) The historical journey of Women's leadership in Kenya. *Journal of Emerging Trends in Education Research and Policy Studies*, 3(6), pp.842-849.

Musembi, C., Kameri-Mbote, P. and Kamau, W. (2010) Gender Audit of Constitution of Kenya 2010. *Unpublished*. Review undertaken for UNIFEM.

Mushtak, N. (2008) 'Politics-Kenya: Taking Up a Women's Agenda.' *Inter Press Service News Agency*. Available at: http://www.ipsnews.net/2008/12/politics-kenya-taking-up-a-women39s-agenda/ (accessed 02 August 2014).

Ngirachu, J. (2014) 'New law allowing polygamy passed.' Daily *Nation*. Available at: http://mobile.nation.co.ke/news/Marriage-Bill-Amendments-Polygamy-MPs-National-Assembly/-/1950946/2252204/-/format/xhtml/-/15g7fat/-/index.html (accessed 2 August 2014).

Njenga, S. (2014) 'Single women headache for men – Kabogo.' *The Star*. Available at: http://www.the-star.co.ke/news/article-152409/single-women-headache-men-kabogo (accessed 2 August 2014).

Nyambura, C. (2013): Election observation report, Unpublished review undertaken for UN Women 2013.

Quota Project (2014) 'Kenya. Quota Project: Global Database of Quotas for Women.' *Online Report*. Available at: http://www.quotaproject.org/uid/countryview.cfm?Country Code=KE (accessed 2 August 2014).

Richardson, A., and Louber, C. (2008) Intersectionality and Leadership. *International Journal of Leadership Studies*, 3(2), pp.142-161.

Simpson, D. (2012) 'Women in Kenya's slums still dealing with post-election sexualized violence.' *Women's Media Center* [online]. Available at: http://www.womenundersiege project.org/blog/entry/women-in-kenyas-slums-still-dealing-with-post-election-sexualized-violence (accessed 2 August 2014).

PART III: GENDER IN THE CONTEXT OF SECURITY CHALLENGES

CHAPTER 10. "BRING BACK OUR GIRLS": CONFLICT AND INSURGENCY IN NIGERIA

===============❖===============

Obadiah Mailafia

Introduction

In April 2014, the world woke up to the shock of the kidnaping of 270 girls from a boarding secondary school in the sleepy town of Chibok, northeastern Nigeria. For years the region had been ravaged terrorism and insurgency masterminded by a brutal Islamist terrorist organisation popularly known as "Boko Haram". Although a few of the girls managed to escape, the fate of over 200 of them remains unknown. The leader of the terrorist group was later to announce that he would "sell" the girls. A few of those who escaped reported incidences of serial rape and other forms of butality. The Nigerian government has been helpless. The world community is outraged. The "Bring Back our Girls" campaign went global, with even American First Lady Michelle Obama being photographed with a campaign poster.

This chapter discusses the politics and economics of terrorism and insurgency in Nigeria set in a global context.[1] The point of departure is that women and children tend to suffer disproportionately from most acts of violence and conflict perpetrated by men. The fate of the Chibok girls brings

---

1. This article is a re-edited version and part reprint of an earlier publication by Mailafia, O., 2012.

into dramatic focus the evil nature of terrorism, Islamic and otherwise, and the gross abuse of Humanity that it entails. The Nigerian case has been particularly savage and its toll on women, children and the family is an affront to human dignity and an evil that must be reversed at all costs.

In this chapter we discuss the nature, origins and impact of terrorist insurgency in Nigeria. We situate this phenomenon not only in the context of globalisation but also in poor governance and the failure to devise effective policies to meet the country's daunting challenges (Cf. Nnadozie, 2012). The presentation is in four main parts. Part one addresses definition and conceptualisation of terrorism as a social phenomenon. The second discusses the global context for the proliferation of terrorist violence. In the third section we analyse the incidence of ethno-sectarian conflict in Nigeria that provides the context for the rise of the Boko Haram insurgency. The fourth part discusses the economic and social consequences of terrorism. We then provide a general summary and conclusion.

Theoretical and Conceptual Considerations

The analytical approach of this paper is premised on the theory of social constructivism. According to this approach, it is not only empirical reality that determines social outcomes. Differences arising from conflicting construction of worldviews, ideas, identities and historical experiences are influential in shaping the structure of politics and public policy. Constructivist epistemology goes back to the renaissance scholar Giambattista Vico, Immanuel Kant, Max Weber and the philosopher John Dewey. According to this approach, human consciousness is shaped by the shared meanings that shape the worldviews of a people and the meanings they give to events and symbols. Reality is thus shaped less by truth than by conditioned learning and received tradition. Socially constructed interpretations of national challenges shape how different segments of society perceive issues and what solutions they proffer. In the words of two co-authors:

> Perceptual differences in terms of relative political and socio-economic issues generate disparate and competing templates for finding solutions to national problems. When one premises these differences on fundamental ideological and cultural foundations, they oftentimes become irreconcilable and hence less amenable to long lasting and durable solutions (Kalu & Oguntoyinbo, 2012: 91).

From the viewpoint of social constructivism, the idea of a universal Muslim 'Ummah', the political categories known as 'The North' or 'The Middle Belt' are socially constructed concepts. While remaining conceptual myths, their potency as idea and rallying banner cannot be under-estimated. Part of the contestations shaping the structure of politics in contemporary thinking relate to the force of these constructed ideas. Solving them will require returning to the fundamentals of nationhood and reinventing the grammar and syntax of political discourse.

Defining Terrorism

Terrorism is a rather emotional topic. Not only do people differ on questions of conceptual definition; they also disagree on interpretation of facts in specific cases of terrorist activity. Noam Chomsky, points out two different and conflicting approaches to the study of terrorism. One is the literal approach and the other is the propagandistic approach. While the first one seeks a rational-scientific understanding of terrorism as a social phenomenon with specific empirical causal factors that lead to particular societal impact, the latter prefers to view terrorism as "a weapon to be exploited in the service of some system of power" (Chomsky, 1991: 56). While the scientific approach is interested in finding lasting remedies, the propagandistic is more interested in labelling and demonising for the sole purpose of deploying hegemonic military power to score strategic advantage over perceived enemies.

The late Charles Tilly pointed out that terrorism as a social phenomenon surfaces in a wide variety of cultures, institutions and political forces. It is certainly not a preserve of Muslims as the American neo-conservatives would have us believe. Indeed, the governments of world powers and developing countries have also practised some form of terrorism or other, not to talk of a whole brigade of environmentalists, liberation fighters and anarchists. According to Tilly, "Terrorists range across a wide spectrum of organisations, circumstances and beliefs. Terrorism is not a single coherent phenomenon. No social scientist can speak responsibly as though it were." (Tilly, 2004: 12)

Terrorism is not just a Nigerian problem; it is a global problem. Nor is it an exclusively Islamic problem. Extremists are to be found in all religions. Our central thesis is that the increasing salience of Islamist terror may be explained by the unique experiences of Arab-Muslim societies and how religion has often been deployed as a weapon of political struggle. Globalisation and the technologies associated with the increasing internationalisation of production, capital and markets have facilitated the capacity of terror groups to mobilise, network and implement their violent projects across nations and communities.

Curiously enough, nobody has ever been known to describe himself or herself as a terrorist. Terrorism is a rather value-loaded term that people often use to describe those who are pursuing goals or deploying methods with which they do not agree. It can even be a term of abuse. Equally problematic is the fact that it is often deployed as a political term to categorise people or countries that have already been identified to be enemies (Kapitan, 2003). A major challenge in seeking to understand terrorism is the fact that perspectives differ, depending on where we stand on a particular issue. The well-worn cliché that "one man's terrorist is another man's freedom fighter" rings as true today as it did when first used in terrorism discourse. For example, both Ronald Reagan in America and Prime Minister Margaret Thatcher in Britain dismissed the imprisoned Nelson Mandela and his colleagues as "terrorists". To their own people and to most Africans, however, they were "freedom fighters"; heroes of a historic struggle for liberation against Apartheid and racial humiliation.

Given these complexities, it is not surprising that there are probably as many definitions of terrorism as there are organisations and governments working to counter the menace.[2] Several definitions have been on offer, most of them expressing nuances and perspectives deriving from the type of agency in question or the historical experiences of the government proffering the definition.

For the purposes of this chapter we understand terrorism to mean all forms of violent action by clandestine and semi-clandestine actors aimed at achieving criminal, military, religious, political or other objectives, with such actions often directed at government and non-combatant populations with the deliberate objective of spreading fear, anxiety and terror.

The Global Context

The resurgence of radical political Islam has been recent key features in Africa. In East Africa, it has been suggested that discrimination against Muslims during the colonial era and after has been a key factor in the radicalisation of Muslim groups (Dickson, 2005). Equally crucial has been Saudi-sponsored Wahabbism in the Horn of Africa and elsewhere. Among the predominant Muslim nations of Africa, Senegal stands out by its unique blend of Islam and modernity and the spirit of tolerance that defines the national culture. This is so despite the prevalence of social and religious conservatism and the widespread influence of the 'mourides' in social and political life (O'Brien, 1971; Trimingham, 1962; Copans, 1988).

Since the 1998 bombing of US embassies in Nairobi and Dar es Salaam by Al-Qaeda, there appears to be an exponential growth in the spate of terrorist attacks, including the kidnapping and killing of Western aid workers. Since the 1990s, the collapse of Somalia has spurred an army of pirates and lawless gangsters who have become a menace to their neighbours and merchant vessels on the Red Sea.

---

2. We could probably avoid these definitional issues by simply defining terrorism as "what terrorists do". But that would be begging the question.

The American military campaign in Afghanistan may have succeeded in breaking the back of the Taliban and their al-Qaeda comrades, but as a consequence they may be turning to Africa. There is evidence that Al-Qaeda has taken a strategic decision to re-locate to Africa as a safe haven for its global operations. The Taliban, al-Qaeda in the Maghreb (AQIM) and al-Shabab from Somalia have joined forces with Tuareg insurgents and drug barons, taking over vast territories in the Sahara desert. Fleeing mercenaries from Libya may have also brought substantial supplies of weapons thereby supplementing what the Sahelian terrorists already possessed.

At the heart of contemporary terrorism is globalisation and how it impacts on national systems, cultures and faith-communities (Coker, 2002). By globalisation, we are referring to the internationalisation of production, markets and capital and the virtual emergence of a single global marketplace. It also entails the trans-border diffusion of knowledge and information through new technologies such as the worldwide web, the Internet and mobile telephony. There are good as well as bad aspects to globalisation.

Most economists would agree that globalisation has been positive in many aspects: in terms of improved international trade and investments; providing an impetus to growth and enhanced global welfare. Indeed, the emergence of new economic powers such as China, India and Brazil would not have been possible without the relaxation of domestic as well as global barriers to the movement of people, goods, services and capital. Thanks to liberalisation and digital technologies, our world has become the proverbial 'global village'. The internationalisation of world markets, the expansion in global trade and the movement of capital through instantaneous communication and the impact of electronic media such as CNN and Al-Jazeera have brought the world closer together as never before. Today information travels at the speed of light. Governments can no longer hide information from their own citizens as they did in the past.

However, globalisation has engendered new forms of vulnerabilities for nations and communities. Financial contagion and the spread of epidemic viral diseases pose greater risks than ever before. Communities that have hitherto lived in cultural cocoons have suddenly found themselves exposed to new habits and mindsets. Terrorist networks such as al Qaeda have become transnational organisations that thrive on the opportunities opened by new technologies and communications channels. Not only are they able to coordinate their activities through such channels, they are also able to raise funds, network and coordinate their activities across national borders and frontiers with greater ease than would have been considered feasible just two decades ago.

Globalisation has to some extent also altered the character of the Westphalian territorial state as we have always known it. In a liberal market economy, the state is expected to restrict itself to playing the role of umpire while looking after public goods such as law and order, transport and infrastructures, education and control of communicable diseases. There is a sense in which globalisation has eroded the traditional 'parental role' of the state while undermining its capacity, authority and legitimacy.[3]

With globalisation, the boundaries between the domestic and the international are becoming increasingly blurred. It has also engendered new inequities between the rich and the poor. In the advanced industrial nations as well as in low-income developing, all the relevant indicators show that income inequalities are reaching alarming proportions.[4]

The National Context

With a population of 165 million, Nigeria is Africa's largest country in terms of demographic size. With a GDP of US$ 415 billion, it is the second largest economy after South Africa. Nigeria holds the record for being the largest oil producer on the continent and the sixth in OPEC. The country is well endowed with petroleum, gas and yet-untapped mineral resources. Its agricultural potentials are considerable, although the country remains a net importer of food. Over the last decade growth has averaged 7.4% (African Development Bank, 2012).

Nigeria remains a paradox, if not an enigma, to many observers. A country of energetic and highly entrepreneurial peoples and with an embarrassment of natural riches, where the bulk of the population remains impoverished. Although per capita income has improved in recent years to about US$ 2,500 (in PPP terms), more than 60% of the people live below the poverty line and income inequalities are widening, with an estimated gini coefficient of 43.7 percent. Unemployment stands at a national average of 24%, with an estimated 54% of youth without jobs. A World Bank study depicts the country's development trajectory in terms of 'jobless growth' (The World Bank, 2009). Massive revenues from oil earnings have gone into consumption and recurrent expenditure, with little left to finance the yawning gaps in physical infrastructures. Corruption is widespread in public

---

3. Of late, we have witnessed the emergence of powerful non-state actors who vie for authority, power and influence with the state. These non-state actors range from transnational firms to non-governmental organisations, drug cartels and international terrorist groups such as Al-Qaeda. Such powerful non-state actors can also seize new opportunities to leverage on their capacity to do good as well as evil.
4. The Occupy Wall Street Campaign in New York in September 2011 emerged as a spontaneous mass movement against what is perceived as the greed and corruption of global bankers and financiers which fuelled inequality as well as the international financial crisis.

life while capital flight is an endemic feature of the political economy. As a result, the vast majority have no access to electricity, water and basic social services. Life expectancy stands at 51 years; well below the average for sub-Saharan Africa.

After decades of military rule, the country returned to democratic rule in 1999. The writer Fareed Zakaria's concept of "illiberal democracy" (2004) perhaps best describes Nigeria's current governance situation, where the culture of impunity reigns supreme and the rule of law and constitutionalism remain very much work in progress. Nigeria is an ethnically diverse country, with some of the most ancient civilisations known to man. In the context of widening inequalities, joblessness and poverty, it is inevitable that social tensions, most of which are exploited by politicians, will tend to find expression in ethno-religious conflict.

Deepening inequalities are, for their part, fostering new forms of anxiety and frustration among dispossessed groups. In oil-rich Nigeria the gap between the rich and the poor continues to widen. Increasingly desperate young, educated and unemployed urban youth, can easily be mobilised for ethnic or religiously inspired violence.[5]

There is no denying that sociological factors deriving from rapid urbanisation and modernisation can and do contribute to spurring alienation and, ultimately, political violence. The French sociologist Emile Durkheim identified 'anomie' as a major psychosocial malady in industrialising societies. The sprawling slums of cities such as Kaduna, Abuja, Lagos and Maiduguri are cesspools of crime, prostitution and violence. When youths drift to cities and lose the traditional moorings that provided meaning and signification to their lives, they can fall easy prey to extremist ideologies. It has been estimated that in Northern Nigeria there are over 9.5 million 'Almajiris' (itinerant youths who attend traditional koranic schools). Most of such children are the cannon fodder for ethno-religious conflicts that spring up from time to time.

There is also the impact of new information and telecommunications technologies (ICT). Such technologies connect disgruntled and alienated groups that may not even know each other. They share information, strategies and tactics and disseminate propaganda materials as a means of recruitment and socialisation into their theology of death. The historian Michael Burleigh observes that the internet "has become the broadband river whereby noxious ideologies...can be accessed in the privacy of the bedroom

---

5. The mere prevalence of poverty cannot be said to engender terrorism. Rather, poverty normally interacts with other variables such as ethnically divided elites, absence of societal cohesion, corruption, political disempowerment and perceptions of horizontal or vertical deprivation.

or study in provincial towns and major cities of the West by young people, of whom significant numbers applaud the actions of al-Qaeda and other Islamic terrorists" (Burleigh, 2006: 468)

It is also evident that a country with historical antecedents of political violence, civil war and dictatorship nurtures an environment that is more susceptible to terrorism. Nigeria's rather long history of civil strife makes it more understandable why terrorism could easily thrive in the country. Over the last decade alone, more than 10,000 people have died as a result of ethnic and sectarian conflict in Nigeria. Nigerians are beginning to accept random violence as their lot and destiny.

Linked to this is the new architecture of global power and the insecurity that it engenders. The Cold War created two major centres of power, one based in Washington DC and the other in Moscow. China and the group of Non-Aligned countries provided a shield for those nations who chose to side with neither camp. Today, we live in a largely unipolar world in which the United States is the dominant economic, military and political power. During the era of George W. Bush, Washington did not hesitate to use its military pre-eminence in pursuit of narrow national goals and purposes. The retreat from multilateralism, the almost religious faith in 'American Exceptionalism' and the pursuit of unilateralist folly has incurred the resentment of many across the world. In the Middle East educated youths, alienated intellectuals and dispossessed communities in Palestine see the fate of their nations as the end result of American 'hegemony'. Most believe that the survival of Israel would not have been possible without American military and financial support.

In November 2001, barely two months after the attack on the Twin Towers, the late French philosopher, sociologist and intellectual Jean Baudrillard, in an influential article entitled "The Spirit of Terrorism", argued that contemporary terrorism has its roots in the contradictions arising from the global system that has emerged with America's Atlantic hegemony (Baudrillard, 2011). Declaring that "terrorism, as a virus, is everywhere", Baudrillard pointed out, quite correctly, that the Bush administration, as late as the summer of 2001, had been fully in touch with the Taliban. He also noted that Washington had over the years provided support to Osama bin Laden and the mujahideen in Afghanistan. He sought to proffer an anti-intellectual antidote to the blind nationalism and wholesale demonization of terrorists that greeted the 9/11 attacks. His own compatriot, the economist and historian Alain Minc, has, however, challenged this view as being in itself a form of 'intellectual terrorism'.[6]

---

6. Minc argues that the real problem is the fact that our globalised post-Cold War international order no longer possesses a moral centre of gravity and represents

In a changing world Robert Kaplan identified West Africa as the signifier in his premonition of a future of chaos and global disintegration (Kaplan, 1994). Kaplan believes "West Africa is becoming the symbol of worldwide demographic, environmental, and societal stress, in which criminal anarchy emerges as the real strategic danger." (Kaplan, 1994: 46) He points to trends such as disease, uncontrolled population growth, criminal violence, resource scarcity, refugees and the "increasing erosion of nation-states and international borders" (1994: 47) as factors likely to speed up the inevitable process of societal collapse in Africa. Kaplan makes oblique references to Nigeria as one of those countries destined to fail, prophesying, in effect, that terrorist groups and criminal bandits are likely to fill the political vacuum that will emerge.[7]

Kaplan paints a rather apocalyptic picture of a new international disorder; a coming age of impending chaos: "To understand the events of the next fifty years...one must understand environmental scarcity, cultural and racial clash, geographic destiny, and the transformation of war" (1994: 54). He is obviously right about the pressures exerted on national systems by demographics, unchecked urbanization and lack of adequate infrastructures, in addition to poor leadership and lack of effective governance. Some of these weaknesses no doubt account for the rise of groups such as Boko Haram. But Kaplan is also the victim of the classic syndrome of "Afro-pessimism" which constitutes the prism from which commentators of his ilk view the continent of Africa. He was writing in 1994 when Liberia, Sierra Leone, Guinea and Guinea-Bissau were enmeshed in violent conflict. Today, West Africa represents one of the regions with the fastest rates of growth in the world. The guns have fallen silent in Sierra Leone as most of the countries in ECOWAS make bold efforts to consolidate their democracies and restore confidence to their people. Nigeria is the leader of West Africa and is bound to be one of the leading countries in the world, if only the leadership could get their act together.

Poverty and youth unemployment

The dramatic unfolding of events in the Middle East at the beginning of 2011 reinforces this hypothesis about the political consequences of economic deprivation. It is evident that deepening frustrations occasioned by poverty and economic stagnation, coupled with the absence of political expression

---

the emergence of a new medievalism, with its chaos and lawlessness. (Minc, 1995)
7. West Africa, he insists, "provides an appropriate introduction to the issues, often extremely unpleasant to discuss, that will soon confront our civilization" (Kagan, 1994: 4).

and dwindling socio-economic opportunities were the key elements that explain the recent upheavals in Tunisia, Egypt, Libya, Syria and Yemen. The countries of the Middle East and North Africa (MENA) have probably the worst records of youth joblessness in the world, averaging some 25% (Kabbani & Kothari, 2005). This largely explains the upheavals that have come to be known as 'the Arab Spring'. The once 'fertile crescent' has remained trapped in the Middle Ages since the end of the Ottoman Empire. According to one account, if you subtract earnings from oil, the entire exports of the Middle East are merely equal to the total exports of Switzerland.

Few developing countries illustrate the spiral of decline in human welfare as Nigeria has experienced in the past four decades. Peter Lewis has undertaken a fascinating comparative study of economic development in Nigeria and Indonesia (Lewis, 2007.) Although both countries began with the same initial conditions in 1960 and both experienced instability and military dictatorships, Nigerian elites bled dry their country while the equally corrupt elites of Indonesia make the critical choice of investing at home. It is clear that poverty is a major factor explaining the current wave of terrorist insurgency.

Poverty in Borno State

On all the poverty indices, it is clear that the North is comparatively more impoverished than the rest of the country. Available studies from UN agencies, the National Bureau of Statistics (NBS) and other relevant institutions point to the fact that poverty is worsening in Nigeria. According to the NBS, over 60% of Nigerians are living below the internationally defined poverty line (National Bureau of Statistics, 2012). It is evident from recent data that poverty in Nigeria wears a predominantly northern face. Borno and the North East comprise some of the most impoverished regions in the country, where the incidence of absolute poverty exceeds 70%.

Borno has one of the fastest growing populations in the country estimated at 4.5 million people, and growing at an average of 2.8% per annum. The rate of urbanisation is estimated at over 4% annually and as people move into the cities, greater pressure is placed on dilapidated infrastructures, social services and housing, and consequently results in a growth of urban slums. Migration southwards is placing additional pressures on scarce fertile land for cultivation and pasture for livestock.

Agriculture, which remains the backbone of the local economy, is hampered by low productivity and access to inputs such as seedlings, fertilisers, appropriate technology and affordable credit. Enhancing farm productivity is critical to eliminating hunger and ensuring food security.

Infrastructure facilities across the State, particularly electricity, transport and water remain in acute deficit with electricity supply largely restricted to urban centres. Water scarcity is probably the single most critical challenge facing ordinary people in the State, much of it due to poor maintenance of dams and boreholes. Ordinary people have poor access to medical services and most cannot afford the charges.

The State remains one of the most educationally disadvantaged regions in the Federation with only one out of seven pupils (13.82%) proceeding from elementary school to secondary education.[8] Most youths have no access and no opportunity to acquire vocational skills that will make them economically self-sufficient. While the State is disadvantaged in terms of western education, it is a magnet for Qur'anic education under the 'Almajiri' system. Of the estimated 9 million 'Almajirai' to be found throughout northern Nigeria, an estimated 1.5 million are said to be in Borno State alone. Such an influx of under-fed, ill-clad and poorly housed youth constitutes a potentially explosive force in the hands of a teacher with extremist ideological views and politicians with an axe to grind with their opponents.

Linking poverty and terrorism

Poverty maybe one direct trigger for terrorism, but we must recognize not all terrorists are poor and not all people in poverty are terrorists. The 19 poorest countries in the world have no recorded incidences of terrorism. A more credible explanation is that the prevalence of poverty makes it easier for extremist groups to mobilise disenchanted mobs in pursuit of their own political goals. In northern Nigeria, where over 70% of the population lives under the internationally defined poverty line, it is easy to see how any demagogue or religious extremist can mobilise the poor and destitute as instruments for his own political goals. Youth unemployment, especially within the growing stratum of university graduates, is an added factor (The World Bank, 2009). When people are pushed to the lowest levels of desperation and hopelessness, they can easy fall prey to religious demagogues who offer them a sense of belonging.

It is equally true that unjust and corrupt governments provide a fertile ground for terrorism. Some would argue that non-democratic governments breed conditions that terrorists can exploit in furtherance of their own objectives. While this is highly probable, social science provides no evidence that undemocratic governments necessarily lead to proliferation of terrorists. In fact, the opposite appears to be the case. The likelihood of terrorism surfacing in countries such as North Korea, China and Cuba is quite remote. What seems obvious is that in fledgling democracies where corruption is rife and institutions are weak, there is a higher likelihood of terrorist activities

---

8. Interview with Borno State Ministry Official in Maiduguri, April 2012.

emerging.

Terrorist movements are always led by well educated and, in some cases, highly privileged people. Osama bin Laden hailed from an affluent Saudi background, having studied economics and engineering at university. His deputy, Ayman Mohammed Rabie al-Zawahiri is a qualified surgeon from an illustrious Egyptian family of intellectuals. It begs the question as to why some of those intellectuals and not others become alienated in the first place. This would suggest other factors relating to individual psychology, personality types, dynamics of socialisation, environmental influences and the specific conditions in which such individuals find themselves.

State failure and the fragility of nations

State failure is another contributing factor. A failed state is defined by the Development Assistance Committee (DAC) of the OECD as a situation where "state structures lack political will and/or capacity to provide the basic functions needed for poverty reduction, development and to safeguard the security and human rights of their populations" (OECD, 2007: 2). State failure can be said to prevail where public institutions are no longer able to deliver positive political goods to citizens and that such failure prevails on a scale likely to undermine the legitimacy and the existence of the state itself. The most critical areas of state failure relate to inability to provide a wide range of public goods, especially in terms of law and order, security, provision of economic and communication infrastructures and supply of basic welfare services (Ghani & Lockhart, 2008). Some of the indicators of state weakness that could potentially lead to state failure include emergence of disharmony among communities, inability to control borders, growth of criminal violence, corrupt institutions and decaying infrastructures. A good number of countries in Africa have been categorised as "failed states", the most obvious cases being Somalia, Central African Republic and Guinea-Bissau.

Nigeria may not be a "failed state", but it is speedily relapsing into the band of failing states. The symptoms of state failure are to be seen in the inability of the state to maintain law and order; in the random outbreak of gratuitous, nihilistic violence; in the widespread practice of cultism among some members of the ruling elites; in the inability to provide stable electricity for all its people; in the parlous state of infrastructures; in the failure to build and maintain refineries and so being a net importer of refined petroleum; in the inability to effectively patrol its borders; in the failure to control corruption; in the high prevalence of lawless violence and criminality; all the carnage on its highways; and in the abject failure to keep the common peace and to secure the lives and properties of its citizens. Millions of youth wonder the streets with no hope on the horizon. A good number are finding succour in cultism, prostitution, kidnapping, robbery and other forms of violent criminality.

State failure provides a good excuse for terrorist groups to question the legitimacy of the state and to seek to impose an alternative vision of political order. With regard to Boko Haram, for example, the writer was surprised to hear from many well-educated 'Northerners' that they sympathise with the movement and would join the group if they had enough guts to do so. In a country that does not offer its citizens any hope and denies its youth all the opportunities, it is no surprise that extremists such as Mohammed Yusuf were able to mobilise such a formidable following.

Equally important is the politics of competitive ethnicity and the dynamics of inter-group relations within the Nigerian federation. The geometry of power places awesome powers in the federal centre. This makes the Presidency the most coveted political prize of all; a zero-sum game in which the winners view state power as an opportunity to corner the nation's wealth for themselves and their small coterie of acolytes. Most development experts have tended to dwell on vertical inequities as measured by the Gini Coefficient as the only real yardstick for determining socio-economic inequality. Important as this is, it is becoming more evident that inter-group inequities are also vital and could actually prove even more politically explosive.

There is also the culture of violence, which has been endemic to Nigerian politics since independence. It has been suggested that the roots of this tradition of violence go back to the colonial state itself, which was founded and maintained by violence. It also took violence to dislodge it. A tradition so established was quite easy to perpetuate in the post-independence period, from the 'Agbekoya riots' in the Western region in the 1960s to the skirmishes between the Northern People's Congress (NPC) and the Northern Elements' Progressive Union (NEPU) to the post-election violence that followed the April 2011 presidential elections.

External influences are also major factors in terrorist activities, particularly in countries such as Nigeria. Muammar Gadaffi in Libya, before his demise, was known to have financed certain extremist groups in Nigeria. There is anecdotal evidence that Iran and Saudi Arabia have provided considerable financial support over the years to Islamic groups in Nigeria. Not all the money has been used for building mosques, schools and clinics. It has been estimated that over the last 30 years Saudi has been spending an annual average of US$ 2.5 billion on Islamic activities across the world. The Islamic Republic of Iran has shown an undue interest in Nigerian politics over the last couple of years. There is no doubting that some of their money has gone into financing terrorist activities in Nigeria. The discovery in October 2010 of 12 containers of highly sophisticated arms that were traceable to Iran was perhaps only the tip of the iceberg.

The roots of ethno-sectarian conflict in Nigeria

Nigeria is a multi-ethnic and multi-religious country. There are some 200 ethnic groups and over 500 dialects within the country. Although national census enumeration exercises have always excluded religion from the headcount, it is generally accepted that the country is almost evenly divided between Christians in the South and Muslims in the North, with the predominantly Christian Middle Belt straddling north and South. The structure of politics in Nigeria has often reflected the fissures, regionalism, identity politics and competitive ethnicity inherent in such a diverse polity (Dudley, 1968).

Most Nigerian Muslims are Sunnis, with some of the elites belonging to rival Qadiriyya and Tijanniya Sufi denominations. Other denominations include the Tariqa, the Malikiya, the Ahmadiya, and the Islamiya. One of the latest denominations to make an entry into the religious landscape in northern Nigeria is the Shi'i religion. Following the Iranian revolution of 1979, several Nigerian students went to study in Iran and returned as Shi'i adherents and proselytisers. One of the new denominations that draw the young educated Muslim intelligentsia is the Jama't Izalat al Bid'a wa Iqamat as Sunna (Society of Removal of Innovation and Reestablishment of the Sunna).[9] Another new group is the Da'awa, sometimes used interchangeably with the Hisba whose role is to enforce Sharia law.[10]

In a country of such diversity, ethnic and religious cleavages can easily be exploited by unscrupulous elites to inflame latent tensions, leading to intercommunal violence. In this respect, Nigeria is no different from other multiethnic developing societies where power elites often prefer to exploit what Crawford Young terms "the politics of cultural pluralism" (1979). Politicians who lose out in power struggles often resort to religion and ethnicity as banners for political mobilisation. This largely explains why violence has been a characteristic feature of the Nigerian political scene since independence.

Political violence has a rather long path-dependent trajectory in

---

9. Also known as Izala or Yan Izala, the movement was founded in Jos by Sheikh Ismaila Idris in 1978 with the objective of purifying Islam from it believes to by Sufi syncretism.
10. It has been suggested that both the Shi'i and the Yan Izala are opposed to the current application of Sharia in Nigeria. They insist that Sharia can only work where the political leaders fully operate an Islamic republic. Among those who hold this view is said to be the Zaria-based Shi'ite leader, Sheikh El Zakzaky, who is said to have opposed the precipitate application of Sharia on the grounds that the prevailing social and economic conditions did not make it feasible.

Nigeria.[11] British occupation was accomplished largely through force and violence. For much of the first decade of independence, politics in Nigeria was characterised by widespread political violence, including violent coups d'état and ultimately civil war during 1967-1970. The traditions of democratic politics have been marked by electoral violence and occasional bloodletting between rival political parties (Anifowoshe, 1981; Cf. Osita Agbu, 2004; Dike, 2003). Succeeding governments, whether civilian or military, have sometimes engaged in what could only be defined in terms of 'state terrorism'.

With the widespread misery occasioned by Structural Adjustment Reforms and the ensuing repression and political decay in the 1980s, Nigerian ethnic communities began to seek succour in new primordial associations. Regional and ethnic militias became the order of the day.[12]

On the specifically religious dimensions of social conflict, northern Nigeria has remained the most troubled region in the country. For much of Nigeria's history since independence, northern elites have found it expedient to use religion as a means of consolidating their power and ensuring their ascendancy over the peoples of the Middle Belt (Kukah, 1994). The latter have felt that the rhetoric of 'One North' rings increasingly hollow and that, in fact, it was never intended to apply to them in the first place. The infamous remarks, rightly or wrongly attributed to the Premier of the Northern Region, Sir Ahmadu Bello, Sardauna of Sokoto, has been a cause of much grief, if not paranoia among middle belt peoples:

> This New Nation called Nigeria should be an estate of our great grandfather Uthman Dan Fodio. We must ruthlessly prevent a change of power. We must use the minorities in the North as willing tools, and the South, as conquered territory and never allow them to rule over us, and never allow them to have control over their future (Bello, 1960).

While the late Premier was actually more liberal in practice than his words would suggest, the near-forcible conversion campaigns towards the end of his life in the Middle Belt further reinforced fears of domination by the peoples of central Nigeria (Paden & Bello, 1986; Tseayo, 1973).

Whatever his shortcomings, Sir Ahmadu Bello was certainly more liberal

---

11. Nigerian political culture has been replete with violence and assassinations. (Ruth Watson, 2003; Shehu Sani, 2007).
12. Notable among these were groups such as the Movement for the Actualization for the Sovereign State of Biafra (MASSOB), Egbesu Boys and O'Odua Peoples' Congress (OPC) in the West, Niger-Delta Volunteers Force, Movement for the Emancipation of the Niger Delta (MEND), Movement for the Survival of the Ogoni People (MOSOP) and the Ijaw Youth Organisation in the Niger Delta.

and more accommodating to others than those pretenders who imagined themselves his legatees. Not only were they infernally corrupt, they were lacking in moral scruples and had absolutely no vision of Nigeria as a nation other than their own narrowly defined class interests. The shadowy group, which came to be known as 'the Kaduna Mafia', was seen as the vanguard and protector of northern interests, essentially defined in terms of elite access to patronage, public appointments and other forms of preferment.[13] The Northern Nigerian Development Company (NDDC) and affiliates such as the former Bank of the North were the economic legacy institutions that provided the financial base for the northern ruling class. During the days of the northern commodity boards, the Middle Belt, which is the breadbasket of the country, felt increasingly short-changed as the commodity boards monopolised the marketing of commodities, imposing prices that amounted to creaming off the profits accruable to local farmers.[14] Rightly or wrongly, the peoples of the Middle Belt felt increasingly treated as second-class citizens by the northern oligarchy, leading to embitterment and alienation.

In the 1980s, the northeast, like the rest of the North, fell under the sway of the Maitatsine sect. Thousands were killed and considerable properties and infrastructures were destroyed during months of mayhem perpetrated by Maitatsine followers.[15] The re-introduction of Sharia criminal law in several northern states during 2000/2001 provoked widespread further unrest. Sharia criminal law was more or less abolished when the British conquered Nigeria. Common law replaced all practices that were deemed to affront the British sense of 'natural justice, equity and good conscience'. The controversy over Sharia had almost threatened to scuttle the political transition process in the late 1970's (Laremont, 2011). Protests by minority Christian communities resulted in the death of thousands. For many, the issue is not whether Sharia should operate, but that the manner of its operation could lead to implicit discrimination and harassment of non-Muslims. The issue has become increasingly entrenched, effectively dividing Nigeria into two separate jurisdictions: one governed by Islamic Sharia and the other by common law tradition (Peters, 2001. Ostien, 2007).

Ethno-sectarian conflicts have continued to characterise the political

---

13. They may have taken too literally Ibn Khaldun's doctrine of 'asabiyya', forging a solidarity based on clannishness centred on the Caliphate and its hegemonic structures. On the role of the 'Kaduna Mafia' in northern politics (Takaya &Tyoden, 1987).
14. The case of cotton may be quite instructive. (Onu & Okunmadewa, 2008).
15. As a young researcher and Fellow of the National Institute for Policy and Strategic Studies, I was part of a team that carried out a detailed study of the Maitatsine phenomenon, carrying out extensive field work in Kaduna, Adamawa and Borno (Gyuse & Mailafia, 1983).

landscape (Suberu, 2001), probably taking the lives of 35,000 Nigerians between 1999 and 2011.

Further complicating the situation has been the emergence of state-sponsored vigilante groups that were purportedly set up to prevent armed robbery and other forms of violent criminality. These often resorted to extra-judicial methods to tackle crime and the meting out of summary justice to alleged criminals. The proliferation of these armed militias reinforced a culture of violence and lawlessness as these groups capitalised on legitimate grievances to justify bank robberies, assassinations and kidnapping.

Under the pretext of keeping the common peace, vigilantes and groups such as the 'Hisba' in the Sharia States have sometimes served as enforcement agents for powerful elements in pursuit of narrow selfish ends. Some of the activities of the occasionally overzealous yan Hisba Sharia law enforcers in places like Kano and other Sharia States have caused concern among Christian communities who feel they are being compelled to subscribe to religious tenets with which they cannot identify. (Olaniyi, undated). From Maitatsine in the 1980s to Boko Haram in 2011, some State Governors have been known to patronise religious teachers with potentially extremist views. We are led to believe that Nigerian political culture does not exert a cost on those who perpetrate acts of political violence.

The Plateau crisis as a metaphor

Perhaps the crisis on the Jos Plateau is the most tragic of these conflicts because of its enduring character, the venom with which it has been fought and, increasingly, the involvement of Islamists from neighbouring countries.[16] Violent killings took place in 1994, 2001, 2002, 2008 and 2010. The Jos crisis has been interpreted variously as a religious, ethnic and political crisis. At the heart of it is the acrimonious question of 'indigene versus settler' that has pitted one group against another. The Hausa-Fulani who have settled in the town would like to lay claim to ownership as much as the Berom, Afizere, Anaguta and others who claim to be the original 'owners' of Jos.13

The creation of Jos North Local Government by the military administration of General Ibrahim Babangida was seen by indigenes as a piece of mischief making. While the area has a substantial population of Hausa traders, it is also the seat of the Gbong Gwom Jos, the paramount

---

16. In a recent email discussion with researcher Jana Krause, she opines that foreign elements, including al-Qaeda, may have been involved in recent episodes of violence on the Jos Plateau. Her study on the subject is probably the most comprehensive so far. (Krause, 2011). See Also (Okpaga, Chijioke and Innocent, 2012).

ruler of the Berom people. The Berom insist that just as no Berom person could ever lay claim to standing for elections in the Local Government which seats the Emir of Kano, they would not accept 'foreigners' lording over them on their own turf (Higazi, 2011). It has become increasingly difficult to provide a dispassionate analysis of the so-called 'Jos crisis'. There is no doubting that the 'settlers' have encountered some form of discrimination by succeeding administrations in the State. Plateau people would insist that it is not a problem peculiar to their State, but rather a problem that is widespread throughout the federation.

Plateau State is located in the central savannah of the Middle Belt of Nigeria, at the confluence between north and south, east and west. Like the rest of the Middle Belt, the vast majority of the people are Christians. This is so by virtue of the fact that, unlike the Hausa city-states of the north, they were never conquered by the Fulani Jihad of the early nineteenth century. The imposition of British colonial rule and its indirect administration foisted the feudal emirate system upon these people who had never been conquered in war and who were themselves heirs of the great Nok civilization of ancient times.[17]

At independence in 1960, it remained part of the old Northern Region, although the area had a reputation for voting for the opposition. For this and other reasons, the Plateau remained largely 'marginalised' by the Northern Region Government.

The Plateau has a rich and fertile soil that supports livestock as well as cultivation of temperate vegetables and fruits. The establishment of the Federal Capital of Abuja under two hundred kilometers away has boosted the demand for agricultural produce from the Plateau. With the worsening crisis of climate change in the far north pastoralists have moved into the Plateau and other parts of the middle belt in search of better grazing land for their livestock.

Historically, the city of Jos was probably the most cosmopolitan urban centre in Nigeria. It was the centre of missionary activity in the Middle Belt, attracting Christian missionaries from different parts of the Western world. The large presence of expatriates meant that physical infrastructures in the city were second to none. This was further enhanced under the late Joseph Dechi Gomwalk, the military administrator of the old Benue-Plateau during 1967—1975. Gomwalk was a master-builder who constructed roads, expanded housing, clinics and schools. He built a newspaper and a new radio

---

17. The Kwararafa peoples of the Middle Belt had conquered Hausa land and were, on and off, the rulers of Kano for the better part of two centuries between the 16th and 18th centuries. On the changing character of identity politics in the Middle Belt, see Mustapha, undated.

house and television station. The northern oligarchy was uncomfortable with these developments, seeing in them a direct challenge to their dominance and hegemony. The Dimka coup attempt of 1976 by predominantly Plateau and Middle Belt officers further soured relations between the Plateau and the core north.

For nearly two decades, the people of the Plateau have known little or no respite from conflict and violence. While some have interpreted the conflict in religious terms, others insist it is all about politics. Many see it in terms of ethnicity and the struggle over land and limited resources. The truth is that most human conflicts are deeply embedded in a complex web of forces. In the case of the Plateau, they may have been triggered by local political factors relating to the willful creation of Jos North Local Government, but they have also taken on the coloration of religion, thanks to the rise of Global Jihad and the re-location of al-Qaeda from Afghanistan to the Maghrib and the Sahel. The demographic movements occasioned by climate change and desertification are also major factors. When all these are linked to dwindling job prospects amongst youth and increasing impoverishment among the general population, you get a fatal cocktail ready to implode at the slightest opportunity.

While much of the conflict may have originated from the problem of political representation, it has snowballed into a religious conflict with global dimensions. It would seem that part of the agenda of Boko Haram and other such jihadist groups is the 'cleansing' of the Christian presence in the north. There are hardly any churches left in Yobe State. Christian communities in Borno have resorted to praying at home instead of meeting at a place of worship. After full success in this 'ethnic cleansing', the next logical step would be to intensify their activities in the Middle Belt so as to break the spirit of those communities through the grand strategy of 'fitna' and to ensure that their ideology prevails throughout the 'Old North'. The fundamental contradiction of this movement is that they entertain a strictly narrow definition of the 'the North', but at the same time they insist that the Middle Belt must also remain in the historic North.

Since they will stop at nothing, it is self-evident that the embattled people of the Plateau and the Middle Belt will have to defend themselves and the values that they hold most sacred. What is at stake is nothing less than the future of Nigeria itself. Given the complete breakdown of trust, the failure of efforts to find a just and lasting solution, and the existential threat which they face, local communities will probably have to resort to self-help to protect themselves and their families – at least until such a time that the government takes concrete steps to protect them.

Governments at State and Federal level have attempted to hold peace summits and institute interfaith dialogues, but these efforts have borne little fruit. Military intervention has only succeeded in maintaining a Carthaginian peace. We have seen neither original thinking nor bold initiatives that would address the situation and rescue the benighted people of Plateau from the jaws of catastrophe. Judicialism has also failed. Between 2004 and 2010 no less than five judicial commissions of inquiry have we established to address the Plateau crisis. None have yielded any meaningful results. For some strange reason, government has not taken bold steps to publish the findings of the commissions as a means of building a framework towards a just and lasting peace (Krause, 2012).

Origins of the Boko Haram Sect

The Boko Haram sect originates from 2001 when a Muslim cleric, Mohammed Ali, succeeded in attracting a large following at his mosque in the northeastern city of Maiduguri. In 2003 its leader and several of its members were killed in a dispute. A charismatic young man by the name of Mohammed Yusuf (Sanusi Aliyu, 2009) took over. The group were known as 'the Nigerian Taliban', on account of their Puritanism, The new mosque they built became known as 'Ibn Tamiyyah Masjid' in honour of the medieval Arab theologian Sheik ul-Islam Ibn Tamiyyah (1263—1328 AD).

Mohammed Yusuf used his charisma and organisational abilities to build a formidable network of followers. His organisation was run almost like a cooperative, where the well off contributed funds that were used to help the poor. He drew a mass following from the elites as well as the masses and was patronised by the wealthy and the politically well connected, including the Governor of the State at the time. From the significant charitable works among the poor the group was increasingly known as a 'State within the State'. (Walter, 2012.)

In 2007 Mohammed Yusuf was accused of having Sheikh Ja'afar Mahmoud Adam, a cleric and regular preacher, assassinated because of his public criticisms of Yusuf and his followers. Bloody confrontations were to follow in Bauchi in July 2009, with the group becoming more radicalised. The highhanded crackdown by the police simply upscaled the level of confrontation, with the group resorting to the use of more sophisticated weapons (CLEEN Foundation, 2011). The conflict soon metamorphosed from being a clash among Muslim groups to a focus on churches and Christians from Yobe to Maiduguri and Bauchi. On 30 July Mohammed Yusuf was arrested while in hiding and was soon reported dead, presumably executed by the police. Also executed was Buji Foi, a former commissioner of religious affairs in Borno State and a known financier of the group.[18]

---

18. In May 2012 a court ordered the Borno State Government and the Federal Government of Nigeria to pay the family the sum of 100 million naira (US$617,000) for the illegal killing of Mohammed Yusuf.

The death of Mohammed Yusuf, far from quelling the rebellion, added more fuel. The April 2011 post-election violence in the north appeared to have enhanced the legitimacy of the Boko Haram sect as an enforcer of northern political interests under the cover of religion.[19] The October 2011 Eagle Square bombings that took the lives of 12 people were the opening salvoes for the current round of terrorist activities. Before then, there were rumours of the massive importation of arms by all sorts of shadowy groups as the country was moving towards an election year. An arms cache coming from Iran was intercepted. The Boko Haram sect, avowedly committed to the forcible Islamisaton of Nigeria, has moved from one audacious act to the other, including attacks on the UN Office and Police Headquarters and military barracks in Abuja.

It would be a mistake to view Boko Haram as being a purely religious problem. Not only are politicians and other influential persons implicated, but it thrives on the increasing misery in which young people, particularly in the impoverished North, find themselves today.

Economic and social consequences of terrorism

In rich as well as poor countries, terrorism exerts a heavy toll on national economies. The economic impact is inevitably felt more in low-income economies. Economists have developed various approaches for analysing the economic costs of terrorism. First, the direct costs resulting from damage to physical infrastructures and economic assets. Secondly the indirect costs associated with long queues at airports and highways due to the security checks that people now have to undergo. A third level derives from the loss of domestic and inward investments associated with terrorism. It is evident that terrorism scares foreign investors and increases the costs of doing business within and between countries.

It has been estimated that the city of New York alone lost US$ 21 billion as a result of the 9/11 attacks. With the establishment of the Homeland Security, the US Government now has to spend a whopping US$500 billion on security alone. Globally, it has also been calculated that world GDP decreased by a massive US$3.6 trillion in 2002 as a direct and indirect consequence of terrorist activities in 2001. Put in perspective it amounts to a third of the GDP of the United States and exceeds the combined GDP of

---

19. Several commentators are of the view that there are not one but several groups that are lumped under the common rubric of Boko Haram. There may well be opportunistic criminals whose activities have been subsumed under Boko Haram.

Argentina, Italy and Britain. Another area of economic cost relates to the impact of terrorism on international trade supply chains, i.e. the sequence of steps that global suppliers of goods take to get products from one area to another.[20]

Linked to this is the increased cost to global supply chain logistics. Substantial costs do accrue to businesses when extra security layers have to be introduced at ports and land borders. According to the OECD, higher transportation costs associated with more security checks have a negative impact on the external trade of emerging economies that, over the last decade, have benefited from reduction in costs in the last decade. This would in turn affect those countries' ability to combat poverty.

Insurance firms revise upwards their actuarial risk projections and premium costs. New market-based instruments such as 'catastrophe bonds' have been introduced to ameliorate risk from terrorist activities. In the industrial economies, the estimated extra spending on security by government and the private sector by 1% of GDP is forecast to result in a 0.7% fall in GDP output, which further complicates national fiscal balances and growth prospects.

For countries such as Egypt, Tunisia, Kenya and Tanzania that are dependent on tourism, any incidence of terrorism is likely to register significant falls in the number of tourist visitors. For such countries, a drop in the number of tourists translates into significant falls in revenue and economic growth. In the case of Nigeria, it is clear that the new focus on tackling terrorism would mean diverting scarce budgetary resources from vital development projects to defence and security.

The association of Nigeria's external image with terrorism and until recently being on the list of 'Terror Watch' countries also means less FDI coming to the country as potential investors reassess their risk options. Some who have already invested in Nigeria may consider relocating their businesses to neighbouring countries such as Ghana, Togo and Benin.

Apart from the economic and monetary costs associated with terrorism, there are also social and psychological costs. Terrorism erodes intercommunal trust and destroys the reservoir of social capital that is so vital to building harmonious societies and pooling community energies for national development. The attendant proliferation of small arms and the militarisation

---

20. It has been estimated that the introduction of additional security measures between national borders may increase the ad valorem cost of trading internationally by 1 to 3 percentage points. With elasticity of trade flows with respect to transaction costs falling within the −2 to −3 range, this could be expected to lead to a significant fall in the volume of international trade, which in turn would have a negative impact on openness, productivity and medium-term global output growth.

of society result in a vicious cycle of violence which hampers national cohesion and stability.

The long-term impact of such violence on cities and regions is best exemplified by the impoverishment that has affected Kaduna and Jos. Kaduna used to be one of the most prosperous cities in Nigeria. It was in many ways the industrial hub of the north, a cosmopolitan city with over a dozen textile firms and prosperous trading companies. The Kaduna of today is a tragically divided city in which Muslims live predominantly in the north and Christians predominantly in the south. Most investors have packed up their businesses. The Jos Plateau is following a similar trend, as it loses its cosmopolitanism and local economies are destroyed. The tragedy is that the collapse of local economies and the erosion of social capital reinforce a downward spiral of further impoverishment, which in itself sows the seeds of further conflict.

For most of the north, the ongoing insurgency impacts on the regional economy. Lebanese and Indian expatriates with established businesses in Kano going back decades relocate to Abuja and the south. Many have left the country altogether. Hotels, banks and other businesses have witnessed significant reductions in their activities. The border towns that once thrived on trade with neighbouring countries have also seen business curtailed because of increasing restrictions on cross-border traffic. In Kano alone, an estimated 126 industries have recently closed down. Another trend is the massive movement of southerners from the north, many of them SME operators and professionals.[21]

The case of Borno is particularly illustrative of the general trend. A State that officially defines itself as "The Land of Peace" has become a by-word for violence and religious extremism. Partly engendered by mass disenchantment born of impoverishment and partly sponsored in the past by misguided politicians, the rising spectre of extremist violence has reinforced a path-dependence of poverty, wiping off livelihoods, undermining societal cohesion and deepening the vicious cycle of poverty.

The terrorist insurgency in Borno and the northeast has not only destroyed the local economy, it has compounded the crisis of poverty in the region. The author visited Maiduguri in April 2011 at the official invitation of the State Governor, Kashim Shettima. Although the Governor gave the impression that he was firmly in favour of finding a lasting solution to the crisis, we also noticed some form of moral ambivalence on his part. Indeed,

---

21. Rumours are rife that the elections of 2014 are likely to lead to another upheaval in which southerners may once again come under attack in the north. Many are therefore selling off their properties and re-locating to the south. (Sunday Sun, 9 September 2012).

it has been suggested that people like him have actually been surreptitiously arming and financing the terrorists as a means of undermining the legitimacy of the Federal Government. We found Maiduguri to be a shadow of its former vibrant self – a city of ghosts where people talk in whispers.

Terrorism and nationhood

It is clear that the current situation portends ominous trends for Africa's most populous nation. In the northern cities of Bornu, Damaturu and Yola, Christian worshippers have been attacked in churches and latest reports indicate house-to-house killings by extremists, far from the eyes of the police, army and security agencies. President Goodluck Jonathan recently alarmed the entire nation when he declared that the Boko Haram sect has infiltrated the military, the police and security services and even the Presidency. He declared the current situation as the worst since the Nigerian civil war of 1967-1970. There are also strong indications that southern Christians - including indigenous Hausa-Fulani northern Christians - are leaving the north en masse. Northern Muslims are also leaving the south by the truckload. What someone has termed the 'spirit of Sudan' has gripped the entire nation, with an unprecedented atmosphere of fear and gloom under what appears like a gathering storm. If Christians were to retaliate, Nigeria's future may hang on a precipice.

The Nobel laureate Wole Soyinka has recently pointed out that Nigeria is already at the verge of disintegration. It is a choice that the current generation of Nigerians must make: whether they want to live together as one country or face the bleak prospects of dissolution. The country stands in that twilight zone where any wrong move or misguided action could spell disaster for the survival of the federation. With the onslaught of Boko Haram and other terrorist groups, the country faces the grim prospects of a disastrous genocidal religious conflict on a scale greater even than Rwanda. The Goodluck Jonathan administration must make very tough choices in the years ahead. Fishing out the kingpins of terrorism and confiscating their assets and prosecuting them is absolutely vital, in addition to decisive military action to defeat the terrorists. He must realise that a government that cannot secure the lives and properties of its citizens has failed in its most elementary duty. In all this, however, efforts must be made to bring Muslims and Christians - north and south – together and heal the bitter wounds of the recent past.

Can we legitimately suppose that some of the political leaders of the north know more about Boko Haram than they are prepared to admit? Could the silence of some of them imply tacit complicity? Are there significant elements in northern society who may not approve of the methods of the insurgents but who nonetheless endorse their objectives?

Whatever the answers that emerge from the foregoing questions, one thing is clear: Boko Haram could not have done a greater disservice to the Muslim cause. Such barbarities seen against defenceless women and children in places of worship are unworthy of any religion. Other Nigerians are more than able to inflict the same, if not higher levels of damage. They have held back, not out of fear, but out of that moral restraint and inner hope that Nigeria must not be allowed to descend into utter darkness. I would urge them to continue to exercise restraint and to forgive those who kill and maim their women and children.

On its part, the international community must rise in wholesale condemnation against the evil that Boko Haram represents. Civil society, government and the international community must join hands to restore hope and to build the foundations for a just and lasting peace. Indeed, the sages of old have taught that light will always triumph over darkness. But it is clear that light can defeat darkness not with the weapons of vengeful violence, but with the arsenals of enlightenment and reason; with that moral force which accords with the spirit of the laws and the conscience of civilised humanity.

The attitude of the United States and the West in general has been rather intriguing. The EU has not expressed a strong position with regard to terrorist violence in Nigeria, beyond the pious resolutions that were passed during the joint ACP-EU Parliamentary Assembly in Horsens, Denmark in May 2012 condemning terrorist violence and urging disarmament and dialogue (ACP-EU Joint Parliamentary Assembly, 2012.) The Obama administration has not placed Boko Haram on the list of terrorist organisations on the pretext that that the link between the sect and al-Qaeda has not been established beyond any shadow of doubt.[22] There are also those who insist that doing so will give Boko Haram undue prominence, expanding its access to international terrorist financing while making it more difficult to engage with the group while providing development assistance to the impoverished North. What has been particularly surprising is that American weapons have been found among the terrorist insurgents. Some Western commentators have tended to blame lack of Christian forbearance

---

22. The seeming coincidence between the EU and U.S. position is rather surprising. This is because the two sides have centred fundamentally on how to confront global terror. Robert Kagan discussed the key elements in the divergence of strategic approaches across the Atlantic. See his "Power and Weakness", Policy Review, No. 113, June/July, 2002. For a critique of Kagan, see Dilling, 2002. Dilling expresses this divergence in terms of "the Hobbesian philosophy of the Americans and the Kantian *Weltanschauung* of the Europeans" (Dilling, 2002: 964).

for prolonging the crisis.[23]

Whilst it is true that it always "takes two to tango" and that aggressive preaching by Pentecostal groups has been offensive to many Muslims, we cannot run away from the statistical fact that the overwhelming number of attacks have often started from one side. The entirety of the north has been undergoing what amounts to a form of low-intensity warfare that fits perfectly with the logic of Global Jihad. The aim appears to be an ethnic cleansing of minority communities in the north through relentless violence, fear and demoralisation.

Some foreign analysts wilfully ignore these realities, in particular, the statistics underlying the slaughter of defenceless women and children in churches and villages that has been a recurrent phenomenon in northern Nigeria since the 1980s. A noted American political scientist and purported 'Nigeria expert', Jean Herskovits, recently wrote an article that seemed to whitewash the atrocities of the terrorist insurgents, putting the blame instead, on the government. Her article amounted to an insult to the families of the thousands of innocent souls who have been lost due to Islamist-inspired terror in Nigeria (Herskovits, 2012)[24] A few years ago a study from the United States predicted that Nigeria would disintegrate by the year 2015.[25] The United States has been in this business of prophesying doom for Nigeria for decades now. The West seems unwilling to lend support to President Goodluck Jonathan because it would not want to offend the Arab-Muslim world by appearing to be taking sides with Nigerian Christians. Some Nigerians see in this attitude a conspiracy to ensure the disintegration of Africa's largest nation. Few understand that if Nigeria does eventually implode, it would result in the bloodiest civil war in Africa's history, an economic disaster for West Africa, a political tragedy for Africa and a catastrophic humanitarian disaster for the international community.

Beyond the loss of lives and the destruction of properties and physical infrastructure, terrorism is even more damaging to the soul of the individual

---

23. An elderly English missionary woman that knew me as a child and taught me Sunday school scolded Christians for retaliating against Muslims. I felt shame and confusion at the same time. I explained to her that as far as I am concerned I could never subscribe to what in the popular parlance is known as 'reprisals'. At the same, I would not be in a position to preach to those who have lost loved ones in terrorist attacks and who insist they have a moral duty to protect their loved ones.
24. Her article prompted a rebuttal by no less than the Nigerian Ambassador in Washington, Professor Ade Adefuye, who happens to be a distinguished historian in his own right.
25. This prophecy was later revised and the date shifted from 2015 to 2030 (Abdallah, 2012).

and the community. Buildings that have been destroyed can be rebuilt in no time. Infrastructures can be rehabilitated. Traumatised souls, sadly, may take a generation to heal.[26]

Summary and conclusions

While globalisation has made the world smaller, it has generated new forms of insecurity among nations and cultural communities that had been cocooned from external influences for centuries. Globalisation has compounded the crisis of governance in some developing countries, deepening the tendencies towards state failure while undermining the capacity to govern at national and international levels. All these factors have weakened the capacity of state authorities, leading to the emergence of transnational terrorist groups that are competing for power and influence with established state authorities. Compounding all these challenges is the absence of multilateral institutions that would ensure effective global governance.

Terrorism is nothing less than the ultimate test of the moral fibre of free societies. In the Nigerian and African context, its rise is not only on account of globalisation and its unequalising tendencies; it is also related to the crisis of development and nationhood, and the failure of the state to provide human security and act as a servant of the people. Tackling terrorism requires a fight to regain the hearts and minds of youth and to foster dialogue among communities. Government must become the servant of the people, not their master. Military action will be necessary, but it must be carefully deployed and it must conform to international humanitarian standards. The security agencies must work more closely together and should be more strategic in their thinking and action. The Federal Government also has to work with its ECOWAS neighbours to prevent terrorists from penetrating the country through its porous borders. The strategy we advocate calls not only for bold action in defeating terrorism; it requires expanding the possibility frontiers of welfare while widening the democratic space for popular participation. Government must provide decent jobs for the teeming millions of youth, steering them from a culture of nihilistic

---

26. In the village of Vwang, outside Jos, a young lad of 11 recounted to me how his uncle lost his only son in Ali Kazaure during a previous conflict. When the next round of violence erupted, the old man came out with a bag full of poisoned arrows. When he brought down his first victim, he crawled to him like a hyena and systematically began to tear off his flesh with his bare teeth. This may not be an isolated case. There have indeed been reports of cannibalism in Jos – of people cooking their enemies and eating them to express their hatred and contempt.

violence to one of tolerance, patriotism and nonviolence. Ultimately, it is about reinventing Nigeria as a compassionate country, a purpose-driven nation with a clearly defined vision of its manifest destiny as the leader of the New Africa.

A generation of Nigerians, tempered by war and tutored by a hard and bitter peace, should appreciate more than any other that civility and restraint are the only true course for the survival of a multi-ethnic and multi-religious democracy. Terrorism is a negation of all civilised values, encouraging as it does such contempt for human life. While violence has been endemic in the Nigerian polity, the leaders of the north have a particular duty to re-examine their readiness to use religion at the slightest opportunity as a weapon of fear against fellow citizens, particularly minorities in the north. The views of Nobel laureate Wole Soyinka may be anathema to some, but his observations on this matter are unassailable:

> When I say that the phenomenon has a very long history, I am talking about a movement that relies on religion as a fuel for their operation, as a fuel for mobilisation, as the impetus, an augmentation of any other legitimate or illegitimate grievance that they might have against society. Because of that fuel, that irrational, very combustible fuel of religion of a particular strain, of a particular irredentist strain....All they need to be told is that this is an enemy of religion and they are ready to kill. No matter the motivations, no matter the extra-motivations of those who send them out, they need only one motivation: that they are fighting the cause of that religion. (The News, 7 February 2012.)

Thinkers as wide apart as Franz Fanon and Maurice Duverger have understood that conflict is endemic in human society and violence merely reflects the existential dilemmas of the human condition. If Boko Haram did not adopt the wholesale murder of defenceless people in the name of Jihad, they would probably have had the majority of Nigerian youth on their side by now. The failures of government and the prevailing culture of impunity have alienated the vast majority of Nigerians from the political system.

In their random and indiscriminate killing of women, children and entire families in places of worship in pursuit of their 'soi-disant' Jihad, Boko Haram have placed themselves outside the pale of civility. If their atrocities continue unchecked and succeed in reaching the south, the inevitable reprisals that will follow will shake the federation to its very foundations. Nigeria's future as a political community will be gravely imperilled as a consequence. Indeed, former aviation minister Femi Fani-Kayode – regarded as an alarmist by some -- insists that the current insurgency represents the greatest threat to Nigeria since the civil war (Nigerian Tribune, 1 July 2012). He likens the Nigerian federation to a marriage in which the 'rich wife' is the South and the 'poor husband' is the North.

The marriage has been strained and turbulent. We fought a brutal and avoidable 3 year civil war from 1967 in which we killed no less than 2 million....Yet today's barbarism and mass killings are far more horrendous than ever and are far better planned, funded, orchestrated and executed by those that are behind them than ever before. The question is how much longer can the "rich wife" and the "poor husband" give and take this sort of thing from one another? For how long can the centre hold before the voices of reason and restraint are completely drowned by the irrational, compulsive outrage that is gradually building up and the uncontrollable outcry for reprisals and revenge? (Nigerian Tribune, 1 July 2012).

To be sure, the insurgents are neither demons nor irrational madmen. They have simply calculated that the payoffs from their activities outweigh the costs. In the words of political scientist David Apter:

Choices by an individual define his moral personality. Choices by governments constitute the moral aims of society and reflect the ambitions of those within it, thus constituting that measure of satisfaction that will lead to a stable order. The efforts to find such a moral condition, however, may lead to the most violent and unstable of human conditions...in such periods, the loftiest human purposes may be expressed in violence. Whatever the situation, it is in such times that men make explicit those core values they hope will lead to both a moral community and moral individuals. Perhaps this is the ultimate secret of political life. (Apter, 1987: 61—62)

Ultimately, Boko Haram may be more about politics than it is about religion. But they have also told us that they are waging a Jihad and have gone ahead to demonstrate it in their praxis. We cannot ignore those realities. But we must not play into their hands. Muslims and Christians are the children of Abraham. Both religions are indigenous to Africa and none can wish the other away. Nigerians will have to learn how to live together or perish. They must therefore create a national system that is all-inclusive and participatory and that encourages the civic virtues of tolerance and social justice. It is said that true love casteth out fear. What the extremists want to do is to impose a reign of fear; fear in turn will force people to retreat to their own tents and prepare for war. Nigerians must deny them the opportunity to render an entire nation captive.

With its vast natural resources, vibrant cultures and energetic peoples, Nigeria has what it takes to be one of the leading nations in the twenty-first century. But she can only fulfil her vocation when she secures a just and lasting peace within her borders, when she is governed by responsible leaders committed to expanding the frontiers of welfare while protecting the liberties of all her citizens without regard to ethnicity or creed. This will entail major constitutional reengineering and reinvention of the very meaning of its nationhood. The ancient Chinese sage LaoTzu famously declared "governing a large state is like cooking a small fish". It is a delicate art requiring skill, dexterity and wisdom. Governing a country such as Nigeria requires the qualities of the highest statesmanship. A vision for Nigeria might just be what is currently lacking in the leadership that is insufficiently capable of demonstrating civic virtue and sense of destiny, the ingredients that would make for the building of a great and prosperous republic.

References

Ahmed, F. (2012) Income Diversification Determinants Among Farming Households in Konduga, Borno State, *Academic Research International*, vol. 2 no. 2, March 2012, pp. 555-561.

Abdallah, N. (2012) *'Nigeria May Become a Failed State in 2030, Not 2015.' African Herald Express*, 18 January 2012.

ACP-EU Joint Parliamentary Assembly (2012) Urgent Resolution on Nigeria: Boko Haram Violence Calls for Specific Answers, *Resolution*. 23rd ACP-EU JPA at Horsens, Denmark, adopted on 28-30 May 2012.

African Development Bank (2012) *Africa Economic Outlook*, Africa Development Bank, Tunis.

Agbu, O. (2004) Ethnic Militias and the Threat to Democracy in Post-Transition Nigeria, Uppsala, *Research Report No. 127*. Nordiska Afrikainstitutet. Sweden.

Aliyu, S. (2009) Religious Based Violence and National Security in Nigeria: Case Studies of Kaduna State and the Taliban Activities in Borno State. *Thesis*. Presented to the Faculty of the U.S. Army Command and General Staff College, Fort Leavenworth, Kansas.

Anifowoshe, R. (1981) *Violence and Politics in Nigeria: The Tiv and Yoruba Experience*, NOK, New York.

Apter, D. (1987) *Rethinking Development: Modernisation, Dependency and Postmodern Politics*, Sage Publications, London and Beverly Hills.

Baudrillard, J. (2011) 'L'Esprit du terrorisme.', *Le Monde*, 2 November 2011.

Bello, A. (1960) Sardauna of Sokoto, quoted in *The Parrot*, 12 October 1960.

Burleigh, M. (2006) *Sacred Causes: Religion and Politics From the European Dictators to al-Qaeda*, Harper Collins, London.

Chomsky, N. (1991) International Terrorism: Image and Reality, in Alexander George (ed.), *Western State Terrorism*, Routledge, London and New York.

CLEEN Foundation (2011) Responding to the Emerging Trends of Terrorism in Nigeria, *Conference Proceedings,* Monograph Series no. 6, Lagos.

Coker, C. (2002) Globalisation and Terrorism, Paper prepared for a seminar on "The Prospects for the Canadian Summit," sponsored by the Canadian Embassy in Tokyo, the Japanese-British Society, the LSE International Social Economic Forum in Japan and the G8 Research Group, Nippon Press, Centre, Tokyo, Japan, 10 June 2002 (mimeo).

Copans, J. (1988) *Les marabouts de l'arachide: La confrérie mouride et les paysans du Sénégal*, L'Harmattan, Paris.

Dickson, D. (2005) Political Islam in Africa: The Need for a New Research and Diplomatic Agenda, United State Institute of Peace, *Special Report*, No. 140, May 2005.

Dike, V. (2003) *Nigeria and the Politics of Unreason: A Study of the Obasanjo Regime*, Adonis & Abbey Publishers, London & Abuja.

Dilling, O. (2002) If I had a Hammer: A Review of Kagan's Power and Weakness, *German Law Journal*, 12 (1) pp. 963-969.

Dudley, B. (1986) *Parties and Politics in Nigeria*, Frank Cass, London.

Fani-Kayode, F. (2012) 'The Poor Husband, The Rich Wife and Boko Haram.', *Nigerian Tribune*, Ibadan, 1 July 2012.

Ghani, A. and Lockhart, C. (2008) *Fixing Failed States: A Framework for Rebuilding a Fractured World*, Oxford University Press, Oxford.

Gyuse, T. and Mailafia, O. (1983) *Religion and Conflict in Nigeria: A Study of the Maitatsine in Northern Nigeria*, National Institute for Policy and Strategic Studies, Kuru.

Herskovits, J. (2012) 'Boko Haram is Not the Problem.', *New York Times*, 3 January 2012.

Higazi, A. (2011) *The Jos Crisis: A Recurrent Nigerian Tragedy*, Discussion Paper, 2 January 2011, Friedrich Ebert Stiftung, Lagos

Kabbanin N & Kothari, E. (2005) *Youth Unemployment in the MENA Region: A Situational Assessment*, The Work Bank, Washington DC.

Kagan, R. (2002) Power and Weakness, *Policy Review* 113

Kalu, K. and Oguntoyinbo, O. (2012) Alternative Explanations of Conflict and Violence in the Niger Delta, Nigeria, *The Air and Space Power Journal*, 1st Quarter, 3 (1), 2012, pp. 85-96.

Kaplan, R. (1994) The Coming Anarchy: How Scarcity, Crime, Overpopulation, Tribalism and Disease are Rapidly Destroying the Social Fabric of our Planet, *The Atlantic Monthly*. February 1994, pp 44-76.

Kapitan, T. (2003) The Terrorism of 'Terrorism', in J. Sterba (ed.). *Terrorism and International Justice*, Oxford University Press, Oxford, pp. 47-66.

Krause, J. (2011) *A Deadly Cycle: Ethno-Religious Conflict in Jos, Plateau State, Nigeria*, Working Paper - Executive Summary. Geneva Declaration Secretariat, Geneva.

Kukah, M. (1994) *Religion, Politics and Power in Northern Nigeria*, African Book Collective.

Laremont, R. R. (2011) *Islamic Law and Politics in Nigeria*, Africa World Press, Trenton, NJ.

Lewis, P. (2007) *Growing Apart: Oil, Politics, and Economic Change in Indonesia and Nigeria*. The University of Michigan Press, Ann Arbor, MI.

Mailafia, O. (26 September 2012), Conflict and Insurgency in Nigeria, *247UReports*, available at: http://247ureports.com/?s=mailafia&x=0&y=0 (accessed 7 September 2014).

Minc, A. (1995) *Le Nouveau Moyen Age*, Gallimard, Paris.

Mustapha, A. (undated) Transformation of Minority Identities in Post-Colonial Nigeria, Queen Elisabeth House, University of Oxford, *Working Paper Series* No. 9.

National Bureau of Statistics (2010) *Annual Macroeconomic Statistics*, National Bureau of Statistics, Abuja.

News, The (2012) "The Next Phase of Boko Haram Terrorism", Interview with Wole Soyinka on 7 February 2012. *The News*, Lagos.

Nnadozie, E. (2012) Managing the Nigerian Economy in an Era of Global Financial and Economic Crises, *Annual Public Lecture* of the Nigerian Economic Society (NES), Transcorp Hilton Abuja, 15 March 2012.

O'Brien, D. (1971) *The Mourides of Senegal: The Political and Economic Organisation of an Islamic Brotherhood*, Clarendon, Oxford.

OECD (2007) *Principles for Good International in Fragile States and Situations*, OECD, Paris

Okpaga, A., Chijioke, U. and Innocent, O. (2012) "Activities of Boko Haram and Insecurity Question in Nigeria," *Arabian Journal of Business and Management* (Oman Chapter), vol. 1 (9), April 2012, pp. 77-99.

Olaniyi, R. (undated) *Hisba and Sharia Law Enforcement in Metropolitan Kano*, University of Ibadan, Ibadan.

Onu, J. and Okunmadewa, F. (2008) What Does the Conduct of the Cotton Market in Nigeria Reveal? *World Journal of Agricultural Sciences* 4 (4): pp. 521-526.

Ostien, Ph. (2007) *Sharia Implementation in Northern Nigeria*, 1999-2006, Spectrum Books, Ibadan.

Ostien, Ph. (2009) *Jonah Jang and the Jasawa: Ethno-Religious Conflict in Jos, Nigeria*, a Study Under the Muslim-Christian Relations Project in Africa, University of Bayreuth, Germany, August 2009.

Paden, J. and Bello, A. (1986) *Sardauna of Sokoto: Values and Leadership in Nigeria*, Hudahuda.

Peters, R. (2001) *The Reintroduction of Islamic Criminal Law in Northern Nigeria*, A Study Conducted on Behalf of the European Commission, Lagos, September 2001.

Sani, S. (2007) *Political Assassinations in Nigeria,* Bookcraft, Ibadan.

Sani, S. (2007) *The Killing Fields: Religious Violence in Northern Nigeria*, Spectrum Books, Ibadan.

Suberu, R. (2001) *Federalism and Ethnic Conflict in Nigeria*, US Institute of Peace Press, Washington DC.

Takaya, B. and Tyoden, S. (1987) *The Kaduna Mafia,* Jos: Jos University Press.

Tilly, C. (2004) Terrorism, Terror, Terrorism and Terrorists, *Sociological Theory*, vol. 22. No. 1, pp. 5-13.

Trimingham, J. (1962) *A History of Islam in West Africa*, Oxford University Press, Oxford.

Tseayo, J. (1973) *Aspects of National Integration in Nigeria: The Tiv Case*, University of Sussex, Brighton.

Walter, A. (2012) What is Boko Haram? *Special Report* No. 308, United States Institute of Peace, Washington DC.

Watson, R. (2003) *Civil Disorder is the Disease of Ibadan: Chieftaincy and Civic Culture in a Yoruba City*, James Currey, Oxford.

World Bank (2009) *Nigeria: Employment and Growth Study*, The World Bank, Washington DC

Young, C. (1979) *The Politics of Cultural Pluralism*, University of Wisconsin, Madison.

Zakaria, F. (2004) *The Future of Democracy: Illiberal Democracy at Home and Abroad*, Norton & Company, New York and London.

CHAPTER 11. OF MULLAHS, RADIO AND RELIGION: THE TALIBAN AND TRIBAL SWAT'S WOMEN IN PAKISTAN

Syed Manzar Abbas Zaidi

The security environment in Pakistan has been dominated in recent years by a fast developing tempo of Talibanisation, which has permeated from the tribal to the urban set-up at an alarming pace. Western socio-political ideology has gradually permeated parts of the urban society, but a clear paradigmatic divide remains between the urban educated mainstream elite and a marginalized tribal populace, where modern ideals are still alien to the behavioural configurations of tribalism (Iqbal, 2006). The Swat area in Pakistan is the epitome of such transmigration, where a full-blown Taliban insurgency took hold before being displaced by the Pakistani army in military operations in 2009. Pockets of resistance still continue to smoulder, but the Swat case study is fascinating as a now historical account of what happens to the local populace, especially women, when such movements gain territorial control of an area. In this context, the author carried out a series of studies on the impact of the Taliban on society, particularly women. These mostly longitudinal, cohort and case studies were carried out during the period February 2006 - October 2013, collectively called the Swat White Papers. These findings of these studies were incorporated in various reports from the area, mostly for the public sector. Most of the findings and first person reportage below are from the various Swat White Paper documents.

❖ WOMEN'S LEADERSHIP IN PEACE BUILDING

The appearance of insurgents in Swat

Once considered a haven for tourists from all over Pakistan, Swat has long depended heavily on the revenue generated through the tourism industry (Rehman, 2008). A rough estimate puts the dependence of more than 60% of the region's inhabitants upon the hospitality industry, which has ground to a complete halt in the wake of violent clashes between militants and security forces, leaving almost 1,200 hotels and thousands of people unemployed. The advent of this pervasive movement can be traced back to July 2006, when Maulana Fazlullah came into the limelight. His religious lineage can be traced to a local cleric Maulana Sufi Muhammad of Tehreek-e-Nifaze-Shariat-e-Muhammadi (TNSM), who is the father in Law of Fazlullah. Sufi Muhammad passed a decree in 1998 declaring military training to be compulsory for every Muslim. Hundreds of TNSM workers, paying heed to this call, reportedly went for military training in Afghanistan. Sufi was imprisoned in 2001 for leading an 'army' of 10,000 men to Afghanistan to fight alongside the Taliban against the US-led coalition forces and the Northern Alliance in the wake of post 9/11 US incursion in Afghanistan. Sufi Muhammad has been in and out of Pakistani jails ever since.

However, the insurgency only reached its zenith under the tutelage of Maulana Fazlullah, who also currently heads the Tehreek e Taliban Pakistan (TTP), the main consortium of anti state terrorist entities in Pakistan. The Tehreek e Taliban Pakistan (TTP) is an organization proscribed by the Government of Pakistan, and is collectively an umbrella body of outlawed militant groups that operate mainly in FATA and Khyber Pakhtunkhwa (KP, the new name for the province of NWFP), but commit nationwide terrorist acts. They operate under leaders who are now household names in Pakistan. The last leader was Hakeemullah Mahsud, who was killed by an American unmanned drone strike, resulting with Fazlullah taking over. Fazlullah was born as Fazl Hayat in 1975; a Babukarkhel clansman of the Yousufzai tribe, he got his early education in Swat. He subsequently joined the seminary run by Sufi Muhammad, who became his mentor and renamed him Fazlullah. He later married Sufi's daughter. This is an aspect of the passive role of women in conservative societies, whereby they unwittingly provide leverage to virtual nobodies like Fazlullah to reach positions of power, through marriage with powerful figures like Sufi Muhammad. Nothing has been heard about Fazlullah's wife since.

Fazlullah, like many other TNSM activists, was arrested after crossing over to Afghanistan in 2001. He was however subsequently released, and took over the organization of his father in law, due to the latter's detention by Pakistani authorities. It seems that he was much more successful than Sufi in concretizing the organization, with the numbers of recruits swelling rapidly. Maulana Fazlullah devised a novel strategy of radical preaching; he installed an FM radio channel in 2004, which he clandestinely operated. His message was simple; anti US and anti-Government rhetoric, interspersed with calls for support of the Taliban in Afghanistan and the establishment of an Islamic state. The title of 'Radio Mulla' given to him is apt; according to an estimate there were about 30 FM Radio channels operated by him and his cronies in Swat, churning out an indigenous mix of Jihadi propaganda. The Government tried to counter this by stepping up the frequencies of the local channels to block this transmission, but these propaganda machines proved quite effective at covert relocation and transmission. Fazlullah was initially quite popular. News reports coming out of the Swat have gauged his meteoric rise to popularity by the fact that when he gave a call for the establishment of a madrassah on banks of the Swat River, Rs. 3.8 million were collected reportedly within 24 hours, and the amount rose to Rs 35 million within a couple of days. His female followers reportedly contributed most of this amount.

Rapid deterioration of security for women in Swat

The Mulla preached an essentialist and Talibanised ideology. This prompted attacks on CD shops, mandatory shaving of beards, and threats to girl's education, all purportedly based on Sharia law. The threat also materialized in the form of the destruction of women's colleges in Swat, which dealt a crippling blow to the educational prospects of women in that area. This area of the country had achieved the highest female literacy rate as compared to neighbouring districts in the conservative province of KP. Even the religious class was tolerant of women's education. There was large-scale destruction of girls' schools in Swat after Fazlullah took over, because the Taliban are firmly opposed to women's education, considering it un-Islamic. By September 2008 some 105 schools had been destroyed in the district, including 71 girls' schools (The News, 2008). The destruction of such a large number of schools in the scenic valley deprived more than 30,000 female students of education.

The situation took an ominous turn when the Fazlullah-led militants joined Tehrik-e-Taliban Pakistan (TTP) formed by top Pakistani militant Baitullah Mehsud in December 2007 in a bid to provide an umbrella to insurgent movements operating in several tribal agencies and settled areas of KP. With this, the movement fell into the hands of tribal-areas-based Taliban, and Maulana Fazlullah lost his authority to make decisions independently. The Swat-based Taliban were previously insisting only on the promulgation of Sharia, but they started making increasingly strident demands of the government. The first peace deal of the Swat chapter of Taliban after being subsumed in TTP was negotiated on 31 May 2008 between the Taliban and the state. It immediately fell to pieces with both sides blaming each other for the failure of the negotiation process. Fazlullah hardened his stance from then onwards, with directions apparently emanating fromm a more centralized Taliban command and control. Fazlullah would eventual emerge as the TTP's central leader, after the deaths of Baitullah and Hakeemullah Mehsud, both by American unmanned drone strikes.

The area has always been conservative, which is presumably why the pervasion of this phenomenon in the guise of Sharia gained traction. A local that I interviewed during the Swat White Paper study remarked: "It is a question of how you look at things. Jirga has long been a part of tribal tradition and cannot be equated with a parallel government. People in tribal areas were already keeping beards. The women were already in purdah. So, you can't say that a Taliban-like Sharia has been imposed". However, the brutal atrocities, which eventually followed on the heels of Radio mullah's sermons erased any ambiguity in the worldview of Swati society that this movement was a missionary one. Currently, anti Taliban opinion prevails almost universally in Swat.

Women were one of the primary targets of the extremists. Women's educational facilities have never been particularly good in the tribal agencies that make up much of Pakistan's frontier with Afghanistan. The female literacy rate for the Federally Administered Tribal Areas, which include Waziristan and Bajaur, is believed to be as low as 3%. Swat was a breath of fresh air compared to these areas, as it tended to be quite progressive in terms of education as opposed to neighbouring district with respect to women's education. This reputation was destroyed, perhaps irreparably, during the Taliban insurgency.

The Taliban in Afghanistan were strictly opposed to women's education, which they saw as an evil. The Taliban in Pakistan, born and bred in refugee camps in Quetta and Peshawar, were similarly brought up to be wary of women as instruments of the devil, as temptations to be strictly resisted. This is the mind-set that was carried by them to Afghanistan, and the same, which is being replicated by the Taliban in Pakistan. One of the most noticeable features of the initial years of conflict involving the Taliban in tribal Pakistan, particularly in Waziristan and Swat, was the Islamist movement's response to the role of women in society. Pakistani Taliban looks upon female education as a social evil. Maulana Fazlullah of Swat declared in one of his broadcasts, "Education of girls will deviate our generations from the right path. They must be restricted to their homes" (Ansari, 2008). His followers destroyed 40 girl's schools in less than a year from July 2007 to May 2008, interrupted only by his ceasefire agreement with the security forces. When hostilities resumed after the ceasefire agreement failed, 24 girls' schools were bombed or torched within a short span of twenty days. Sardar Hussain Barbak, Education

Minister of NWFP, mentioned at the time that 64 girls' schools had been destroyed in Swat valley alone.

As the only alternative, parents of female students in these agencies and Swat sent their daughters to private schools using their own resources, some moving to suburban cities like Peshawar. There was continuing blackmail on the part of the militants, through handbills thrown in girls' houses and schools warning that "we have decided to bomb the school building. If any student shows up, she will be responsible for her own death" (Ansari, 2008). In the face of such threats it was not possible to resume any semblance of female education, though militants sometimes showed discretion to the extent that they did not kill the students, often only tying up watchmen and setting the buildings on fire. There are many harsher instances as well. In one such instance, a female teacher in Mohmand Agency was shot at random for not covering herself from head to toe. She was in a Hijab at the time, which completely covers the hairline.

Initially, the Taliban in Swat denied that they were involved in these attacks on women's institutions. Mullah Noor Allam, an earlier spokesman for the Taliban in Swat, reiterated many times that the militant group was not responsible for destroying the schools. "We did not burn schools in Swat; that was someone else, probably splinter groups. They certainly do not fight for Maulana Fazlullah," he said in a propaganda video (TTP Swat No. 3, 2006). "In fact we support women having an education, such as nurses and doctors. But there are some fields in which a woman should not work, like the armed forces and engineering." The Pakistan Taliban movement blamed "foreign elements" for the school burnings, which they said were calculated to discredit them as a political movement. "We don't oppose education for women, but (we) want a favourable environment for them. We don't want Western-style co-education without dupatta (veil)," Noor Allam said (TTP Swat No.5, 2006). However, the school destruction campaign was wholly owned by the militants later. Malala Yousafzai, the now universally famous child education activist from Swat, was also shot at by the Swat TTP Chapter who initially denied that they had done it. Later, Adnan Rasheed, one of the major commanders, 'sent' a letter to Malala explaining why she 'had to be shot' (Khan, 2013).

In the grip of fear

This had a deep psychological impact on women throughout Pakistan's tribal areas, even in regions not controlled by the Taliban. "There are no Taliban here (but) I'm afraid to go to school," explains 10-year-old Sehrish, a student at Chukdar High School in the Kurz area of Dir Agency, a tribal area controlled by the government that lies half an hours drive south of Swat. I interviewed Sehrish during the Swat White Paper study. "What if they burn the classroom while we are inside?" he said. It is not just the students who are risk; the teachers that I interviewed shared the same terror. "Once a young man jumped into our class with his face covered. We all screamed in panic, we thought he was Taliban," recalls Mrs. Nizhad, who teaches fine art at Chukdar. "In the end it was just a local boy doing some silly practical joke but he got us very worried. I've been teaching for nine years and I've never felt this scared," she says. "I don't enjoy my job very much anymore. After the school burnings (in Swat) we have all been very scared."

Many other students that I interviewed in different localities in Swat shared similar sentiments. Sara, a high school student from Swat now living in Kurz Dir, says she doesn't know who is trying to stop girls going to school. "The conflicts in Bajaur and Swat will only be stopped if the terrorism is eliminated. But to do that (the Pakistan authorities) need to address the root causes," she adds. Sara complains that the most difficult thing about life is going outside to work "especially because you have to wear the Burka and there are strict rules (about where women can go and with whom)."

Fazlullah also regularly ordered the murder of adulterers by stoning. This 'punishment' was being regularly meted out by FATA based TTP militants, and Fazlullah ostensibly wanted to emulate them. There are a few quasi-judicial channels in the FATA region run by Pakistan government, but their services have seldom been useded by the Waziristanis who preferred approaching TTP for the dispensation of primeval forms of justice. In these areas, these men were the law. Fazlullah wanted to be seen as upholding these values in Swat as the supreme commander from the area.

Unfortunately, the brunt of these adultery punishment decisions fell on women. Most of the so called adultery cases were instances in which an adult man and woman had decided to marry each other, which purportedly went against the tribal customs as perceived by their family. Even though the married couple had carried out a nikah (Islamic consecration of marriage), were of adult age of consent, and had formally and legally married according to the country's legal systems, such marriages were abhorred usually by the woman's family. This is the long standing debate in Pakistan whereby the male patriarchs of the family consider it only their privilege where and with whom a woman would be married, sometimes much like a commodity to be exchanged for position or kinship alliance making (termed the 'biradri' system). When the male patriarchs in the family oppose such a marriage, many women decide to get married themselves, and many have perished at the hands of 'honour killing' because of the 'affront' to family honour. In Swat, many families would approach Fazlullah saying their daughters had affronted family honour by getting married by themselves. A sham court would be convened by the terrorists, in which the nikah as above would be declared null and void. The couple were not considered married because permission had not granted by the male patriarchs (wali). The couple would then be deemed adulterers because they would have presumably had sex without 'being married', and then stoned to death.

It was only after some time that it was realized by the Policy echelons of Government that a FATA type situation was developing in Swat. Ironically, it was the plight of women as identity markers of extremist violence in Pakistan that highlighted the extent of pervasive extremism in Swat. The Swat Taliban released a video in 2009 in which a young woman was shown as being whipped, which stirred up huge anti Taliban sentiment in Pakistan. Even though there had been rumblings, this video aroused a huge domestic and international outcry, and is presumably one of the main reasons that lead the state to mobilized its forces against the Taliban in Swat. Even more surprisingly, it has been clearly documented that despite all the atrocities on women by terrorists in Swat, support from local women was one of the primary reasons why Taliban became entrenched in the area. This will be considered below.

Pashtun Code of Conduct

There have been many pieces of research into the causes of growth of militancy in Swat, identifying a number of factors that were responsible for the breakdown of governance and the loss of control that promoted a fully-fledged Taliban insurgency. However, before examining this cause in detail, it is important to grasp some nuances of tribal system of Pashtunwali, tribal honour, and its dynamics. This is because this tribal code has been merged into the Taliban worldview, which affects women directly.

Pashtunwali is the pre-Islamic Pashtun code of conduct that regulated the intra and inert tribal dynamics of the tribal Pashtuns. It is more a set of principles, rather than codified laws. Honour and chivalry occupy a central theme in this tradition, along with undying loyalty to the tribe, and fierce opposition to occupation. This code consists of core elements of Nang, Badal, Melmastia, Nanawatay and Hamsaya. Nang (honour) implies the use of every conceivable means to shield and protect the tribesman's honour and the honour of his family. The 'honour' rests upon a multitude of codes of conduct demanded of others in the community and outside, which, if infringed, are to be avenged at all costs, even at the costs of one's own life. Badal (revenge) refers to vendettas arising from a family member's death, or the violated honour of a woman in the family. A "revenge killing" is deemed obligatory in order to restore the violated honour, which can be immediately carried out, or occur after generations if the victim family of the perceived dishonourable act is not in a position to react immediately to the infraction.

Badal is apparently a critical tool used by the Taliban to indoctrinate and recruit new fighters, alienated by counter insurgency operations or drone attacks in the tribal areas. Melmastia (hospitality) is the offering of unconditional hospitality to all visitors, without any hope of remuneration or favour; protection is also to be offered unconditionally to any Pashtun by another. This is also has the advantage for the Taliban who can gain asylum in most places within the Pashtun belts. Nanawatay (forgiveness) is the only alternative available to Badal, in which a perpetrator goes to ask the forgiveness of the victim's family. The Hamsaya (neighbour) device is a broadly defined concept, which implied servitude for protection from stronger tribes, which is a kind of protection status accorded to an affiliated or neighbouring tribe from a stronger enemy, from which they are incapable of protecting themselves. This can include military service in exchange for land (mlatar). The rules of engagement cannot be defined easily in terms of 'you are either with us or against us,' alliances being in a constant state of flux in Pashtun society. Pashtun history is thus replete with heroes and legendary figures, which tended to play with both (or multiple) sides for the benefit of tribe, family, and honour. This code of conduct can compel a Pashtun to place all his hospitality at the door of the guest, while 'unwelcome guests' are treated with violence equally passionately. Revenge is a central theme in Pashtunwali, with honour demanding a vendetta sometimes lasting for generations, due to some perceived wrongdoing usually related to honour. Honour (perceived to be infringed) is in turn, unfortunately often related to women, if not most of the time, in Pashtun tribal society.

A woman is pivotal to the family structure of society, considered as a homemaker who raises the children. She is also the main focus of Badal. Badal in Pashtunwali is one of the central pillars of tribal Pashtun socio cultural values, but is also a very violent principle. Any perceived insult or 'Tor' to male honour generates the badal process, and only death of both the males and female who brought upon this perceived dishonour will satisfy the 'wrong'. Pashtunwali had been undergoing a metamorphosis in KP before the advent of the Taliban whereby it was getting more relaxed, allowing the women to go out, get education, do jobs and household chores etc. In time, consensual marriages might have been accepted into the fabric of Pashtunwali, though it would have been a long drawn out process. Talibanisation of the tribal belt has reversed all this progress, whereby militants have modified Pashtunwali by selectively mixing it with their own version of Sharia, which is much more stringent. Pashtunwali itself has morphed into an organic entity, which is called into play whenever the militants need a reference point. The literalist versions of Sharia that Taliban enforced in Swat and Waziristan was actually a hybrid of Pashtunwali as they understood it, and their own perception of religion as learnt from ideologues or seminaries. Thus, it is understandable that this would be unduly focused on regulating the personal and private sphere of women, since so much presumably hinges on honour, tor and the female.

The Regime of 'Replicate, Close, Capture'

However, even despite these brutal measures against women by Fazlullah's Taliban in Swat in the guise of enforcement of Sharia, many women still supported him and were in fact pivotal in elevating him to the position that he gained. This is the paradox that may confuse an observer of the phenomenon, but the answer perhaps lies in the regime of 'replicate, close, and capture' that is explained below.

The almost obsessive zeal of the Taliban in Afghanistan to start implementing penal laws and to control unruly elements in society was driven by using the jihad as a means to 'correct' society. The newer Pakistani Taliban have done the same. Even when Pakistani military operations were proceeding against them, they have engaged in organizing penal punishments against offenders. Baitullah Mehsud engaged in these tactics, and so has Fazlullah. It seems that the inherent structural imbalances in distributive social justice in Pakistan have left gaping wounds, which the extremists are quick to exploit.

People in KP province as a whole and FATA in particular, have tended to feel left out of Pakistan's development processes. With clearly documented widespread poverty, a provincial GDP that is only 60% of the national GDP, and achievements in the education and health sectors well below the national average, KP had the highest infant mortality rate in Pakistan of 56 deaths per 1,000 live births. Only 58% of the total households received clean drinking water. The NWFP seemingly does not get its fair share even in judicially determined shares of governmental gross net profits. One of the reasons for militancy in tribal areas may very well be the lack of legitimacy felt towards both the political and economic fronts; for instance the unemployment rate for the age group 15-25 years in Waziristan is above 80%. With such abysmal statistics, it hardly needs a huge stretch of imagination to conceptualize that unemployed youth may be attracted towards militancy as a way of venting their grievances. It also partly explains how the extremist project was able to capture their target audience by 'replicating' the state processes of providing justice, when the state seemed incapable of doing so.

Real life examples illustrate how the militants try to fill in the socio-economic vacuum. "He has restored law and order in the area. Dacoits and thieves have left the area fearing harsh punishments," Hussain Khan, a local told us. According to him, "Some people also believe that there are many bad people in his militia", citing the killing of 13 family members of the federal government's political agent in Khyber agency, an adjacent tribal area, in an armed attack by Baitullah's militia about four months before. "He (Baitullah) publicly apologized for the incident," Khan said. "The Taliban involved in the attack have been languishing in (his) jail for the last four months. They would have been punished if anti-security sentiments against military action had not been aroused and military option had not been exercised." (Latif, 2008).

Aslam Awan, a journalist working with the Jihadi publication Weekly Takbeer, cites the setting up of a 'special task force' in June 2007 to purportedly crack down on criminals in South Waziristan. "This force launched a number of crackdowns and successfully urged a feared kidnapper Abdul Rashid Bakakhel to free some of his hostages. Baitullah also collected donations from the local people to establish peace. It was a kind of protection money," Awan continues (Shehzad, 2006). Similarly, Fazlullah seemed to be playing out the Robin Hood theme too as mentioned above. Public lashings in Imamdheri resonated to the media images emanating from Afghanistan during the Taliban heydays. It is pertinent to mention here that many of these acts were at the time endorsed by the local populace. These were seen as non-discriminatory acts aimed at punishing criminals masquerading as Taliban and committing acts of robbery. In an area where the locals have traditionally complained of ineffective governance by successive governments, which allegedly indulged in nepotism and inadequate resource allocation, a heightened local sense of security may have been a driving factor swelling the ranks of Taliban. This supports the notion that an imbalance in governance in a 'closed' society (like Waziristan), where the mechanisms of the state are weak, may be one of the various causes of extremism in the area. In any case, this replication of roles of the state (whereby it was perceived not to be working properly) has been a hallmark of the entrenchment of Taliban insurgency both in FATA and Swat. It is therefore not surprising that this was the first phase of the Taliban entrenchment that usually preceded mass violence, and also the time when locals could be seen to be supporting the Taliban. The movement would inevitably turn violent, and the knee jerk local mass support would fade away. This process of replication would set the scene for the next stage, since it would have already aroused the interest of the masses.

Perhaps the absence of distributive social justice and the remnants of feudalism in the shape of the 'Maliks' has also had an effect on the promotion of militancy. Some analysts suggest that the social vacuum was generated by the apathy of the Maliks of Swat towards the conditions of the peasant class. This apathy, and delays in obtaining speedy justice from courts, prompted the locals to look to TNSM as an organization that seemed to be at least agitating for reforms in the shape of Sharia. TNSM gradually became unpopular as the movement lost steam, and the Taliban neatly stepped into its shoes as an effective substitute (the replication phenomenon again, or rather a re-replication). This analysis is bolstered by the fact that the Taliban movement initially became popular in the rural areas of Khwazakhela, Matta and Kabal. All three areas are characterized by a strong feudal system and what is widely considered to be downtrodden peasantry. It is only after the Taliban had consolidated their hold in these relatively less affluent localities, that they started turning in strength to other more prosperous areas like Babozai and Barikot. Thus, the Taliban seem to have started as a grass roots movement in feudal dominated areas, which is perhaps the main reason why they have not been able to gain a stronghold in the neighbouring district of Buner. Buner is characterized by an absence of Malik feudal system, and paradoxically, has a poorly developed system of agriculture as opposed to Swat. If poverty alone is considered as the main variable in generating militancy in these areas, then Buner should have been the district giving birth to the phenomenon of Taliban, since it is nearly identical topographically to Swat except for being poorer. However, the distinguishing feature of absence of feudalism has perhaps saved Buner.

The role of radio-broadcasting

The Taliban set up illegal FM radio stations to campaign for funds and recruits to fight alongside the Taliban. These radio stations played an active role to gain followers of their ideology, inform on decrees, address rallies in support of the Taliban, and serves as a tool for fundraising. Maulana Fazlullah became known as "Mullah Radio" for his repeated use of radio for frequent broadcasting in the region. These broadcasts helped greatly insurgency to gain a foothold in the Swat Valley as they proved to be instrumental in gathering support for the militants. Other Taliban radio broadcasters, popularly known as "FM Mullahs", continuously transmitted anti-American and anti-government sermons, calling democracy "un-Islamic" and those practicing it "infidels". They encouraged local youth to rise for jihad against foreign forces and urged the elderly men and women to lend their moral and financial support to the cause of jihad. In their fiery speeches on radios, the Taliban demanded that non-Muslim minorities in Malakand pay the jizya (protection fee) or face jihad. In the same tone, they issued warnings to NGOs, musicians and anyone else involved in "anti-Islamic" activities. Later, those defying their orders were brutally murdered and daily announcements of the details of their death broadcasted on FM transmissions.

However, in the earlier phases of consolidation, these channels became very popular with women especially who tend to be at home most of the time. Listening to these stations became a favourite pastime with Swati women. Since women in these areas spend most of their time at home, watching television or listening to radio accounts forms a huge part of the entertainment and information based activities open to them. The Taliban were extremely active against the few TV cable channel operators in Swat, since according to their brand of Sharia, TV was 'haram' (sacrilegious) since it purportedly showed images of women. All the TV cable channel operators and CD shops selling movies, dramas or other forms of entertainment were bombed or forced to shut down, many of the owners of such establishments assassinated. This resulted in a virtual shutdown of televised media for the Swat women, who were forced to resort to listening to FM radio. In this way, by 'closing' the options for the women in the area, the Taliban effectively set the stage for audience 'capture' of Swat's women.

Through these channels, the Taliban demanded that parliamentarians, security forces and other government officials should resign their positions as a mark of protest against the military operations, otherwise they should be ready to face 'jihad'. An important aspect of the radio broadcasts was its effect on women. The militants won loyalties of the women by presenting messages through religious interpretations. They were encouraged to give money and also put pressure on their families to join the movement. Many women gave away all their jewellery and money to the Taliban. Sometimes, the authorities tried to block broadcasts, but radios were back on the air after some time. Most people in Swat become regular listeners of FM radio stations as they wanted to know about new threats or decrees issued by the militants. Transmissions at night were also heard in some areas outside the district of Swat. This had allowed the Taliban to spread their influence into the regions of Upper and Lower Dir districts of Dir and Malakand.

FM Programs such as the one run by uber militant Shah-e-Dauran from Qambar exhorted the Swati women to force their husbands and sons to go for Jihad. The Taliban relied on a clever strategy; they did not underplay the importance of women in Islam, but on the contrary purportedly espoused it. Sermon after sermon stressed the importance of women in Islamic society, how staying at home was critical to the upbringing of their children and how women could play a critical role in society by carrying out their religious obligations to their husband and family. Women were enjoined to even forcibly send their sons and family for jihad, and in doing so they would fulfil their own obligations in lieu of actually going for jihad. This was deemed to be the jihad for women. A lady told us in one of our focus groups during the Swat White Paper Research: "I felt so important for the first time listening to him (the FM mullah) – I had always felt that I was just a useless part of society since all I did was stay at home and look after the family, which was not actually acknowledged by my husband at all. In fact he used to treat my contribution to the family chores with contempt. The (mullah) made me realize my importance, and even my husband was impressed when I started exhorting the principles of jihad to him. I felt elevated."

Other observers have observed this audience capture as well. In the Pakistani context, Ahmed Rashid in his authoritative book on the Taliban stated that the Taliban command preferred young men between 16-25 years of age who were unbound by 'family strings', or paradoxically, had spent most of their time with mothers. A recent empirically conducted psychosocial analysis characterises these kinds of boys as being pulled by matriarchic strings, when mothers have the burden of raising these children in conservative and patriarchal societies where fathers are often absent.[1] The mothers pass on their 'burden' of despondency to these boys, who are prone to look for symbolic figures in order to join the mythological ranks of these heroes (Merari, 2005). The violent end to an otherwise unremarkable life becomes the final glorifying act of such individuals who go to their deaths imagining themselves to be achieving a kind of legendary status. Thus, there is no feeling of despondency in many of the 'will letters' of suicide bombers, which indeed seem to radiate even a positive jubilation at going to meet the creator. Not surprisingly, many such letters talk of 'making their mothers proud' (and not their families).

Conclusions

Despite studies, which have been carried out, this is only the tip of the iceberg. Time will tell how future generations of young Swati boys under strong matriarchal influences will turn out. There are many different variables, which act upon individuals to radicalize them, and so the causality of extremism in Swat are numerous. If this is the case, any negative extremist influence which women exercise on the upbringing of young children may very well be offset by the now almost universal distaste for the Taliban times. People of Swat have just seen too much bloodshed in the name of religion to trust such radio mullahs again. Since the reasons behind the rise of militancy are many fold, an analysis utilizing any single variable would be nothing short of empirical, and largely misleading. Contemporary literature reviews have suggested that that the post 9/11 presumed link between a reduction in poverty, or an increase in educational attainment and a simultaneous de-escalation of international terrorism is quite tenuous. The connections between poverty, education and terrorism have been suggested to be ephemeral, inasmuch the recent profiles of terrorists suggest that they are not the stereotypical impoverished and uneducated youth as was generally presumed. Instead it is the result of years of frustrated political aspirations and indignity, which inculcates an acute sense of insecurity and consequently hatred towards those who are ostensibly perceived to have brought about these conditions. These findings may further vary according to the local socio-cultural contexts of the national or sub national theatre under consideration.

However, qualitative and quantitative studies still indicate nostalgia for

---

1   There are many reasons for their potential absence, from having been killed in conflict, working away from the district, or simply just staying away from the house.

radio mullahs by a significant number of Swati female respondents. The Taliban attempted to win the sympathies of the target populations by exploiting the lacunae in distributive social justice, thereby bypassing the formal governance framework with improvised local economic 'pumps' catering to the masses, particularly the landless poor. Interestingly, this seems to have won them sympathy and a certain legitimacy amongst cross-sections of society, including many women. These women then became converts to the ideology, notwithstanding the fact that the Taliban seemed to be closing their access to education and media. Many women forced the males in the household to listen to these FM programmes, forcing children under matriarchic influence to conform to the transmitted Talibanized ideals. It seems incredulous that despite the clearly harsh anti women ideology of the Taliban there was still considerable support for the Taliban from women. These complex dependency relationships have just been elicited during the Swat White Paper Study but it is clear that much still needs to be done to analyse these pervasive phenomena.

References

Ansari, M. (2008) The Ticking Bomb. *Herald*. 1 August.

Anwar, I (2006) Taliban command structure in Fata alarms US. *The Dawn*. [Online] 28 December. Available at: http://www.dawn.com/2006/12/28/top1.htm. (accessed 21st January 2012).

Khan, T. (2013) Taliban leader advises Malala to return, join madrassa. *The Express Tribune*. [Online]17 July 2013. Available at: http://tribune.com.pk/story/578128/taliban-leader-advises-malala-to-return-join-madrassa/. (accessed 13 July 2013).

Latif, A. (2008) Pakistan's Most Wanted. *On Islam* [Online] 29 January. Available at: http://www.onislam.net/english/news/3339/433768. (accessed 9 March 2014).

Merari , A. (2005) 'Social, Organizational and Psychological Factors in Suicide Terrorism' in *Root Causes of Terrorism*, T. Bjorgo (ed.), Routledge, London.

The News (2008) Seven more killed in Swat violence. [Online] 10 September. Available at: http://www.thenews.com.pk/TodaysPrintDetail.aspx?ID=17154&Cat=13&dt=9/9/2008. (accessed 17 March 2013).

Rahman, T. (2008) Swat hotel industry on verge of collapse. *The News* [Online] 14 May 14. Available from http://www.thenews.com.pk/TodaysPrintDetail.aspx?ID=112457&Cat=7&dt=6/4/2008. (accessed 17 March 2013).

Shehzad, M. (2006) Why is the Pakistan Army Scared of This Man? *Rediff News*. [Online] 10 March. Available at: http://www.rediff.com/news/2006/mar/10pspec.htm. (accessed 9th March 2014).

TTP Swat No.3 2006, (Video recording), Swat, Al Umer media Taliban Propaganda Video.

TTP Swat No.5 2006, (Video recording), Swat, Al Umer media Taliban Propaganda Video.

CHAPTER 12. NATIONAL SECURITY: NAVIGATING THE COMING ROUGH SEAS BETWEEN THE USA AND CHINA

=============❖=============

Andre Zaaiman

"The first, the supreme, the most far-reaching act of judgment that the statesman and commander have to make is to establish […] the kind of war on which they are embarking." (Clausewitz, 2007, p.61)

Will China and America cooperate, compete or go to war?

The emerging geo-political great game between the USA and China is of great importance to the world in general, and to Africa and South Africa in particular. How this great power relationship unfolds will have a commanding influence on the 21st century. As it intensifies, it will remind us that ideology, politics, strategy, money and geography matter; that history has not ended.

The future cannot be known, but probability and prediction can be improved as well as surprise avoided if we are assisted by facts - by a proper understanding of what is going on - as well as by quality information, good theory and of course, secrets. However as the renowned Stellenbosch academic Paul Cilliers (1998) demonstrated, complex and dynamic contexts cannot be properly understood using the classic tools of analytic reductionism. Complexity science with its emphasis on the non-linearity of relationships between multiple components in a system may provide a methodological escape and a way to deal with the uncertain, the unexpected and the sudden.

In statecraft, the purpose of intelligence is to provide a competent decision-maker with an informational advantage in the context of national security and the pursuit of national goals. As before, events and decisions made by others on distant shores will have a critical impact on Africa and South Africa. Since the world has become hyper-connected and interdependent, events elsewhere will reverberate across the system faster and more directly. The smooth and orderly flow and exchange of goods, information, money, food, energy and people is now of critical importance for the domestic stability of each country. Movement becomes as important as access and relationships. Albert O'Hirschman of National Power and the Structure of Foreign Trade (1980) made compelling arguments to demonstrate how dependency and domination can arise out of foreign trade relations and how the power to interrupt or disrupt commercial or financial flows or relations with other countries, is a determinant of a country's power position. In other words, a country trying to make the most out of its strategic position with respect to its own trade will try to create conditions which make the interruption or disruption of trade of much graver concern to its trading partners than to itself.

According to Hudson Institute naval expert Bryan McGrath in an article entitled "A new look at an old Maritime Strategy", he stated that the central proposition of the US Naval Strategy is:

> That there is a global system in place that works to the benefit of the people of United States and all other nations who participate in it. The system consists of tightly interconnected networks of trade, finance, information, law, people and governance, and the strategy posits that U.S. maritime forces will be deployed to protect and sustain the system. (McGrath, 2014)

Some American maritime strategists already worry that the Chinese People's Liberation Army's (PLA) can now field robust anti-access/area-denial (A2/AD) capabilities along their key maritime trade routes, that are threatening to make US power projection increasingly risky and, in some cases and contexts, prohibitively costly.

The control over these flows and exchange – until now enforced and policed by the USA and its Western allies through norms, rules and institutions created by themselves and backed up by the coercive power of the globally-deployed US Military – is increasingly contested and some would argue, breaking down. The launch of the New Development Bank (NDB) and of the Contingency Reserve Fund (CRF) by the emerging countries of Brazil, Russia, India, China, and South Africa (BRICS) in July 2014 is a powerful signal that developing countries are no longer willing to play second fiddle on the global stage. A senior official of the ruling African National Congress in South Africa, Obed Bapela, commenting in the ANC

Today newsletter noted that:

> The Sixth BRICS Summit just concluded in the picturesque coastal city of Fortaleza. This was a historic and seminal moment in the post-Bretton Woods era since the BRICS Leaders witnessed the BRICS Finance Ministers signing the two founding agreements on the New Development Bank (NDB) and Contingent Reserve Arrangement (CRA). President Zuma has hailed the establishment of the NDB as 'an everlasting legacy that will change the face of global economics and the face of all the developing world for better'. (Bapela, 2014)

The desired post-Bretton Woods era does not only contain different global financial institutions – not controlled by the USA – but some analysts believe also rests on different values. In an article published on The Huffington Post entitled, "New BRICS Bank a Building Block of Alternative World Order" Parag Khanna notices that:

> The New Development Bank was therefore not just born out of resentment over the World Bank and IMF's main donors stubbornly clinging to their over-weighted voting shares. It also reflects a difference in philosophy over the need to prioritize physical infrastructure over other priorities (such as education, healthcare, women's rights, etc.) towards which the World Bank has been drawn in recent decades. From a holistic point of view, all such investments are crucial for equitable national prosperity and wellbeing, but nothing creates jobs and literally drives 'state-building' like infrastructure. (Khanna, 2014)

As the current global architecture decomposes, the resultant vacuum and ideological contestation in the interregnum may lead to adventurism, friction and conflict. The world therefore also needs new political institutional arrangements that are representative of the shifts in the balance-of-forces. For theorists of hegemonic wars such as A.F.K Organski, Jacek Kugler and George Modelski, this coincides with a high-risk and dangerous moment in world history when a rising power starts to challenge an existing hegemon; a historical moment that when viewed from the longue durée, frequently ended in vicious trade disputes and eventually in large-scale war.

President Barack Obama has made it clear that America does not want its relationship with China "to become defined by rivalry and confrontation". Rejecting the basic premises of the theorists of hegemonic wars he, in the words of his National Security Advisor Tom Donlin disagrees "with the premise put forward by some historians and theorists that a rising power and an established power are somehow destined for conflict. There is nothing preordained about such an outcome." (Donlin, 2013)

In an interview with David Remnick in The New Yorker (January 2014), Obama confirmed that what he needs isn't any new grand strategy: "I don't really even need George Kennan right now"—but, rather the right strategic partners. "There are currents in history and you have to figure out how to move them in one direction or another," Rhodes said. "You can't necessarily determine the final destination [...]The President subscribes less to a great-man theory of history and more to a great-movement theory of history—that change happens when people force it or circumstances do." [Later, Obama told me (that is Remnick) 'I'm not sure Ben is right about that. I believe in both.'] (Remnick, 2014).

This private denial is revelatory and provides us with important information. It also raises an important question: which currents and waves are America riding in the advancement of their goals and the implementation of their strategy? The correct answer to this question will unlock a treasure trove of information and needs to be probed further.

For American scholars like John Mearsheimer according to his work "The Tragedy of Great Power Politics" (2001) there is a limited role in international affairs for either intelligent leadership or for diplomacy, because in his view, as powers gain economic strength, they will pursue the acquisition of coercive, military power. And this in turn will lead to conflict making the idea that economic interdependence contributes to peace, a delusion. Currently China, India, Japan and Russia are all in the process of rapidly modernizing their military forces.

President Barack Obama reconfirmed the main currents of his thinking in his 2014 West-Point speech:

> In such circumstances, we should not go it alone. Instead, we must mobilize allies and partners to take collective action. We have to broaden our tools to include diplomacy and development; sanctions and isolation; appeals to international law; and, if just, necessary and effective, multilateral military action. In such circumstances, we have to work with others because collective action in these circumstances is more likely to succeed, more likely to be sustained, less likely to lead to costly mistakes. (Obama, 2014)

Grand Strategy declares long-term intentions and how all instruments of national power will be wielded over time in the pursuit of specific goals. Whilst rejecting rivalry and confrontation with China, Obama at the same time, reconfirmed his adherence to the Doctrine of American Preponderance – albeit articulated softly as "global American leadership". In other words, his intent is to arrest the decline in US hegemony that started with its disastrous military invasions of Iraq in 2003 – the latter an inflection point in post-Cold War history correctly read as such at the time by a small team of South African national security experts working with then President Thabo Mbeki that included Lindiwe Sisulu, Aziz Pahad, Welile Nhlapo, Super Moloi, Thembi Majola and myself. South Africa took an unusually strong and public position against that invasion and it was precisely Shock-and-Awe in Iraq that woke the Chinese and Russian military from their complacency and aroused their suspicions of American grand-strategic encirclement and containment. That invasion and the manner in which it was conducted, is directly linked to the unfolding great power dynamic between the US, China, Russia and India.

Giovanni Arrighi in his New Left Review article entitled "Hegemony Unravelling", refers to the works of David Harvey including "The New Imperialism", and Thomas Mccormick's "America's Half-Century: United States Foreign Policy in the Cold War and After" and remarks:

> The attempted implementation of the (Neo-Conservative) plan through the unilateral decision to invade Iraq, Harvey argues, 'created a bond of resistance [...] between France, Germany and Russia, even backed by China'. This sudden geopolitical realignment made it 'possible to discern the faint outlines of a Eurasian power bloc that Halford Mackinder long ago predicted could easily dominate the world geopolitically'. In light of Washington's longstanding fears that such a bloc might actually materialize, the occupation of Iraq takes on an even broader meaning: Not only does it constitute an attempt to control the global oil spigot – and hence the global economy – through domination over the Middle East. It also constitutes a powerful US military bridgehead on the Eurasian land mass which, when taken together with its gathering alliances from Poland down through the Balkans, yields it a highly significant geo-strategic position with the potential to disrupt any consolidation of a Eurasian power; and which could indeed be the next step in that 'endless accumulation of political power' that must always accompany the equally endless accumulation of capital. (Arrighi, 2005, p.34)

As far back as in 1997, Zbigniew Brzezinski, writing in Foreign Affairs, asserted that:

> Eurasia is home to most of the world's politically assertive and dynamic states. All the historical pretenders to global power originated in Eurasia. The world's most populous aspirants to regional hegemony, China and India, are in Eurasia, as are all the potential political or economic challengers to American primacy. After the United States, the next six largest economies and military spenders are there, as are all but one of the world's overt nuclear powers, and all but one of the covert ones. Eurasia accounts for 75 percent of the world's population, 60 percent of its GNP, and 75 percent of its energy resources. Collectively, Eurasia's potential power overshadows even America's. Eurasia is the world's axial supercontinent. A power that dominated Eurasia would exercise decisive influence over two of the world's three most economically productive regions, Western Europe and East Asia. A glance at the map also suggests that a country dominant in Eurasia would almost automatically control the Middle East and Africa. With Eurasia now serving as the decisive geopolitical chessboard, it no longer suffices to fashion one policy for Europe and another for Asia. What happens with the distribution of power on the Eurasian landmass will be of decisive importance to America's global primacy and historical legacy. (Brzezinski, 1997)

In the same article of 1997, Brzezinski went on to say:

In the short run, the United States should consolidate and perpetuate the prevailing geopolitical pluralism on the map of Eurasia. This strategy will put a premium on political manoeuvring and diplomatic manipulation, preventing the emergence of a hostile coalition that could challenge America's primacy, not to mention the remote possibility of any one state seeking to do so. A sustainable strategy for Eurasia must distinguish among the more immediate short-run perspective of the next five years or so, the medium term of 20 or so years, and the long run beyond that. Moreover, these phases must be viewed not as watertight compartments but as part of a continuum [...] By the medium term, the foregoing should lead to the emergence of strategically compatible partners which, prompted by American leadership, might shape a more cooperative trans-Eurasian security system. In the long run, the foregoing could become the global core of genuinely shared political responsibility." (Brzezinski, 1997)

In other words, he proposed making regimes compatible with US values and interests whist pursuing counter-alliance disruption, building (co-) dependence that must lead to (inter)-dependence. Brezezinski expanded on these ideas in his subsequent two books: "The Grand Chessboard: American Primacy and Its Geo-Strategic Imperatives" in 1997; and "Strategic Vision: America and the Crisis of Global Power" in 2013.

This exposes a major and long-standing American anxiety: the biggest medium term threat to US hegemony and preponderance, lies – from a US perspective – in a deepened rapprochement between Germany and Russia. It also tells us why the US government so actively pursues the destabilization of the Ukraine: it wants to maintain friction between Germany and Russia; prevent rapprochement from deepening and build a geo-political buffer. And it explains why America, through its NSA, is spying in such a comprehensive manner on its own ally: Germany.

Obama therefore aims to restore the traditional sources of American hegemony – US economic, financial, rule-making and ideological or soft power. Tom Donlin goes on to say that "the United States is implementing a comprehensive, multidimensional strategy: it is an effort that harnesses all elements of U.S. power—military, political, trade and investment, development and our values" (Donlin, 2013). In as far as Asia is concerned "the overarching objective of the United States in the region is to sustain a stable security environment and a regional order rooted in economic openness, peaceful resolution of disputes, and respect for universal rights and freedoms" (Donlin, 2013).

This Strategy rests on five pillars:

- Strengthening US alliances particularly with Japan
- Deepening partnerships with emerging powers particularly with India

- Building a stable, productive, and constructive relationship with China;
- Empowering regional institutions;
- Helping to build a regional economic architecture that can sustain shared prosperity.

In trying to read and interpret the current context correctly – and starting with the American side – the above facts create an interesting analytical dilemma: Obama has publicly rejected the Data Modelling and warnings of the theorists of hegemonic wars on the one hand; but on the other hand, he has clearly stated his intention to not only continue to pursue American hegemony but to restore and rebuild it.

The progressive American scholar Noam Chomsky argues that successive US Governments are all pursuing the same objective; they just develop new pretexts and enemies as they go along – unintentionally affirming Obama's claim that American Grand Strategy remains unchanged (TomDispatch, 2014). Chomsky hones in on the ideological and argues that US security policy does not aim to secure "the people" but rather the US ideology of private sector capitalism built around an elite group of banks, financial institutions and the military-industrial complex. He refers to the Snowden revelations and quotes the prominent liberal scholar and government adviser Samuel Huntington: "The architects of power in the United States must create a force that can be felt but not seen. Power remains strong when it remains in the dark; exposed to the sunlight it begins to evaporate" (Huntington, 1981). Huntington wrote that in 1981, when the Cold War was again heating up, and he explained further "you may have to sell [intervention or other military action] in such a way as to create the misimpression that it is the Soviet Union that you are fighting. That is what the United States has been doing ever since the Truman Doctrine" (Huntington, 1981).

In trying to solve our analytical dilemma and without revealing any secrets, it might be useful to start by looking again at the facts.

The impact of the incipient US-Chinese and Western-Russian contestation and ongoing strategic re-positioning, is already starkly visible in regions across the globe stretching from Ukraine or Crimea; the South and East China Seas; or in the Middle East. The African continent has not been spared with the large-scale but diffused physical American military and economic presence across the whole continent as part of a far-reaching American manoeuvre ironically known as the Pivot to Asia, now the most visible red flag. This American military deployment in Africa has until recently, largely gone unnoticed but its scale and depth has caused some policy-makers to call this US geo-strategic manoeuvre "the Pivot to Africa" instead. Its landward presence is constantly and stealthily being expanded through leadership training, anti-terrorism, anti-poaching and anti-organized crime or joint military-exercise "partnership" initiatives in all regions of Africa.

US Defence and its public and private security arms are re-positioning themselves for new and not-so-new forms of kinetic and non-kinetic interventions aimed at shaping environments, building or breaking alliances and weakening adversaries. This will include complex informational and media warfare; economic, trade and currency interventions; as well political subversion. In a hyper-connected world, the maritime capabilities for anti-access and area-denial, flow throttling or systems control and disruption, become critical. For example world trade, conducted in US Dollars via digital informational platforms, moves and happens through shipping and therefore seas, sea lanes, harbours, coastal borders and navies – both commercial and military –are key elements in the new mix of challenges confronting us. Destabilizing adversarial regimes or alliances through economic warfare, disrupting trade flows and support for tech-savvy youth groups, efforts at regime de-legitimization and strengthening oppositional forces, will be escalated.

The 2013 book of Juan Zarate "The Treasury's War: Unleashing a New Era of Financial Warfare" which lifted the lid on these new national security tools developed and deployed by the US government since 2011, is a warning of things to come. In July 2014, Reuters reported that the French bank BNP Paribas had pleaded guilty to two criminal charges laid against it by the US Treasury, and agreed to pay almost $9 billion to resolve accusations it violated U.S. sanctions against Sudan, Cuba and Iran, a severe punishment aimed at sending a clear message to other financial institutions around the world. Behind this lies an even more important fact: the US will go to extraordinary lengths to maintain the supremacy of the US Dollar as the world's reserve currency - a critical element in maintaining US hegemonic control.

Whilst the Pivot – often called "re-balancing" – has lead America to build its presence in the Asia Pacific region, it is also trying to extend its North Atlantic hegemony southwards towards the Central Atlantic region, making the entire Western Rim of Africa a critical part of this geo-political shift – a practical manifestation of the Roosevelt corollary to the Monroe Doctrine.

This will prevent or disrupt the emergence of a BRICS-oriented, Brazilian-lead South American and South African-lead African security community developing in the Central Atlantic. And it will make Nigeria, not a BRICS member, a more important geo-strategic player. The Northern African Rim, following the 2011 Franco-American military intervention in Libya in particular, already forms part of a broader European-led Mediterranean security and influence zone as articulated in the Lisbon

Concept adopted by NATO, also in 2011.

This new focus on the seas and oceanic Rims is neither limited to Africa nor is it a coincidence as it is all part of a deliberate US-European geo-political repositioning. Although both pivoting and the modern variant of geo-strategy is often traced back to the 1904 article of the British geographer Harald Mackinder titled "The Geographical Pivot of History" in which he proposed a land-based, heartland theory of geo-politics, it was his critic Nicholas Spykman who drew on the work of the American naval theorist Alfred Mahan and his work, "The Influence of Sea Power upon History, 1660–1783", which was an influential study on the role of the navy and of sea-power on the rise of the British Empire, that developed a complementary counter-argument of a sea-based, rim land theory of geo-strategy. Whilst Mackinder argued that Eurasia – incorporating both contemporary Russia and China – were the heartland around which world domination pivoted; and therefore whoever controlled it would control the world –Spykman in turn argued that the sea-lanes and ocean Rim around the heartland, in particular the South and East China Seas, were the key geographical areas from which the heartland and thus the globe could be dominated. From a South African perspective, this would make the Eastern Rim of Africa, as important as its Northern and Western Rims.

It is therefore not insignificant that not only the US and China but also India, Russia, Japan and Brazil have all heavily invested in their naval capabilities over last five years. Chinese stability depends on peaceful development and American preponderance on military domination and control over the Dollarized global financial system. Both China and Russia fear that the US is busy with an elaborate and incipient manoeuvre of encirclement and destabilization as part of a broader strategy of containment. South Africa fears that Africa and South Africa itself, will get embroiled in this American manoeuvre with negative consequences for our key national security goal: political-economic transformation as part of a broader African revival. America fears that China – with or without its Allies – will rival and pose a threat to US Preponderance or hegemony; or that West and East Europe would unite.

Whilst the physical and material consequences of US-Chinese repositioning are visible, the much-less visible political and ideological dimension that undergirds this may not be less important.

The American scholar Charles A. Kupchan argues that:

> Understanding and managing international change requires examining not just shifts in material power, but also the associated contest among competing norms of order. Transitions in the international distribution of power produce not only novel hierarchies, but also novel brands of international order that rest on the social and ideological proclivities of newly powerful states in the system. [This is because] as great powers rise,

they, as a matter of course, seek to extend to their expanding spheres of influence, the norms that provide order within their own polities. (Kupchan, 2014, p.220)

In September 2002, then US President George W. Bush articulated the Grand Strategy of the United States of America as follows: "We will defend the peace by fighting terrorists and tyrants. We will preserve the peace by building good relations among the great powers. We will extend the peace by encouraging free and open societies on every continent." (Bush, 2002)

Following his announcement in November 2011 of an American Pivot to Asia in a speech in Canberra and later rephrased as re-balancing, President Barack Obama has consistently maintained that the core elements of the existing Grand Strategy – US Preponderance and the defence, preservation and extension of the values of "freedom, liberal-democracy and free enterprise" – remain intact. These three components, and the way it has been turned into a global hegemonic praxis through constructs such as "globalization" and US coercion immediately after the end of the Cold War, have come together under the term "neo-liberalism".

The 20 March 2003 American "Shock-and-Awe" military invasion of Iraq was precisely the start of this hegemonic praxis based on neo-liberal ideology, geo-strategy and coercion.

This particular brand of liberalism – now known as anti-statist neo-liberalism – lead Henry Giroux to remark that:

> Neoliberalism has become the most dangerous ideology of the current historical moment. It assaults all things public, mystifies the basic contradiction between democratic values and market fundamentalism, and weakens any viable notion of political agency by offering no language capable of connecting private considerations to public issues. Under the rule of neoliberalism, politics are market driven and the claims of democratic citizenship are subordinated to market values. What becomes troubling under such circumstances is not simply that ideas associated with freedom and agency are defined through the prevailing ideology and principles of the market, but that neoliberalism wraps itself in what appears to be an unassailable appeal to common sense. As Zygmunt Bauman notes, 'What [...] makes the neo-liberal world-view sharply different from other ideologies – indeed, a phenomenon of a separate class – is precisely the absence of questioning; its surrender to what is seen as the implacable and irreversible logic of social reality.' Also lost is the very viability of politics itself." (Giroux, 2002, p.428)

Peter Mair subsequently noted in his essay "Ruling the Void" (2006), that under Tony Blair:

> The role of 'progressive' politics was not to provide solutions from above, by exercising the 'directive hand' of government, but to bring together 'dynamic markets' and strong communities so as 'to offer synergy and

opportunity'. In Tony Blair's [a key proponent and advocate of the 2003 Iraq invasion] ideal world, politics would eventually become redundant. As one of his close cabinet colleagues was later to remark, 'depoliticizing of key decision-making is a vital element in bringing power closer to the people'. At one level, this was a simple populist strategy—employing the rhetoric of 'the people' in order to suggest that there had been a radical break with past styles of government. At another, however, it gelled perfectly with the tenets of what were then seen as newly emerging schools of 'governance' and with the idea that 'society is now sufficiently well organized through self-organizing networks that any attempts on the part of government to intervene will be ineffective and perhaps counterproductive'. In this perspective, government no longer seeks to wield power or even exercise authority. Its relevance declines, while that of non-governmental institutions and practices increases. In Ulrich Beck's terms, the dynamic moves from Politics, with a capital 'P', to politics with a lower-case one, or to what he has called 'sub-politics'. (Mair, 2006, p.26)

Anti-political sentiments were also becoming more evident in the policy-making literature of the late 1990s. Mair continues:

In 1997, an influential article appeared in Foreign Affairs expressing the concern that government in the US was becoming 'too political'. Its author, Alan Blinder, a leading economist and deputy head of the Federal Reserve, suggested extending the model of independent Central Banks to other key policy areas, so that decisions on health, the welfare state and so on would be taken by non-partisan experts. The role of politicians in policy-making would be confined to those areas in which the judgement of experts would not suffice to legitimize outcomes. Similar arguments were emerging in the European context. In 1996, for example, Giandomenico Majone argued that the role of expert decision-making in the policy-making process was superior to that of political decision-making in that it could take better account of long-term interests. (Mair, 2006, pp. 26-27)

South Africa was not spared from this Western hegemonic coercion then and it will not be spared from it in the future. The ANC Government under Presidents Mandela and Mbeki had to chart a very careful path amidst dangerously constrained external and domestic environments. The global environment has significantly changed, despite American grand strategic intentions remaining the same, and the international balance-of-power has very slowly begun to shift. Whilst we need to use the opportunity to domestically reintroduce the state, politics and political debate in South Africa – the anti-politics machine must be stopped – we need to do so with wisdom and as part of a broad national consensus or compact. There can be no democracy without the demos; and in national security when the chips are down, there still remains only two final arbiters: capabilities and the national will of the people.

As the ANC government under President Zuma pursues our path in

BRICS and builds a democratic developmental state aimed at fast sustained, sustainable and inclusive growth, we need to bear in mind that internationally, the intricate sets of competing great power interests and grand strategies create fertile conditions for misperception, miscommunication and miscalculation. Nonetheless nothing should deter us from enhancing the competitiveness and performance of our economy, building equity in our society or the deepening of our democracy and national will; this can only occur through the comprehensive transformation and realignment of our current dysfunctional political economy and skewed social realities.

South Africa should remain an active, constructive and consensus-building participant in the ongoing process in which the phenomenal potential of our continent and its people is finally being realized – our future and the future of our continent can never be separated. This in turn will require us to be wise shepherds in shaping new, progressive global governance architecture – financial, political, economic, security and culture – and an ideological praxis in which people and politics will claim their rightful place.

References

Arrighi, G. (2005) Hegemony Unravelling – 1. *New Left Review,* [online]. Available at: http://newleftreview.org/II/32/giovanni-arrighi-hegemony-unravelling-1 (accessed 10 September 2014).

Bapela, O. (2014) BRICS New Development Bank's Africa Regional Centre In South Africa: Impact And Outlook. *ANC Today,* [online]. Available at: http://www.anc.org.za/docs/anctoday/2014/at13.htm#art3 (accessed 10 September 2014).

Brzezinski, Z. (1997) A Geostrategy for Eurasia. *Foreign Affairs,* [online]. Available at: http://www.foreignaffairs.com/articles/53392/zbigniew-brzezinski/a-geostrategy-for-Eurasia (accessed 10 September 2014).

Chomsky, N. (2014) Tomgram: Noam Chomsky, America's Real Foreign Policy. *TomDispatch.com,* [blog] 01 July 2014. Available at: http://www.tomdispatch.com/blog/175863/tomgram%3A_noam_chomsky_america's_real_foreign_policy/ (accessed 10 September 2014).

Cilliers, P. (1998) *Complexity And Postmodernism: Understanding Complex Systems*. Routledge, London.

Clausewitz, C. von., (2007) *On War*. Oxford University Press, Oxford.

Donilon, T. National Security Advisor To The President: The United States And The Asia-Pacific In 2013: White House Press Statement, 11 March 2013*,* [online] Available at: http://www.whitehouse.gov/the-press-office/2013/03/11/remarks-tom-donilon-national-security-advisory-president-united-states-a (accessed 10 September 2014)

Giroux, H.A. (2002) Neoliberalism, Corporate Culture And The Promise Of Higher Education: The University As A Democratic Public Sphere. *Harvard Educational Review*, 72(4), pp. 425-464.

Harvey, D. (2005) *The New Imperialism*. Oxford University Press, Oxford.

Khanna, P. (2014) New BRICS Bank A Building Block Of Alternative World Order. *The Huffington Post*, [online]. Available at: http://www.huffingtonpost.com/parag-khanna/new-brics-bank_b_5600027.html>(accessed 10 September 2014).

Kupchan, C.A. (2014) The Normative Foundations Of Hegemony And The Coming Challenge To Pax Americana. *Security Studies*, 23(2), pp. 219-257.

Mackinder, H.J. (1904) The Geographical Pivot Of History. *The Geographical Journal*, 23(4), pp. 421-437.

Mahan, A.T. (1987) *The Influence of Sea Power Upon History, 1660-1783*. Dover Publications, Mineola

Mair, P. (2006) Ruling the Void? The Hollowing of Western a Democracy. *New Left Review*, [online]. Available at: http://newleftreview.org/II/42/peter-mair-ruling-the-void (accessed 10 September 2014).

McGrath, B. (2014) A New Look at an Old Maritime Strategy. *War on the Rocks*, [online]. Available at: http://warontherocks.com/2014/06/a-new-look-at-an-old-maritime-strategy/ (accessed 10 September 2014).

Obama, B. (2014) Remarks by the President at the United States Military Academy Commencement Ceremony. [*press release*] 28 May 2014. Available at: http://www.whitehouse.gov/the-press-office/2014/05/28/remarks-president-united-states-military-academy-commencement-ceremony (accessed 10 September 2014).

Remnick, D. (2014) Going the Distance: On and off the road with Barack Obama. *New Yorker Magazine*, [online] Available at: http://www.newyorker.com/magazine/ 2014/01/27/going-the-distance-2 (accessed 10 September 2014).

Zarate, J. (2013) *Treasury's War: The Unleashing of a New Era of Financial Warfare*. PublicAffairs, New York.

PART IV – WOMEN'S LEADERSHIP IN RE-INVENTING A GLOBALIZED WORLD

CHAPTER 13. TECHNOLOGY AND THE POWER TO CONNECT: PARTICIPATION OF WOMEN IN SUPPORTING ACTIVITIES THROUGH INTERNET COMMUNITIES

Gerard van Oortmerssen

The development of technology and how it changes our world

History of technology

Homo sapiens is the first species to employ technology to make life easier and increase possibilities for survival and progress. Throughout history of mankind we have seen a continuous development of tools of increasing sophistication, from fire, the wheel, literacy, the steam engine, to the computer in our times. Technological development took place in waves. Every now and then a new technology emerged with considerable impact, heralding a new era with new impulses to economic and cultural progress. Examples are literacy, which made it possible to accumulate information and knowledge in documents, and book printing, which subsequently made this knowledge accessible to large numbers of people. Other examples are the steam engine, which started the industrial revolution and made relatively fast transportation over larger distances possible by steamships and railways.

Next came electricity, mass media and the use of hydrocarbons as a source of energy, which subsequently enabled fast air transportation. In our era it is Information and Communication Technology (ICT), which has a disruptive influence on life and society. The waves of technological development appear to happen at ever-shorter intervals. Nowadays, the amount of change that happens during the lifetime of a person is unprecedented, and the pace of change seems to accelerate even further.

Considering the ubiquity of ICT in terms of global penetration, as well as the multiple aspects of life in which it plays a role, it is hard to believe that it is only just over half a century ago that the first computers were developed. The single property of ICT that is essential for its success is the fact that it is a digital technology. The technology uses zero's and one's to represent any kind of data, making it possible to transfer and copy information indefinitely without errors and to perform computational operations on information. The value of this property can hardly be overestimated.

The first computers were built around the end of the Second World War. They were very big machines, expensive, and could be operated by specialised staff only. There were only a few, operated by government (defence) agencies, universities, and a few major corporations. They were mainly used for scientific computations and automation of administrative processes. Over the years computers became more powerful, cheaper and smaller. A major step was made in 1983 when the first personal computer came on the market. Working with a computer was no longer the privilege of specialists in a Computer Department. Anybody in an organisation could have a computer on his or her desktop, and soon even non-professional consumers could buy a PC. The democratisation of ICT started, bringing this digital technology to everyone who could afford it, and with prices going down, more and more people were able to afford the technology over the years.

In the early years computers were stand-alone machines, but in 1969 the first network was built by connecting computers at three American universities. The idea was to make more efficient use of the computing capacity by "time sharing". Soon the network was also used for sending messages and this eventually became the most important application of networks. Over the years more and more computers were connected, and interconnections were built between the various networks, thus creating a single worldwide network of computers, the Internet. Personal computers at homes could be connected to this Internet via public telephone services. The Internet got its real value in 1989, when Tim Berners Lee developed the World Wide Web (WWW) at CERN in Geneva. The WWW made it possible to easily access information on websites, navigating by just "clicking" on a word or icon, and ignited an explosive growth of the Internet. At just about the same time digital mobile phones made their entry on the market, growing at a similar rate. In just two decades the number of mobile phones grew to 7 billion, which means that there are as many mobile phones as people in the world. The mobile phone evolved from a device for talking and sending SMS text messages to a powerful pocket computer with full Internet functionality. People in high-income countries possess various devices such as smart phones, tablets, notebooks and desktop computers all of which give access to the Internet. The way we interact with these devices has evolved as well: from punch tape in the early days, via keyboard and mouse to touch screens and voice control, which are intuitive and easy, aligned with human nature and not requiring any special training.

Trends

When considering the development of ICT we can identify a number of trends.

The first one is the compression of space and time at exponentially growing velocity. This is the so-called Moore's law, stating that the number of transistors on a computer chip is doubling every 18 months. Effectively this means that computers become smaller, more powerful, with more memory space at an amazing speed. The price of digital devices is also going down continuously. It is difficult to fully grasp the significance of exponential growth, but doubling every 1.5 years gives a very steep growth curve after a decade or so.

It is not just the number of transistors on a chip that exhibits this growth. It is also characteristic for the amount of data on the Internet, the number of devices connected to the Internet, the number of websites, etc. etc.

The second trend is increasing connectedness. ICT is the technology that connects: it connects devices (computers, websites, information) into a global network. ICT also connects people, facilitating communication and collaboration. In its report, "Measuring the information Society 2013" the International Telecommunication Union (ITU) (2013) estimated that by the end of 2013, 2.7 billion people (40% of the world's inhabitants) were using the Internet. (The number is growing rapidly as just a decade ago this was only 10%.). All these people can connect to each other, building new communities, local as well as global. This is typically realised by using social networks like Twitter and Facebook. At this moment Facebook has around 1.3 billion active users, a significant part of the world population and one out of two Internet users.

Associated with the trend of connectivity is the phenomenon of convergence. Various previously separate technologies such as radio, television, telephone, computers, photography, all converge and are embraced within Internet technology.

The third trend is increasing complexity. A modern smartphone or tablet is more complex than a mainframe computer from the early years of ICT, and nowadays all these complex devices are connected to the Internet, together constituting an ensemble of tremendous complexity, with a multitude of interactions between devices, information and people. Just imagine that this complex system is growing every day. So does its complexity.

Some traits described in these trends are not exclusive to ICT but can be discerned in other technological developments as well, and can even be associated with the process of evolution itself. As the waves of technology seem to accelerate, the waves we see in the process of evolution have been accelerating as well: it took two billion years for life to emerge on earth, in the next several billion years many more complex forms of life emerged, mammals appeared around 100 million years ago, while homo sapiens dates back just a million years.

The future of ICT

How will ICT develop from here? It is important to recognise that development will continue, at an accelerating pace. Think a moment about how your life was 10 years ago, and about the changes that took place due to ICT. Then, realise that for sure you will experience far more change in your life in the next 10 years to come! The phenomenon of exponential growth means that for a growth from 1 to 20 in the past 10 years, we will see a further spurt to almost 1000 in the next decade. We ain't seen nothing yet! How exactly our lives will change cannot be predicted, but some of the new things that are ahead can be identified with great probability.

One of the new developments we can already see is that of 'wearables', like smart watches and Google Glass. Devices are getting continuously smaller and are attached to our body, integrating Internet in our life even more than is already the case now. The data we generate are increasingly stored in the 'cloud', on servers somewhere in the Internet rather than on our own devices. This has the advantage that we can access our information anywhere, on any device, and easily share it with other people. It also means that all data can in principle be connected.

Another important development is that of sensors. There are already many sensors in our smartphones: microphones, cameras, position measuring equipment, compass, accelerometers. Sensors are also increasingly integrated in our environment and in infrastructure, to measure all kind of properties: temperature, moisture, material integrity, air quality, etc. etc. Also, RFID[1] chips and sensors are attached to all kind of objects and products,

---

1   Radio Frequency Identification (RIFD) it is a simple chip that allows the tracing and tracking of objects to which the chip is attached;

enabling continuous tracking and monitoring. In this context the concept of the 'Internet of Things' is emerging. Sensors are connected to the Internet and are feeding a continuous stream of data about the physical world into the 'cloud'. Thus, a digital description of the world around us, including all infrastructure, houses, cities, objects and the real time position and properties of these assets, is built. Google maps, which besides geography and roads may already contain pictures of streets and houses and other assets, may be seen as a rudimentary form of this digital description of the world. The digital description will also contain information about people, where we are, what we do, maybe even about our pulse, blood pressure etc.

What we see emerge is one global system consisting of the Internet, all the connected intelligent devices and computers containing all information, and all sensors that generate data. One global 'cloud' that begins to resemble a living organism, with intelligence, a nerve system and senses. An organism that grows and evolves, becoming more and more complex.

It is important to note that this development is a rather autonomous process. The resulting system is not designed by humans (although its components are). It is growing and evolving because we all buy new stuff and connect it to the Internet. While the complexity of the system is increasing, we may expect new emergent behaviour of the system. We cannot predict this future behaviour, but one of the main questions is whether this system with increasing intelligence and complexity may develop some kind of consciousness, and to what extent it will control us instead of us controlling the system.

ICT is a disruptive technology, changing our behaviour and values

Not just enabling but disruptive

ICT is often regarded as an enabling technology, a technology that automates existing actions and processes, making these actions cheaper and more efficient. ICT is doing that, for sure, but ICT is much more. It is a disruptive technology, creating completely new possibilities and causing fundamental change to our lives and to our society.

ICT is truly a 'disruptive' technology. We see creative destruction. Automation means many people are losing their jobs, while on the other hand new jobs that did not exist before are created. The success of web shops, a completely new way of shopping, means the end of many retail shops. Digital music and video have brought tremendous changes in the entertainment industry. Consumers are empowered to express themselves through blogging, music recordings and video's and get exposure to a global audience, thus becoming so-called 'prosumers': producers and consumers of content at the same time.

Internet has brought new ways of learning, like Massive Open Online Courses, Kahn Academy, Hole-in-the-Wall, blended learning, gaming, developments that most certainly will disrupt traditional educational institutions in the coming years. Internet empowers children and adults who are truly motivated to learn by themselves, with amazing results.

We can access expert information on any subject. Patients can learn a lot about their disease from the Internet and interactions with other patients on Internet fora, enabling them to have informed discussions with medical staff and manage their own medical treatment.

ICT is challenging existing institutions like our legal system. Digital technology made it very easy to share information and make multiple copies of material that is protected by copyrights. New types of criminal behaviour emerge, cybercrime, which requires adequate counter actions.

Since so much digital information is stored on the Internet, our world is becoming fully transparent. This has huge advantages. Adverse behaviour of our political leaders becomes apparent and people can denounce this behaviour and protest against their government. Social media are a great help in this respect, as we have seen during the so-called Arab Spring. On the other hand, the Internet can also be used by dictators to find protestors and suppress actions that threaten their position of power. These two sides of the Internet have become quite obvious from the revelations made by Wikileaks and more recently by Edward Snowdon.

ICT changes our behaviour

On the one hand ICT is empowering the individual, while on the other hand it helps us to build and maintain relationships with others. This is one of the paradoxes of the Internet. Will this lead to more individualism, or to a more social world? Hopefully to a social world consisting of strong individuals. There does not have to be a contradiction.

Internet and mobile devices have created a world in which we are always online, always connected, wherever we are. As a result, the boundaries between work and private life, and between the here and now of real life and the digital world are blurred. The online world is addictive; we still have to learn how to live in this new reality. Internet makes us aware of what is happening in other places in the world, what is happening to our friends, and we can share with the world what we are doing and thinking. But how do we combine the real world with cyberspace? We often see people in a meeting, or having dinner at a restaurant with friends, who are more involved with their screen than the people they are with. Attention is a limited resource. How do we use it? Social media enable us to establish relationships with hundreds, or thousands of people. But with how many can we maintain a really meaningful relationship? There is so much information coming to us that it becomes difficult to handle. The Internet is screaming for attention, and it is sometimes difficult to resist. It becomes difficult for us to take time to concentrate and contemplate. Many young people find it difficult to read a book, being so accustomed to short bites of information. In his book The Shallows Nicholas Carr (2010) analyses this aspect of ICT. There are indications that frequent use of Internet has an effect on our memory and maybe even affects our brains.

ICT and Values

It is obvious that the new technology offers very powerful tools that have a profound effect on the way we live. A quote from Marshall McLuhan says: "First we build the tools, then they build us". As described in the previous paragraph, ICT is changing our behaviour, is changing maybe even our brain, our physical existence. ICT interacts with our values and our ethics. Our values determine our actions, our behaviour. We use tools, technology, to enhance our actions. If we do good, technology can help us to have a greater beneficial effect. By the same token, technology will amplify evil actions. We remain responsible for the choices we make, what we do and how we use technology, but we also have to be aware that technology may influence our choice. Some ICT tools will stimulate our creativity or our social behaviour, while other tools will stimulate controlling behaviour. ICT can assist in peace building, but also in making war. ICT empowers the individual, but can also be used to strengthen relationships. It is important that we become aware of what is really important to us, what our most precious values are, and consequently calibrate the way we use ICT to these values. For developers of ICT it is important to take user values into account when designing new technology (Van Oortmerssen, 2014). Users should make conscious choices of which ICT tools to use, and how and when to use them. We are all still in the process of adapting to ICT and the way we adapt depends on who we are, where we live, our culture and our values.

The digital divide and the gender gap

The digital divide

ICT with the new possibilities of e-learning and m-health brings a lot of hope for improving the standard of living and possibilities for economic growth and progress in low-income countries, in particular in rural areas without infrastructure, adequate schools and proper healthcare in place. The obstacle met here is called the digital divide, the lack of ICT infrastructure and skills in many developing regions. This has been recognised by many, resulting in initiatives for so-called ICT4D projects -- ICT for Development. The established development aid community, however, has never been too enthusiastic about ICT. They believe the priority should be given to clean water, food and health care. In the short term that might be so, but for the longer term it seems more effective and respectful to provide the tools to empower local people to take responsibility for their own lives.

When comparing the regions of the world, the African continent is the one with the least access to Internet. According to the International Telecommunication Union (2013) Africa has the lowest ICT Development Index (IDI). The IDI is based on three variables: ICT readiness (ICT infrastructure and access), ICT skills and ICT use. Its theoretical value is between 0 and 10. The most advanced countries in terms of ICT, South Korea, Scandinavia, the Netherlands, have IDI's typically between 8 and 9. In 2012 the IDI for Africa was 2.

ICT4D projects have been hampered mostly by lack of fixed network infrastructure, in particular in rural areas. Consequently Internet access often depended on satellite connections, which are prohibitively expensive. In addition, major barriers are presented by a lack of equipment, availability of components, lack of ICT skills needed to manage computer networks, and no or intermittent electric power supply.

An example of a successful project is Macha Works (Van Stam, 2010) that brought Internet to rural communities in Zambia using an approach of empowerment of local talented young people while paying attention to, and respect for the local cultural context.

There have been justified fears that the digital gap would be hard to close, or that it would even get wider, mainly because high income countries could enjoy wideband access at decreasing cost while in regions like rural Africa the access situation was stagnant. Fortunately the situation in Africa is changing rapidly, thanks to the advent of the mobile phone, which has spread over the continent at an incredible rate. Several countries show a double figure growth rate of mobile phone penetration. Consequently Internet access is changing dramatically within a short space of time.

Devices will continue to get cheaper and more abundant, which means that this new technology will increasingly become available to anyone in the world, including in low-income countries. Where in the past equipment sent to developing countries was often out-dated, the new smaller and cheaper devices, like smartphones, become available with smaller time lags.

The backlog in development and lack of resources to stimulate the take-up of disruptive ICT technologies in innovative ways can sometimes become an advantage, leading to a phenomenon called leapfrogging. One example is mobile payments. In Africa, which lacks a well functioning financial system, the possibilities of mobile networks for making payments has been readily recognised and systems for making payments with mobile phones have been developed. A well-known example of such a system is m-Pesa that is operational in several African countries. At present, Africa is leading the world in mobile payments. This successful innovation may lead to more examples. We begin to see centres of ICT-based innovation and business creation emerging in various places in Africa.

Notwithstanding this positive development there remain many challenges. Information on the web is predominantly available in English, not in local vernacular. In order to really empower people in rural areas it would require a "re-narration" of the web, using vernacular and adapting information to local contexts. Interesting work on this has been done by Dinesh (2012). In the re-narration model, a web page is rewritten to make it accessible to a target audience of users in a completely decentralised way. The notion of re-narration is completely general. It could, for example, mean translating a page automatically to another language. Or it could mean creating a more accessible version of a technical (or legal) document for laymen. There is also the possibility of text-to-speech to make written information accessible for illiterates.

The gender gap

According to Intel's report Women on the Web (2012): "On average across the developing world, nearly 25% fewer women than men have access to the Internet, and the gender gap soars to nearly 45% in regions like sub-Saharan Africa."

Though Africa has recently seen rapid growth in Internet access, women are vastly underrepresented in technology. The rise of cybercafes has benefited men more than women because boys and men have more freedom of movement to get to the cafes and have more access to make and spend money.

Furthermore, there is a disturbing trend of cyber bullying experienced by young women.

Because women face barriers such as poverty, illiteracy, and discrimination when getting training and education, we are witnessing the rise of a second digital divide according to Sow (2014). It is important to understand that technology and access to the Internet is essential to women's empowerment and it is therefore key to overcoming these barriers. Becoming technologically skilled can play a major role in getting jobs, being competitive in the job market and enable these women to pull themselves out of poverty.

The mobile phone may also prove to be a vast advancement with respect to the gender gap. Mobile phones are more accessible to women than computers, are user friendly and women do not have to leave their home to get Internet access. A recent study by Velghe (2013) in a township in South Africa has shown the amazing potential of mobile phones for literacy acquisition and informal learning. Women use the social network MXIT, which is quite popular in Africa, and they help their illiterate friends to use the phone and learn to read and write.

As Intel's report concludes: "The expansion of broadband and explosion of Internet-enabled mobile phones have begun to erode some of the toughest barriers to Internet access. They will continue to do so, and stakeholders must support these structural shifts and even help them to accelerate".

When women do have access, their use of the Internet is different compared to male users. Women spend more time on online shopping and are more active on social media. The active role of women in social media can be observed worldwide (Lee, 2011).

Challenges we are facing

Adverse effects of technological development

Technology has brought tremendous progress for mankind in all realms of life. Thanks to medical technology the average life expectancy has changed considerably; the world population has grown and continues to grow, while agricultural technology has made it possible to feed this large population. Technology has enriched our life, making it possible to live a comfortable life. Physical work has been alleviated or taken over by machines, computers automate many tasks, thus creating time for us to develop ourselves and do things that we find more meaningful. Long distance travel gave the possibility to experience other countries and cultures and to collaborate internationally.

At the same time this technological development has created new problems. Automation has resulted in a rise of unemployment. Industrial activities and use of hydrocarbons has created environmental problems and is changing climate at a frightening pace. The climate change in itself is a threat for agriculture, but also causes additional problems like rising sea level, extreme weather, tsunami's etc.

The continuing rise of life expectancy results in demographic changes, a need for more elderly care and the challenge to feed a still growing world population. Obviously there is a limit to how many people can live a decent life on our earth, but we do not know exactly where the limit lies.

The demand for energy is growing, while the end of supply of fossil fuel is coming in sight. Natural resources of all kind of metals and chemicals vital for technology are limited and some are nearing depletion.

The recent financial crisis has raised doubts about the adequacy of our economical system for the future.

Some may feel these problems are so severe that we should stop with further development of technology. This is no option. On the contrary, we will need more and smarter technology in order to be able to control and solve the problems caused by technology in the first place.

Regional inequalities: a potential cause for conflicts

As was mentioned in the first section of this chapter, technological evolution came in waves of increasing frequency. These waves, however, were not uniformly distributed over the globe. The waves in the various regions of the world were not in harmony, resulting in imperialism, exploitation and oppression. The picture of the world of today is that technology has enriched the life of many. But it is not equally available to all. Many people in low-income countries do not benefit from all the advantages technology can bring. The problems that result from the technological development are basically global problems. Climate change affects people wherever they live but its effects will probably be even more severe for farmers in low-income countries in Asia, Africa and South America.

Although people in less privileged regions may not have a car, modern agricultural tools, high standard health care etc., the one technology that comes within reach now is the most modern one: ICT. The digital mobile phone has penetrated most of the globe at an unprecedented speed. Mobile phones have brought the possibility for communication with family members away from home, and the technology helped many to improve their business. At the same time it has connected people in rural areas to the world, creating awareness of what is beyond the horizon, creating awareness of the inequalities in wealth and living conditions that exist in today's world. Differences in wealth, opportunities, access to resources, access to technology, living conditions, all these differences become obvious to everybody in a transparent, connected world and may lead to large scale migration, resentment and tensions and thus are a potential cause for conflicts.

Conflicts abound

As I write this, we commemorate the start of the First World War, the Great War that was said to end all wars. We now know how naive was this thought. When we look around we see fighting all over: in the Middle East, Africa, Europe, Asia. The character of armed conflicts has changed. In World War I the great nations were fighting each other, through soldiers shooting at each other on a rather confined battlefield. Now we often see situations where groups of rebels or fanatics take up arms. Anybody can join the fighting, sometimes even children. In many cases we see fighting within rather than between nations, typically between different ethnic or religious communities. Fighting is no longer taking place on confined battlefields but often in cities and villages, causing many casualties among civilians, in particular women and children. Terrorist actions can pop up anywhere, with the assault on the World Trade Centre in New York as a terrifying example.

Many believers in the blessings of Internet thought that the Internet would help to bring worldwide democracy and peace and that the so called Arab Spring, in which social media played an important role, were heralding this new era. I am optimistic myself about the opportunities that the Internet provides us with in this respect, but it is obvious that we need more time. Our ability as human beings to change and adapt to the new world order is a limiting factor. Change is rapid, so rapid and intrusive that we are confused and have difficulty to adapt, even in parts of the world that have experienced technological development for centuries. Many people living in remote rural areas with a traditional culture, however, did not have this experience and are now suddenly exposed to modern communication technology, connecting them to the world, confronting them with different values and belief systems. We have to recognise these differences and invest in promoting mutual understanding, building relationships and finding common values.

The grand challenge

One thing what we have in common is that we all live on this earth. We have to share finite resources. We have to share wealth, land, and opportunities. We are also facing the same challenges of climate change, pollution and conflict. How can we share in a fair way and live in peace? What is the future we will share? We come from a past with many communities, each with their own narratives about who we are, where we come from, and about the meaning of life. We are now entering an era with a new reality. Together we become aware that we are part of a global community. That does not mean that the old communities will no longer exist; they transcend into the global community. We have to reconcile the differences between the existing communities in order to make it possible that this new global community will prosper. We need a narrative for a common future. We have no alternative; time cannot be reversed.

Building a global community: the role women can play and how ICT can help

A global community, a new reality

We live in an exciting time. Technology is changing the world in an unprecedented way. Modern ICT is creating a connected world. The breakthrough of the Internet took off with the creation of the World Wide Web in 1989, the year that marked the fall of the Berlin wall. Mark Taylor (2001) suggested that this is no coincidence. In a connected world, the situation of two large power blocks divided by an iron curtain is not sustainable. Thus, the year 1989 can be seen as the start of a process of transition towards a really connected global community. This new reality that we cannot yet fully grasp, will be a complex one. The new world community will not be a single monolithic super 'nation' which ends all existing nations, but a community which includes a multitude of smaller communities. These constituent communities will have different scales. Some will live together in one location. Some will be spread out over the world but connected through Internet. Each community will have its own culture, its own narrative. Everybody will simultaneously be a member of several of these communities (as we already are), as well as of the global community.

The role of women and ICT

Violent conflicts have a great impact on women. It is estimated that women and children make up 80% of the worlds refugees. Male members of their families are often missing or detained in connection with hostilities. Therefore women bear increased responsibility for their children and elderly relatives. Women are often at the forefront of conflict prevention and resolution, post-conflict healing and reconciliation. ICT is a powerful tool for supporting women in peace building activities. As Jensine Larsen, founder of the women's network and online forum World Pulse formulates: "Being connected, heard, and externally validated within a global community provides many women the courage and support they need to become change agents at home." (Larsen, 2012: 40).

In October 2005, on the occasion of the 5th anniversary of the adoption of the UN Security Council Resolution 1325, the International Women's Tribune Centre launched the Peacebuilding Cyberdialogue which brought together women from Asia and Africa, representing 40 women's organizations through a 'real time global town hall meeting' using Internet. It connected women working on peace building and conflict resolution at country and community levels with gender advocates, policy makers and diplomats (Cabrera-Balleza, 2006). The Peacebuilding Cyberdialogue represented an important link in 'grounding' the connection between policies proposed at a global level and realities confronting women at the local level. It was an effective exercise in making local voices heard in a global space and bringing back that global discussion to make sense at the local level. Moreover, the Peacebuilding Cyberdialogue is an example of innovative usage of ICT. It should be remarked that in addition to Internet, local radio can also play an important role in reaching local communities.

There are many examples of grassroots initiatives where women come into action and use ICT to report local violence, mobilise local people, organise public actions. In Zambia, ICT has been used in the fight against gender-based violence. Organisations combating violence against women have used social media to help raise awareness and educate the public about gender-based violence. Access to social media is a particularly effective way to reach youth and mobilise them in campaigns against gender-based violence (Banda, 2012).

ICT also gives the means to reach out across borders to mobilise international support.

A recent case that illustrates this phenomenon is the international mobilisation around Boko Haram's kidnapping of schoolgirls in Nigeria (Morse, 2014). Across the continent, women's groups mobilised on social media through the hashtag #BringBackOurGirls to campaign for the release of the schoolgirls.

There are many empowerment organisations for women that use the power of ICT. One example is Make Every Woman Count (2014), which uses ICT as a tool to train women in Africa so that they are able to access the political arena more easily.

Peace building has to start at local scale, among neighbours. But our goal must be to achieve global peace, by building the global community and start a dialogue about the global challenges in order to mitigate tensions and prevent potential conflicts. Women have a special role to play here, with their focus on relationship, care and responsibility and ICT provide the means that can empower them to do this.

References

Banda, L. (2012) *Zambian teens learn Twitter & Facebook to stop violence against women* [online]. Available at: http://womennewsnetwork.net/2013/04/12/zambian-teens-twitter-and-facebook/ (accessed 22 August 2014).

Cabrera-Balleza, M. (2006) *Reclaiming women's space at the peace table: the Peacebuilding Cyberdialogue as a model of using ICTs for peace building* [online]. Available at: http://www.genderit.org/content/reclaiming-women%E2%80%99s-space-peace-table-peacebuilding-cyberdialogue-model-using-icts-peacebuild (accessed 22 August 2014).

Carr, N. (2012) *The Shallows: What the internet is doing to our brains* W.W. Norton & Company, New York, NY.

Dinesh, T. Uskudarli, S., Subramanya S., Deepti A. and Venkatesh C., (2012) "Alipi: a framework for re-narrating web pages", *Proceedings of the International Cross-Disciplinary Conference on Web Accessibility*, ACM, New York, NY.

Intel, Dalberg and Globescan (2012) Women and the Web: Bridging the internet gap and creating new global opportunities in low and middle-income countries Intel [online]. Available at:

http://dalberg.com/documents/Women_Web.pdf (accessed 22 August 2014).

International Telecommunication Union (2013) *"Measuring the Information Society"* ITU [online] Available at: http://www.itu.int/en/ITU-D/Statistics/Documents/publications/mis2013/MIS2013_without_Annex_4.pdf (accessed 22 August 2014).

Lee, A. (2011) Why Women Rule The Internet *TechCrunch* [online]. http://techcrunch.com/2011/03/20/why-women-rule-the-internet/ (accessed 22 August 2014).

Make Every Women Count (2014) [online] Available at: http://www.makeeverywomancount.org/ (accessed 22 August 2014).

Morse, F. (2014) "The Bring Back Our Girls Campaign is working: Boko Haram should be scared of a hashtag" *The Independent* [online] Available at: http://www.independent.co.uk/voices/comment/the-bring-back-our-girls-campaign-is-working-boko-haram-should-be-scared-of-a-hashtag-9360830.html (accessed 22 August 2014).

Oortmerssen, van, G. (2014) "Ethics and ICT: beyond design ». *2014 IEEE International Symposium on Ethics in Engineering, Science, and Technology,* IEEE, Chicago.

Sow, R. (2014) "Women and ICT in Africa: A new digital Gap", *Aljazeera* [online]. Available at: http://www.aljazeera.com/indepth/opinion/2014/05/women-ict-africa-new-digital-ga-201452210244121558.html (accessed 22 August 2014).

Stam, van, G. and Oortmerssen, van, G. (2010) *'Macha Works'. Proceedings of the WebSci10: Extending the Frontiers of Society On-Line, April 26-27th, 2010,* Raleigh, NC.

Taylor, M. (2001) *The Moment of Complexity.* The University of Chicago Press, Chicago.

Velghe, F. (2013) "Literacy acquisition, informal learning, and mobile phones in a South African township", *ICTD '13 Proceedings of the Sixth International Conference on Information and Communication Technologies and Development,* ACM, New York.

CHAPTER 14.
WOMENLEADERS4PEACE: FINDING AN AUTHENTIC AND MEANINGFUL CONTRIBUTION IN A CONFLICTED AND SEXIST GLOBALIZING WORLD

Ineke Buskens

> In the course of history there comes a time when humanity is called to shift to a new level of consciousness. To reach a higher moral ground. A time when we have to shed our fear and give hope to each other. That time is now.
>
> Wangari Maathai's
> Excerpt from Nobel Peace Prize Acceptance Speech, 2004

Introduction

On 31 October 2000, the United Nations Security Council adopted Resolution 1325 which gave a commitment to

> reaffirming the important role of women in the prevention and resolution of conflicts and in peace-building, and *stressing* the importance of their equal participation and full involvement in all efforts for the maintenance and promotion of peace and security, and the need to increase their role in decision-making with regard to conflict prevention and resolution (UNSC 2000 Preamble).

Since that moment, the world has seen what seems an escalation of violent occupations, revolutions, sectarian violence and civil war. At the same time 'a growing body of literature has painted a less optimistic picture of the resolution and its implementation', which is "portrayed as yet another 'trick' played by the members of the Security Council in an effort to appease women activists" (Tryggestdad, 2009). It is therefore timely and pertinent, in the light of the abovementioned comprehensive commitment to women's equal participation and full involvement in matters of peace and security, to consider what leadership qualities women could bring to efforts for alleviating, mediating and possibly preventing more conflict and violence, and what they would need in order to contribute fully and meaningfully.

This chapter seeks to explore the relationships between female leadership, peace and justice in a globalizing world. Justice is brought in relation to peace in the sense that absence of justice implies absence of peace, even when open conflict has not erupted (yet). Leadership is understood as the capacity/power to change realities, ideas, and people (including oneself) emerging in response to a situation and not exclusively defined by a position or personality characteristic. Paramount to the type of leadership our globalizing and conflicted world seems to ask for are first, the capacity to align tasks, organisations, persons, thoughts and emotions to a purpose of social justice; secondly the capacity to collaborate instead of dominate, which implies the capacity for dialogue and for creating opportunities for dialogue; and thirdly the capacity to establish credibility as a leader, which is grounded in establishing coherence between intentions and actions, between ideologies and interventions and between doing and being.

After discussing leadership capacities for a globalizing world, grounded in recent examples of war and political unrest, this chapter will sketch the specific leadership gifts women can bring to conflict resolution and peace building. It will touch on the specific challenges they would have to overcome as women and women leaders given almost ubiquitous sexism and gender discrimination. It will conclude by suggesting that enhancing self and gender awareness will enhance women leaders' capacity to make an authentic and meaningful contribution to conflict resolution and peace building efforts, in our globalizing and conflicted world.

Leadership, justice, globalization and peace

The world we live in is a deeply unjust and hence conflicted place. The structural inequalities that are embedded in relations of domination between and within countries, institutions, peoples and persons have given rise to endemic injustice in access to and control over resources and wealth distribution. The inevitable and seemingly perpetual conflict makes the world a very unstable and volatile place. Arguing that our particular econcentric global worldview is deeply elitist, as it "works to the benefit of the few and penalizes masses of people today and in the future". Willis Harman, futurist and past president of the Institute of Noetic Sciences, characterizes our time as follows:

> At one time, it was a dominant belief in western society that if you behaved pretty well here on this plane you'd go to heaven; that belief system held the society together in certain ways. Then we changed that belief and essentially said if you can trample on others and succeed then you'll get the most toys in the end and you'll win the game, and people behaved accordingly (Harman, 1995).[1]
>
> Because the underlying value system of our global civilization is grounded in an economic ideology that has made monetary value its king pin and keystone, human beings and the natural environment do not hold intrinsic value (Buskens, 2013: p. 329).

In order to embark on a coherent trajectory towards sustainable development, peace is pertinent: peace between persons, people, organizations and countries. Human history has however given us ample opportunity to realise that peace needs to be grounded in justice and that measures of justice need to be backed up by truthful reporting.

Facilitated to a large degree by the use of Information Communication Technology (ICT) and social media, global collaborations and solidarities have emerged that cut across the boundaries of nation states and other human divides. How global relationships and solidarities effect existing leaders and give rise to emerging leadership acts can be illustrated through two recent events: the Ferguson Incident and the latest war on Gaza.

On 9 August 2014, an unarmed African American teenager, Michael Brown, was killed by a white police officer for no apparent reason in Ferguson, St Louis, Missouri, United States of America (USA).[2] The unrest that was caused by this incident was treated heavy-handedly by the police with journalists covering the protest demonstrations, assaulted, tear-gassed and arrested (Taibi, 2014). The incident evoked responses from Palestinians

---

1. It will invariably be the most powerful institution in our society that will determine the parameters in which we think, act and find our meaning as human beings in relationship to each other. In this era, this institution is what we have come to understand as The Global Economy and hence the term econocentric worldview or paradigm. In the words of Willis Harman: "Every society has some kind of an organizing myth; traditional societies had one, medieval society had one, we have one. Very central to our modern myth is the idea that it's perfectly reasonable that the economy should be the paramount institution around which everything else revolves, and that economic logic and economic values should guide our decisions" (Buskens, 2013: p.329).
2. The reason given by the police officer and the friend accompanying Michael Brown, was the fact that Brown was walking in (the middle of) the street. Ferguson protests. (McCarthy, 2014).

who tweeted to Ferguson citizens with advice on how to deal with teargas attacks and expressing empathically that they know from experience how it is to be attacked because of one's ethnicity (Times of Israel, 2014; United States Hipocrisy, 2014). This incident brought into sharp focus the unresolved issue of racial discrimination and injustice in the United States.[3] President Obama acknowledged this and urged the various stakeholders to listen to and attempt to understand each other, so that justice and peace could be brought about.[4]

The incident also raised pertinent questions regarding the militarization of the US police force and the role Israel has played and still plays in the training of US police (Dail Kos, 2011.[5]

The Ferguson Incident happened at a time that Israel received intense international attention and increasing critique because of its latest attack on Gaza. When it became apparent that certain US weapon deliveries were dispatched to Israel without approval of the White House, this evoked strong negative local and global reaction and a halt to the transfer by President Obama (Ravid, 2014). It needs no explanation why the lack of clear political oversight had dismayed the US President, but this issue also became a concern for quite a few global citizens. The arms trade is big business (Shah, 2013) and what this means in a neo-liberal capitalist world economy where monetary value is kingpin and human lives do not hold intrinsic value, should in itself be cause for grave concern. But the fact that

---

3. The show of military-style force in an American city has created a huge backlash because the underlying concerns for justice have not been addressed. (Kucinich, 2014).
4. "And that requires we listen, and not just shout. That's how we're going to move forward together -- by trying to unite each other and understand each other, and not simply divide ourselves from one another. We're going to have to hold tight to those values in the days ahead. And that's how we bring about justice, and that's how we bring about peace." (Washington Post, 2014).
5. It is alleged that the New York Policy Department has opened a branch in Tel Aviv, and that there is regular training given to U.S. Police personnel by Israeli military (Ashkenzi, 2011; Daily Kos, 2012). See also the Jewish Institute for National Security Affairs (JINSA) (http://en.wikipedia.org/wiki/Jewish_Institute_for_National_Security_Affairs), a neoconservative think tank, that claims to have hosted some 9,500 law enforcement officials in its Law Enforcement Exchange Program (http://www.jinsa.org/events-programs/law-enforcement-exchange-program-leep/all) since 2004. Not only does LEEP take "delegations of senior law enforcement executives to Israel to study methods and observe techniques used in preventing and reacting to acts of terrorism", it also "sponsors conferences within the United States, bringing Israeli experts before much larger groups of law enforcement leaders (http://www.jinsa.org/files/LEEPbookletforweb.pdf).

political oversight and due regulatory process regarding major arms deals were lacking also raised questions pertaining to democracy and governance: "Has globalization become a threat to democracy? Can democratically elected leaders fulfill their mandate in a globalizing world within the current economic dispensation?"

At the same time, the transnational solidarity that sprung up after the Ferguson Incident prompted the emergence of unexpected leadership. The first Palestinian citizen to tweet to Ferguson initiated him or herself as a global leader through this act. In our networked world we are all global citizens, no incident is merely local anymore, (cyber) dialogues on happenings in places as far apart as Ferguson and Gaza inspire reflections on justice as a necessary condition for peace and leadership emerges 'from the bottom up' (Towil, 2014).

Leadership4Peace: Purpose-alignment, Integrity and Dialogue

The capacity for social justice, i.e. the capacity to understand structural inequality and mitigate and/or act towards correcting it, needs translation in the here and now into specific purposes. Effective leaders present visions, or higher purposes that appeal to peoples' values and function like a moral compass for the people who have come together for a specific purpose. A higher purpose could be: "A world where all people are free" or "a world that works for all."[6]

Purpose-alignment

Purpose-aligned leadership is effective because it can adapt to a complex and fluid reality. The shared alignment creates an open system where the learning gained along the way forms and informs objectives, goals and operations; where newcomers can be included as long as they are aligned to the shared purpose; where leaders do not exclusively rely on best practices or past blueprints but are committed to a process of discovery, design and deciphering rather than of engineering, dictating and presupposing (Pascale, Milleman and Gioja, 2000: 171-195). Purpose-aligned leadership is however also a complex capacity that requires a deep and empathic understanding of the socio-political-economic-religious-historical context from a local and

---

6. Berret-Koehler Publishers is 'dedicated to an ambitious mission "Creating a World that Works for All"'. The Berrett-Koehler Story; http://www.bkconnection.com/static/story.asp. The GRACE Network's higher purposes are: "a loving, just and sustainable world" and "a world where all people are free" Buskens 2014a: p. 3 and Buskens 2014b: p.295.

increasingly global perspective as well; a firm belief that the envisaged future is humanly possible; a tolerance for uncertainty; the confidence to resist the temptation to fall back on tried recipes because 'they worked in the past' and a talent for facilitating people's thinking and acting through open ended processes.

Integrity

For leadership to be effective it has to be credible and hence integrity is another important requirement of leadership. In our connected and globalizing era, every moment is a 'photo-moment' and every saying and every act of leadership will inevitably be shared with the world. Secrecy is not what it was been anymore. The bulk document released by whistle-blowers such as Bradley Manning and Edward Snowden into mainstream media have established a political climate of radical openness and transparency. If there is something that the current crises in our globalizing world show, however, it is that lack of integrity in leading figures. Discrepancy between words and deeds, incoherence between proclaimed intentions and actions will sooner or later be revealed through the use of Information Communication Technology. The contributions of amateur journalists in conjunction with the ubiquitous use of social media, the easy availability of camera enhanced mobile phones make it ever more pertinent for leaders to be authentic and coherent in order to stay credible.[7]

In recent cyber dialogues for instance, the US president and government have come under stark condemnation for the discrepancy between their continued military and diplomatic support for Israel whilst at the same time criticizing Israel for the increasing number of Palestinian civilian deaths in Gaza (Waters, 2014). The Israeli government has been criticized for its proclamation that it wants peace whilst acting contrary to that through continuing the occupation of the West Bank, expanding the illegal settlements, pursuing the blockade of the Gaza strip and more recently, its 50 day bombardment of Gaza (Levy, 2014; Glazebrook, 2014; Hedges, 2014).

Integrity however not only speaks to the sense of coherence between intention and action and between ideology and intervention in the sense of "meaning what you say, saying what you mean and doing what you say," but it also refers to the coherence between doing and being. The person of the leader her or himself communicates directly what her/his leadership is about.

---

7. "But once the testimony of the activists became available and the blogosphere got its teeth into the visual evidence, from whatever source, an alternative picture quickly emerged and the mainstream media struggled to keep up." (Lerman, 2010).

The quality of being that leaders would need in order to be convincing, especially in striving towards conflict resolution or peace building, can be described as having 'peace within'. Peace within does not necessarily mean that one is (able to) live a peaceful life, live in a peaceful environment or be without emotional turmoil. The 'peace within' can be understood as the authentic coherence one has created within oneself between ones purposes, thoughts, emotions, actions and behaviour. This 'peace within' flows from authentic self-acceptance and from the joy one experiences when one can freely express who one is (becoming), in actions that are meaningful in relation to what one values in life. Authenticity is an important characteristic of leadership (Helgesen & Johnson, 2010). To have 'peace within' is pertinent when one wants to contribute to peace: you cannot 'give the peace that you do not have' yourself. [8]

Dialogue

Capacity for dialogue is paramount for any leader in any situation. The type of communication that seems very suitable for leaders4peace in the context of the maintenance and promotion of peace and security, seems to be the mode of communication which Marshall Rosenberg (Rosenberg, 2003) calls Non-Violent Communication (NVC) and which Kazanka Comfort and John Dada formulate as a home-grown mode of peace mediation traditionally used by African elders (Comfort & Dada, 2014). Crucial in this form of dialogue is to stay compassionately focused on the observed needs of people and communities (Comfort & Dada, 2014: 114) and refrain from judgment or diagnosis (Rosenberg, 2003). The NVC imperative to express honestly and receive empathically resonates with the open-heartedness and open-mindedness that Adri Smaling recommends for research dialogues. Open-mindedness implies being open to the partner and her/his sharing and open-heartedness means not holding back issues, feelings, insecurities or embodied experiences when they are relevant to the conversation (Smaling, 1995: 29). Both speaking and listening are grounded, in the NVC approach, in the four elements or key pieces of information, which are shared in dialogue: observations, feelings, needs and requests (Rosenberg, 2003).

Characterizing NVC as a language of the heart, Rosenberg affirms that this approach to communication frees one from cultural conditioning; allows one to break patterns of thinking that lead to argument, anger and depression; enables one to resolve conflicts peacefully, whether personal or public, domestic or international; that it creates social structures that support

---

8. Leaders such as Martin Luther King and Mahatma Gandhi chose the path of peace to accomplish justice. Acting from coherence between beliefs and actions, did grant them inner peace.

everyone's needs are being met and that it will lead to the development of relationships that are based upon mutual respect, compassion and cooperation. He admits however, that it can make one feel vulnerable in situations where not all partners are committed and/or versed in this type of communication but asserts that, as it leads us to give from the heart, it will connect us with ourselves and with each other in a way what allows our natural compassion to flourish. Rosenberg affirms that he uses the term 'nonviolence' in the way that Gandhi used it "to refer to our natural state of compassion when violence has subsided from the heart" (Rosenberg, 2003: 8).

Women and leadership for peace: a match made in heaven?

Women's leadership accomplishments would understandably be under reported (because unacknowledged) in a male-dominated world and much female leadership would remain un and under-developed. Yet, a variety of discourses seem to suggest that women's leadership would not only be different and complementary to that of men, but that it would be very much in tune with the needs of our globalizing world and very valuable in relation to sustaining and creating peace. At the onset of this section however, I want to note that the following observations and reflections do not speak to all women in an absolute and essentialist sense, but I do suggest that there are enough indications that they would pertain more to women than to men, given the way women and men are currently socialised and that they would be true in various degrees to a majority of women.

Women's capacity as life-givers and care takers seems to predestine women as natural peace makers and women seem to have contributed to peace making efforts in Africa and elsewhere across times and cultures in sacred and ritualized ways (Isike and Okeke Uzokike, unknown).

Speaking to the way women have been able to fulfill top political positions in Asia, Amartya Sen recommends "to pay more attention to the part that women have been able to play, given the opportunity, at diverse levels of political activities and social initiatives" (Sen, 1999: 200). Discussing how empowerment of women contributed directly and indirectly to the well being of their families, communities and societies, Sen concludes that, "nothing, arguably is as important today in the political economy of development as an adequate recognition of political, economic and social participation and leadership of women" (Sen, 1999: 203).

Women seem to develop their self-in-relationship, which is different from the male focus on the self as an independent, separate and autonomous unit. The capacity for relational expression therefore co-constitutes their core-self (Jordan et al, 1991) and this predisposes women to develop the capacities for caring for others and for creating nurturing environments. Women's moral development has been described by Carol Gilligan (1982) as the development of an ethic of care and her work endeavours to explain why 'a morality of rights and non-interference may appear frightening to women in its potential justification of indifference and unconcern' (Gilligan, 1982: 22).

These observations resonate with those of Sally Helgesen and Julie Johnson, who have found that women's leadership style is different from men not only in what they do, but in what they value and therefore notice. Discussing the absence of senior women executives in the firms that caused the 2008 financial crisis in the US, and interviewing women that had raised early, albeit unheeded, concerns about their firms' risky behaviour, they concluded that women leaders differ from men in that they care deeply about the social fabric of their companies and society at large and are thus less enamoured with risks and short term gains at the expense of a sustainable future. Because women value the social fabric of their world and want to align their work with their vision of how best to serve this, they found it very disturbing to see their companies compromise on those visions. Furthermore, women's capacity for 'broad spectrum notice' and empathy, and their tendency to being focused in the present moment instead of mainly oriented towards a potential future, would have alerted them to danger signals before men would become aware of such (Helgesen & Johnson, 2010).

When women engage processes of personal change and transformation, their families, communities and societies change with them. When women change, they seem to 'change-in-connection', with their connections changing with them and growing stronger in and through the processes of change they have set in motion (Buskens, 2014a). As Helgesen and Johnson confirm, women experience themselves in the centre of a web of relationships rather than on top of a hierarchy (Helgesen & Johnson, 2010).[9]

Transferring these observations about female leadership to the earlier discussed needs of leadership in our globalizing world and to the area of conflict resolution and peace making, it can be postulated that women are eminently suitable to develop the kind of leadership4peace that our conflicted globalizing world seems to ask for: women's capacity of broad

---

9 These two authors deplore the fact, that whilst women leaders have much to give in the current era, the world of business does not seem ready to accept what they have to offer: women leaders are not defining the 'what' and the 'why' yet; whilst more and more organizations value what women do, they do not appreciate fully women's greatest gifts: their vision and their ideas (Helgesen and Johnson, 2010).

spectrum notice would facilitate purpose aligned, adaptive leadership; women's capacity for empathy and their tendency to value the relational aspect of situations and events, would facilitate their capacity to appreciate context and engage effective dialogue. Because women value the social fabric of their world and want to align their work with their understanding on how best to strive towards accomplishing this, women have the mental equipment to become coherent and hence credible leaders.

Regarding the area of conflicts resolution and peace making, women's talent for empathy and relationship would bring relational and caring qualities to the various processes, from decision-making level to execution procedures, and this would make it easier for people to reach each other across the various divides. The fact that women tend to embody the relational aspects of change processes seems particularly relevant and appropriate in the fields of conflict resolution and peace building since processes of peace, especially where they are grounded in and aligned with seeking to establish social justice, are inevitably processes of social change.

Whilst women leaders' leadership capacities thus seem to be particularly suited for purposes of peace in our conflicted globalizing world, the following questions present themselves: How can womenleaders4peace establish their credibility as leaders in a sexist world? How can they give what is authentically theirs against the sexist tide and contribute fully and meaningfully? How can they experience and hence radiate their peace within?

WomenLeaders4Peace: Challenges in a sexist world

As a first step in taking up the challenge of contributing fully and meaningfully as womenleaders4peace, it is important for women to take full cognizance of the reality of sexism and patriarchy in their environments. Without acknowledging this reality they will not be able to equip themselves to overcome and where possible transform the challenges they might face because of their gender. Such an understanding needs to comprise several aspects:

> Since women will be inclined to bring an empathic and relational openness, and need for connectedness to the various situations they face, they are particularly vulnerable to sexist and discriminatory situations. They would thus need to recognize the ways sexism and patriarchy are mediated in and through social relations. This will help them to accept such realities and relationships without taking such personally and allowing them to define situations, projects and purposes.
>
> Since women have learnt to develop their dreams according to what was deemed desirable in accordance with their traditional role in society, they may have developed an 'in-authentic' understanding about female well being

and hence their own personal well being in the situations they find themselves. Having 'adapted their preferences' (Nussbaum, 2000) to a sexist and discriminatory environment, they may have become active participants in their own disempowerment as women. Therefore, in order to understand and express their more authentic self, they may have to develop their 'capacity for voice' in conjunction with their 'capacity to aspire'.

Appadurai (2004: 63) brings the 'capacity to aspire' into dialogue with Hirschman's (1970) concept of voice. Whilst his treatise focuses on the poor, his reflections can be extended to women: "The posture of 'voice,' the capacity to debate, contest, inquire, and participate critically" (2004: 70) is the capacity to engage social, political and economic issues in terms of the ideologies, doctrines and norms that are widely shared and credible, and hence this capacity is reflexively related to the capacity to aspire. "It is through the exercise of voice that the sinews of aspiration as a cultural capacity are built and strengthened, and conversely, it is through exercising the capacity to aspire that the exercise of voice by the poor will be extended" (2004: 83). Women may have to go through a process of revelation to fully appreciate how their deepest understandings of themselves as women and their ways of negotiating their needs may actually be expressions of their subaltern position in male dominated societies. Subordinate groups have been socialised to think for, and in support of, the dominant group and its interests even when this would disadvantage themselves. In the same vein, women have learnt to think for and in support of the male gender and its interests and so may have become part of, and agent in, their own oppression (Baker Miller, 1991). Women may have limited their preferences and choices as to what they have learnt is socially acceptable (Nussbaum, 2000) and they have learnt to see many of their authentic aspirations for themselves as 'selfish' (Gilligan, 1982). In order to flourish as WomenLeaders4Peace they would have to see, acknowledge and transcend the ways in which they give their power away by adhering to traditionally accepted norms, beliefs and practices. Having fully acknowledged this, they can embark on a journey of authentic self-discovery, empowering themselves to contribute to their personal life trajectories and that of their families, communities and societies in more authentic and sustainable ways.

Given that women's personal experiences and perspectives have been formed and informed by the fact that they are human beings that are living as women in a sexist world, it is perfectly understandable that women may have developed coping strategies that make them more judgmental of women than of men and even discriminate women because they are women (Chesler, 2001). How will women learn to see, acknowledge and deal with their own inevitable and probably partially unprocessed sexism versus women and men? These questions are pertinent to all women, yet they are pivotal for WomenLeaders4Peace because of the responsibility women leaders have and because of the impact their sexism will have on people and on processes of conflict resolution and peace building.

Since peace in a sexist and unjust world has to be grounded in social and gender justice, WomenLeaders4Peace that are aligned with justice need to question themselves as to what 'peace' actually means: the absence of blatant and bloody conflict, or the absence of justice and mutual respect? It seems more sound theoretically, strategically and humanely to understand open conflict and injustice as different points on the continuum of 'absence of peace'. They would thus be wise to investigate themselves and other women as to what degree they have come to accept gender injustice as normal. Subordinated groups have been socialised to expect unjust treatment and when they experience anger or bitterness they will tend to suppress this or otherwise express it in ways that will not threaten the social 'harmony'. But a situation of endemic injustice is not reconcilable with sustainable peace.

Finally, WomenLeaders4Peace have to realise that their society's perspectives on aggression and power have been formed and informed by a male dominated society where generally men get to be dominant and aggressive and women get to do the caring, repairing and nurturing work. With society generally placing a higher priority and reward, monetarily and otherwise, on dominance and aggression than on the caring and nurturing that women are groomed for, women need to ask themselves what it means for them to take up a role as peace makers in such a dispensation. It would be important to question this issue, so as not to perpetuate an imbalanced gender dispensation by and through their peace building efforts.

It has become obvious that WomenLeaders4Peace are undertaking a complex and involved endeavour in this deeply sexist, unjust and conflicted world. Relations of dominance create a complexity in society where a superficial layer of social harmony between various groups co-exists with a deeper layer of seething dissent about the inequality and injustice underneath. The impact this all has on the self may be partly unconscious. This would make it more difficult for oppressed and dominated groups, such as women, to find a coherent and authentic relationship with oneself and come to joyful self-acceptance. Experiencing 'the peace' within and being able to communicate this, is possibly the most powerful and enduring leadership quality in times of conflict when peace-making capacity is most pertinent. And whilst women may have special gifts in this regard as women because of evolutionary development and / or through gender socialization, they also face the biggest challenges in this regard because of the pervasive reality of male domination, which is not only present in external social structures but also is embedded in the deeper recesses of the personal self.

Self and gender awareness as part of WomenLeaders4Peace training

Since situations of conflict resolution and peace making will inevitably create delicate situations where people could be exposed and vulnerable a special leadership training for WomenLeaders4Peace would have to include the following elements: purpose-aligned, adaptive leadership capacity, empathic dialogue such as for instance grounded in the Non Violent Communication approach and a discipline of enhancing personal self and gender awareness in conjunction with engaging women's capacity to aspire and their capacity for voice.

In order to be good leaders to both women and men, and to lead processes of conflict resolution and peace building, WomenLeaders4Peace have to take their own gender socialization seriously and strive towards becoming aware how the internalization of gender beliefs and practices has affected their sense of self and their relationship with themselves and with others (Buskens 2014 b, 2014c). Since leadership is grounded in women's agency, it stands to reason that women leaders could and should become agents of their own processes of becoming aware of their gender socialization and the degrees in which, and ways in which, this socialization predisposes them to self-limiting beliefs and behaviours and sexism towards self and others.

As has been argued earlier in this text, women have learnt to adapt themselves to sexist and patriarchal environments and have learnt to reflect on themselves and their aspirations, conditioned by these impeding cultural factors. As women's capacity to reflect on and conceptualize their feelings, experiences and perspectives may be formed and informed by the dominant culture to the degree that they have become agents of their own discrimination and oppression, they have to become aware of these processes and transform the mental dynamics of self-limitation into dynamics of self-liberation. This will not only support them in coping with and transforming their personal gender discrimination experiences and patterns, but it will also make them better leaders of women and men.

The clarity and confidence women leaders would gain through such a process would help them to establish coherence between their intentions, purposes and the processes they set in motion. Expressing themselves with joy in who they are and what they do and aligning themselves with the values they cherish, in words and deeds, will enable them to enact their relational leadership capacities, effectively and sustainably in a conflicted world.

Summary: FemaleLeadership4Peace: capacities and challenges

Since women, because of evolutionary development and gendered socialization, have a capacity for 'broad-spectrum notice', relationship and empathy, the kind of adaptive leadership style that a conflicted globalizing world requires, will suit them well. WomenLeadership4Peace capacity has a preventative and a management function: since women tend to be concerned about the social fabric in their environments and notice threats to social harmony, it is less likely that systemic injustices would emerge and be continued when they could pursue their authentic concerns and perspectives and when their suggestions would be given full authority. Because of their 'caring' socialization and relational capacities women would be able to create the kind of nurturing environments that would make it possible for people to reach out to each other over the various 'divides', which would make eruption of conflict less likely. Furthermore, because women very likely have had the experience of gender injustice, being 'othered' and discriminated against because of their gender, they may be better able to empathise emotionally with oppressed and excluded groups and persons than men might be. When women could translate their concern for the well being of the social fabric, into effective responses and measures, the emergence of injustice-induced conflict would be reduced. Because of women's capacity for empathy and relationship, women would also be eminently suitable to mediate in conflict situations and create opportunities for the various parties to communicate with each other and resolve their mutual grievances.

Female leaders however, face specific challenges as women in a male dominated and patriarchal world. In the first place, women's leadership (capacity) may not be given sufficient authority because of their gender and in the second place, women may also find it hard to voice their perspectives, thoughts and experiences coherently and confidently because they have adapted their being, doing, thinking, feeling and relating to a male dominated conceptual universe.

In order for femaleleadership4peace potential to become a feasible reality, the challenges women face in a sexist and male dominated world should therefore not be under estimated and women should be supported on how to deal with such in the most fruitful and growth-enhancing way. Opportunities should be created for women with leadership potential or needs to develop, besides the above mentioned leadership capacities, the capacity for self and gender awareness (Buskens, 2014b, 2014c).

Conclusion

The eighteen provisions of Resolution 1325 of the United Nations Security

Council, whilst covering a broad range of issues and concerns that apply to the levels of the headquarters and member states of the United Nations, as well as to the operational level of the organization's activities, can "roughly be separated into three main categories (Tryggestad 2009):

1. Representation. The resolution urges member states to increase the representation and active participation of women at all decision-making levels in national, regional, and international institutions and mechanisms for conflict prevention, conflict management, conflict resolution, and peace building.
2. Gender Perspective. A gender perspective should be adopted in the planning and implementation of peace operations and peace negotiations, including gender-sensitive training of personnel, an expanded role for women as peacekeepers, and increased attention to local women's peace initiatives, needs, and interests in mission areas.
3. **Protection.** The resolution emphasizes the need for increased attention to the protection and respect of women's rights, including protection against gender-based violence in situations of armed conflict and initiatives to put an end to impunity for such crimes."

In this chapter, women's potential leadership capacities and challenges in conflict resolution and peace making have been discussed. It is suggested that in order for women leaders to optimize their capacities and overcome their challenges, it would be good for them as part of a leadership training for peace, to engage a discipline of self and gender awareness. This is different from, and in addition to, the second category of Resolution 1325 perspectives: the Gender Perspective category. Whilst support for women leaders in a sexist environment is absolutely necessary, it would not be sufficient. Leadership capacity is grounded in agency and hence women leaders have to develop their capacity for agency, which, in a male dominated world is grounded in the capacity for voice and the capacity to aspire.

Women who have developed their capacity for voice and their capacity to aspire, and have learnt how gender discrimination has affected their awareness of self and their social world, will be better equipped to deal with the inevitable sexist and discriminatory experiences and relations they will be confronted with in their efforts to mediate conflict and make peace. They will not only be better able to protect themselves, but through becoming more empowered and socially confident (because they know they can affect their world) also have more impact on their environment and their society and consequently be more effective in their peace making work. Being able to be and act more authentically as WomenLeaders4Peace, their contributions will thus be more authentic and hence more meaningful.

References

Appadurai, A. (2004) 'The Capacity to Aspire: Culture and the Terms of Recognition' in V. Rao & M. Walton (eds.), *Culture and Public Action*, pp. 59-85, Stanford University Press, Palo Alto, CA, pp. 59-85.

Ashkenazi, A. (2012) NYPD Opens Branch in Israel, *Al Monitor*, 5 September 2012 [online]. Available at: http://www.al-monitor.com/pulse/security/01/09/nypd-kfar-saba-branch-new-york-p.html# (accessed 24 August 2014).

Baker Miller, J. (1991) 'The Construction of Anger in Women and Men' in J. Jordan, A. Kaplan, J. Baker Miller, I. Stiver and J. Surrey (eds.), *Women's Growth in Connection - Writings from the Stone Centre*, Guilford Press, New York.

Buskens, I. (2014a) 'Introduction', in I. Buskens and A. Webb (eds.), *Women and ICT in Africa and the Middle East: Changing Selves, Changing Societies*, Zed Books / IDRC, London, pp. 1-21.

Buskens, I. (2014b) 'Research Methodology for personal and social transformation: purpose- aligned action research, intentional agency and dialogue', in I. Buskens and A. Webb (eds.), *Women and ICT in Africa and the Middle East: Changing Selves, Changing Societies*, Zed Books / IDRC, London, pp. 275-291.

Buskens, I. (2014c) *Developing the Capacity for Gender Awareness in Development Research: Some Thoughts and Suggestions – A Think Piece for the IDRC's Information and Networks Team*, International Development Research Centre, Ottawa.

Chesler, P. (2001) *Woman's Inhumanity to Woman*. Thunder's Mouth Press/Nation Books, New York.

Comfort, K. and Dada, J. (2014) 'ICT in a time of sectarian violence: reflections from Kafanchan, Northern Nigeria' in I. Buskens and A. Webb (eds.), *Women and ICT in Africa and the Middle East: Changing Selves, Changing Societies*, Zed Books, IDRC, London, pp. 111-122.

Daily Kos (2011) Are U.S. Police training with the Israeli Military? Daily Kos, 12 December 2011 [online]. Available at: http://www.dailykos.com/story/2011/12/12/1044508/-Are-U-S-Police-training-with-the-Israeli-Military# (accessed 22 August 2014).

Glazebrook, D. (2014) Israel's target is not Hamas, but Palestinian statehood, Middle East Eye 8 August 2014 [online]. Available at: http://www.middleeasteye.net/columns/israel-s-target-not-hamas-palestinian-statehood-1483362297 (accessed 22 August 2014).

Harman, W. (1995) Transformation of Business – The evolution of consciousness, culture, and business from the foundations of structures that will replace the crumbling old order. An Interview with Willis Harman by Sarah van Gelder – One of the articles in

Business on a small planet. *Context Institute*. [online]. Available at: http://www.context.org/ICLIB/IC41/Harman.htm (accessed 15 July 2014).
Hedges, C. (2014) Why Israel lies, *Truthdig*, 3 August 2014 [online]. Available at: http://www.truthdig.com/report/item/why_israel_lies_20140803 (accessed 22 August 2014).
Helgesen, S. and Johnson, J. (2010) *The Female Vision – Women's Real Power at Work*, Berrett-Koehler Publishers, San Francisco.
Hirschman, A. (1970) *Exit, Voice and Loyalty: Responses to Decline in Firms, Organizations, and States*, Harvard University Press, Cambridge, MA.
Isike, C. and Okeke Uzokike, U. (2011) 'Towards an indigenous model of conflict resolution: Reinventing women's roles as traditional peacebuilders in neo-colonial Africa' in *African Journal on Conflict Resolution* 11(2) pp. 32-58.
Jordan, J., Kaplan, A.,Baker Miller, J., Stiver, I. and Surrey, J. (1991) *Women's Growth in Connection – Writings from the Stone Centre*, Guilford Press, New York.
Kucinich, D. (2014) Militarized Police and the Threat to Democracy, *Huffington Post*, 18 August 2014 [online]. Available at: http://www.huffingtonpost.com/dennis-j-kucinich/police-militarization_b_5687598.html (accessed 24 August 2014).
Lerman, K. (2010) Israel PR machine won Gaza flotilla media battle, *The Guardian*, 4 June 2010 [online]. Available at: http://www.theguardian.com/commentisfree/2010/jun/04/israeli-pr-machine-gaza-flotilla-media-battle (accessed 22 August 2014).
Levy, G. (2014) Israel does not want peace, *Haaretz, 4 July 2014* [online]. Available at: http://www.haaretz.com/news/diplomacy-defense/israel-peace-conference/1.601112 (accessed 22 August 2014).
Nussbaum, M. (2000) *Women and Human Development: The Capabilities Approach*, Cambridge University Press, Cambridge.
McCarthy, T. (2014) Ferguson protests: Michael Brown family calls for calm amid criticism of video release – as it happened *The Guardian*, **15 August 2014 [online]. Available at: http://www.theguardian.com/world/live/2014/aug/15/ferguson-police-officer-michael-brown-darren-wilson (accessed 16 August 2014).**
Pascale, R., Milleman, M. and Gioja, L. (2000) *Surfing the Edge of Chaos – The Laws of Nature and the New Laws of Business*. Texere, London.
Ravid, B. (2014) U.S. halts missile transfer requested by Israel, *Haaretz, 14 August 2014* [online]. Available at: http://www.haaretz.com/news/diplomacy-defense/1.610493 (accessed 22 August 2014).

Rehn, E. and Johnson Sirleaf, E. (2002) *Women, War and Peace – The Independent Experts' Assessment on the Impact of Armed Conflict on Women and Women's Role in Peace-Building*, United Nations Development Fund for Women, New York.

Rosenberg, M. (2003) *Nonviolent Communication: A Language of Life*, 2nd edn, PuddleDancer Press, Encinitas, CA.

Sen, A. (1999) *Development as Freedom*, Oxford University Press, Oxford.

Shah, A (2013) The Arms Trade is Big Business, *Global Issues, 5 January 2013* [online]. Available at: http://www.globalissues.org/article/74/the-arms-trade-is-big-business (accessed 22 August 2014).

Smaling, A. (1995) 'Openmindedness, open-heartedness and dialogical openness: the dialectics of openings and closures', in I. Maso, P. Atkinson, S. Delamont and J. Verhoeven (eds.), *Openness in Research: The Tension between Self and Other*, Van Gorcum, Assen, pp. 21–32.

Taibi, C. (2014) Ferguson Police Use Tear Gas On Al Jazeera America Team, *Huffington Post, 14 August 2014* [online]. Available at: http://www.huffingtonpost.com/2014/08/14/al-jazeera-ferguson-tear-gas-journalists_n_5678081.html (accessed 16 August 2014).

Tawil, S. (2014) No justice, no peace – in Gaza of Ferguson, *Mondoweiss, 20 August 2014* [online]. Available at: http://mondoweiss.net/2014/08/justice-peace-ferguson.html (accessed 22 August 2014).

Times of Israel (2014) Palestinians tweet support for Ferguson protesters, *Times of Israel, 15 August 2014* [online]. Available at: http://www.timesofisrael.com/palestinians-tweet-support-for-ferguson-protesters/ (accessed 15 August 2014).

Tryggestad, T. (2009) *Trick or treat? The UN and implementation of security Council resolution 1325 on women, peace, and security*. Free Online Library [online]. Available at:
http://www.thefreelibrary.com/Trick+or+treat%3F+The+UN+and+implementation+of+security+Council...-a0215069791 (accessed 17 July 2014).

United Nations Security Council (2000), Res. S/RES/1325/2000; Refworld | Security Council resolution 1325 (2000) [on women and peace and security] [online]. Available at: http://www.refworld.org/cgi-bin/texis/vtx/rwmain?docid=3b00f4672e; 31 October 2000; (accessed 26 August 2014).

United States Hypocrisy (2014) Palestine's Letter of Solidarity With Ferguson, Missouri, *USHipocrisy,* 18 August 2014 [online]. Available at: http://ushypocrisy.com/2014/08/18/palestines-letter-of-solidarity-with-ferguson-missouri/ (accessed 22 August 2014).

Waters, R. (2014) Pink Floyd's Roger Waters: Why moral perversity of U.S. position in Gaza is stunning, *Salon, 25 August 2014* [online].

Available at: http://www.salon.com/2014/08/25/pink_floyds_roger_waters_why_moral_perversity_of_u_s_position_in_gaza_is_stunning/ (accessed 25 August 2014).

Washington Post (2014) Full Transcript: Obama's Remarks on Ferguson, MO and Iraq, *The Washington Post,* 18 August 2014 [online]. Available at: http://www.washingtonpost.com/politics/running-transcript-obamas-remarks-on-ferguson-mo-and-iraq/2014/08/18/ed29d07a-2713-11e4-86ca-6f03cbd15c1a_story.html (accessed 24 August 2014).

CHAPTER 15. A RELIGIOUS DEDICATION TO COMMUNITY: THE LASTING PROMISE OF THE CONCEPT OF CARITAS IN A PLURALIST WORLD

Erik Borgman

In this article, I will try to show why and how religious attitudes and religious concept, in particular the Christian concept of caritas, charity, is important in our thinking about community, both locally and globally. It is well known that religious traditions can exclude the contribution of other traditions, religious or secular, from the necessary attempts to find common ground in a world of differences. However, religious concepts can also bridge gaps and make connections, thus building a community of people from a wide diversity of cultures. Here, I will argue that the concept of caritas is directed towards a community of people aware of the fact that they depend on one another and that we are responsible for each other's wellbeing.

Religious dedication and openness

In December 1957, then Secretary General of the United Nations Dag Hammerskjöld (1905-1961) wrote a text meant to consecrate the United Nations Meditation Centre, referred to by him as 'A Room of Quiet'. Hammerskjöld explains that given the fact that people of many faiths will use the room none of the usual symbols expressing religious identity could be used in the room. For that reason the architects have found some "simple things which speak to all of us with the same language". For instance, there is a stone in the middle of the room, a large block of iron ore, symbolizing the earth as an inheritance, a gift and a responsibility to human beings:

> We may see it as an altar, empty not because there is no God, not because it is an altar to an unknown god, but because it is dedicated to the God whom man worship under many names and under many forms.

But the Room of Quiet itself, "dedicated to silence in the outward sense and stillness in the inner sense" in Hammarskjöld's formulation, is the ultimate symbol:

> There is an ancient saying that the sense of a vessel is not in the shell but in the void. So it is with this room. It is for those who come here to fill the void with what they find in their centre of stillness. (Hammarskjöld, 1957)

Some four years earlier, at the beginning of his first term as Secretary General, Hammarskjöld had personally given his wholehearted support to the people that were lobbying for a Meditation Room in the U.N. building:

> I do not believe in the possibility of such cooperation as we are engaged in [in the U.N.] without the deep inspiration of faith in ideals which we all share. 'Ideals' in itself is a general word. What I mean here are the ideals established by our deepest faith and highest longings. (Lispey, 2013: 325)[1]

At that moment in time, hardly anybody was aware of the fact that Hammarskjöld himself lived from a deep religious commitment that was fundamental to what he considered to be his task as a Secretary General.

For the general public the Christian mysticism that at least according to his own conviction enabled Hammarskjöld to bear the heavy responsibilities of his office, only came to light with the posthumous publication of *Markings* (Swedish original: *Vägmärken*), the diary reporting on what he called his 'journey inwards'. It has become recognised as a spiritual classic. Only in these personal notes it becomes fully clear how much the imitation of Jesus Christ's life of dedication and self-sacrifice until the end meant to Hammarskjöld, as he had to find his way to the ever uncertain and dangerous landscapes of international politics, in which he eventually would lose his life. [2]

However, in November 1953, in a statement made on an American radio show called 'This I Believe', produced by the then famous journalist Edward R. Murrow, Hammarskjöld had already said:

---

1. 'Summary of remarks by Dag Hammarskjöld on 12 August 1953'
2. Hammarskjöld was killed in a diplomatic mission to Congo, under circumstances that never were fully clarified. (Williams, 2011).

... the explanation of how a man should live a life of active social service in full harmony with himself as a member of the community of the spirit, I found in the writings of those great medieval mystics for whom 'self-surrender' has been the way to self-realization, and who in 'singleness of mind' and 'inwardness' had found strength to say yes to every demand which the need of their neighbours made them face, and to say yes to every fate life had in store for them when they followed the call of duty, as they understood it. "Love' – that much misused and misinterpreted word – for them meant simply an overflowing of the strength with which they felt themselves filled when living in true self-oblivion. And this love found natural expressions in an unhesitant fulfilment of duty and in an unreserved acceptance of life, whatever it brought them personally of toil, suffering – or happiness.

I know that their discoveries about the laws of inner life and of action have not lost their significance. (Hammarskjöld, 1954)[3]

In Hammarskjöld view, there was no contradiction whatsoever between religious commitment and openness to the unknown and ability to learn from it should it reveal itself. Strictly speaking, there was not even a tension. For him, firm religious rootedness made it possible to be open to the different expressions others cultivated to feed their dedication. His mystical Christianity enabled Hammarskjöld, as he wrote in *Markings,* to purify longing into openness: "each action a preparation, each choice a yes to the unknown". (Hammarskjöld, 1957)

The same line of thought led Marga Klompé (1912-1986) in 1948, then the only female member of the Dutch delegation to the negotiations on the Universal Declaration of Human Rights who would eventually become the first female government Minister in the Netherlands. [4] As a devoutly practicing Roman Catholic, Klompé was convinced that human rights was rooted in the creation of human beings in the image of God. However, when it became clear to her that this was not the consensus among those dedicated to passing the Universal Declaration, she wrote in her personal diary: "Can we enforce a conflict of consciousness on others? I think not."[5] Therefore

---

3. A recording of the programme is available at: http://thisibelieve.org/essay/16608/.
4. See the article of Mirjam van Reisen in this volume.
5. Cf. Erik Borgman e.a. (ed.) (2012), *In Liefde en Rechtvaardigheid: Het dagboek van Marga Klompé 1948-1949,* Hilversum: Verloren, 51: 'Mogen wij anderen een gewetensconflict opleggen? Ik vind niet' (entry 8 October 1948). For further background, see Erik Borgman (2012), '"Iemand die... de liefde centraal heeft gesteld": Het geloof van Marga Klompé', in: Erik Borgman and Mirjam van Reisen (ed.), *De verbeelding van Marga Klompé: Perspectieven op de toekomst,* Zoetermeer: Klement, 43-68, here esp. 55-60.

she did not insist on bringing the Divine origin of human dignity into the declaration. For Hammarskjöld and Klompé the personal and deep adherence to the Christian tradition was a bridge to connect to people dedicated to others traditions of faith and culture. Because for them the lives of human beings had an inherent quality of sacredness, they considered it their obligation to be open to the longings and visions expressed in other traditions and cultures, religions and philosophies than their own.

A charity as wide as the world

Both Hammarskjöld and Klompé drew inspiration from the mystical tradition within Christianity. One of Klompé's favorite mystics was Saint Catherine of Siena (1347-1380). As she traveled to Rome in 1948, Klompé jots down in her diary that she prays on St. Catherine's grave. The body of Catherine of Siena was – and still is today – located in the Santa Maria Sopra Minerva in Rome. During Klompé's first visit to Rome in 1948 that church was 'opposite my hotel room' (7 Sept. 1948). Klompé was in the habit of attending Mass daily and during her stay in the Eternal City she probably did that in this Church. Be that as it may, the presence of Catherine of Siena so close by meant a great deal to Klompé. She noted in her diary:

> This morning in Church something became very clear to me. If I want to do something good in politics, I shall have to be totally an instrument, that is to say that spiritual deepening has to come before everything else. This has been made clear to me by Catherine of Siena, I think (10 Sept. 1948).

Catherine of Siena had been living a retired and reclusive life in one room at the house of her parents. From a life of contemplation and fasting, at a certain moment she came to become feverishly political – she succeeded in convincing the Pope that he should return from Avignon to Rome – and to charitable activity. It gave her a large group of followers. It is probably her freedom and her dedication to the welfare of the world and the Church that spoke to Klompé.

We do not know what exactly Marga Klompé had read from the writings of Catherine of Siena. But as a matter of fact Catherine wrote rather eloquently on the love of community that was at the heart of Klompé's commitments all her life. In one of her many visions, Catherine of Siena heard God explain to her how He had bound human beings with 'the chain of charity':

> Thus, that you may practice charity in action and in will, I in my providence did not give to any one person or to each individually the knowledge for doing anything necessary for human life. No, I gave something to one, something else to another, so that each one's need would be a reason to have recourse to the other. So though you may lose your will for charity

because of your wickedness, you will at least be forced by your own need to practice it in action. Thus you see the artisan turn to the worker and the worker to the artisan: each has need of the other because neither knows how to do what the other does. [...] Could I not have given everyone everything? Of course. But in my providence I wanted to make each of you dependent on the other, so that you would be forces to exercise charity in action and will at once (Catherine of Siena, 1980: 311-312).

We need *caritas,* we have to love one another and care for one another in order to survive. We tend to limit our charity to those we know. We need, however, to love especially those who really differ from us.

After her political career Marga Klompé dedicated her life to building, consolidating and securing the Dutch branch of the Ponticial Council for Justice and Peace, a global Roman Catholic organisation to promote social justice and mutual responsibility, established in 1967 in the aftermath of the Second Vatican Council. Embodying Christian love and trying to help a little to realise God's plan with the world was, in her view, the task of the council. And God's plan, in her view, was a decent and dignified life for all people.[6]

In a more political vein, the usually very diplomatic Dag Hammarskjöld indicated on 4 May 1959, speaking at the University of Lund in his native Sweden, the provincial character of what had long been seen as 'universality' in European culture. With a striking boldness, he stated:

> Goethe's 'universality' was combined with a firm conviction of the supremacy of the European man of culture, a supremacy which erected invisible walls around the spiritual life in relation to other parts of the world.

This European alleged supremacy not only lead to colonialism as an expression of an attitude Hammarskjöld called 'untenable' – which in 1960 was certainly not generally excepted – but also to a closing of the spirit. It was only after the First World War that 'the whole closed European circle was broken up'. What strikes us, Hammarskjöld said, about European views on other cultures dating before this breakthrough, is:

> in the first place, perhaps,... how much they did *not* see and did *not* hear, and how even their most positive attempts at entering into a world of different thoughts and emotions were coloured by an unthinking, self-assured superiority...

In Hammerskjöld's view, he and his contemporaries are the lucky ones

---

6. Cf. Victor. Scheffers and Gerard Swüste (ed.) (2006), 'Mensen kunnen de wereld veranderen': Over de inspiratie en de bewogenheid van Marga Klompé, Den Haag: Justitia et Pax.

for having the possibility of the 'richest satisfaction in meeting different spiritual traditions and their representatives', thus attaining the biggest possible treasures to achieve what he considered 'the common future goal', a world of both universality and unity on the one hand and a deep understanding and respect for difference and diversity on the other. Building this future means, Hammarskjöld's feels, walking in the footsteps of "askers of questions like Socrates or the carpenter's son from Nazareth". With this reference to Jesus, Hammarskjöld makes clear how being religiously committed does not contradict openness for ideas originating from outside one's own tradition. The ultimate embodiment of the Divine in Christianity, Jesus Christ himself, in his view exemplified openness.

Three year earlier, on 3 February 1956, Hammarskjöld had given a clear example of how his interpretation of the Christian tradition could lead to conclusions that may be considered surprising. Addressing the Indian Council of World Affairs in what he characterised himself as a speech from notes made in the plane coming to New Delhi, he made the surprising point that we should not understand support to poor countries from rich countries as 'aid' or 'help'. We should consider them as 'charity'. He was fully aware that he was on thin ice here, and not just because he relied on a specific, highly profiled Christian idea. He tackled the possible misunderstanding without much ado:

> Now I want to be very clear from the very beginning so that nobody, when I use the word 'charity', misunderstands it. I mean it in the original sense as something a brother does for a brother, not as a handing-out operation with the benevolence of the 'haves' in the relation to the 'have-nots'. I mean charity in the sense of mutual cooperation in a well-understood common interest. (Hammarskjöld, 1954: 659)

Gender inclusivity in language was not yet invented in the 1950s, but we can assume that to Hammarskjöld 'charity' was also what 'a sister does to a sister'.

Hammarskjöld starts from the idea that, as he admits himself is 'no news to anybody', namely that today's world is 'more than ever before one world'. This situation, he argues, does not mean the end of solidarity and charity and the start of a situation in which every nation and every people has to fight for itself and its own. On the contrary, in this interdependent world charity is needed more than ever:

> The weakness of one is the weakness of all, and the strength of one – not the military strength, but the real strength, the economic and social strength, the happiness of the people – is indirectly the strength of all. Through various developments which are familiar to all, world solidarity has, so to say, been forced upon us". (Hammarskjöld, 1954: 661)

We have to be charitable to one another, because in that way we can all receive abundantly from each other's riches and it will be clear that in the ultimate analyses there are no 'haves' and 'have-nots'.

Caritas as core concept to understand society

In contemporary societal and political debates, charity, *caritas,* has become a problematic concept. *Caritas* is considered to be something additional, an 'extra'. It is generally taken for granted that *caritas* would not be necessary if society would function well. *Caritas* is seen not as something a brother does for a sister and a sister for a brother, as Hammarskjöld saw it, but as additional support for those who need help and cannot properly support themselves. *Caritas,* charity, is understood in a way exactly opposite to how Hammarskjöld wanted it understood: as 'aid', 'help'. As a consequence, the debates about *caritas* focus on whether peoples or countries applying for it really need it, and whether the help that can be given will really solve their problems. This is the situation within nations, but also between nations. *Caritas* is seen as a favour of which individuals, peoples and countries should prove themselves worthy.

There is, however, a different tradition of thinking about the relation between *caritas* and society. In the tradition of Catholic Social Thought, canonized in a whole range of documents originating from members of the hierarchy, theologians and social philosophers within the Roman Catholic Church and more or less systematised in the *Compendium of the Social Doctrine of the Church* (2004), but also a living tradition of reflecting on social questions from a Christian point of view close to social practices, *caritas* is considered as an integral and essential aspect of being human. *Deus caritas est* was the first sentence of the first encyclical of now Pope emeritus Benedict XVI in 2005, quoting from the first letter of John (4:16): 'God is love', charity. The document explains how the Catholic tradition takes as its starting point that human beings are created in the image of God. God is love and therefore their natural human *eros* is intrinsically directed towards *agape;* their desire is for love, love to give and love to receive.[7] The natural inclination of human beings is to connect with one another, to be cared for by one another and to care for one another. Therefore, from this point of view, *caritas* is not something that can or cannot be added to society, as an addition that should not be necessary. Society comes into existence and is maintained because people are inclined to *caritas*. Living together in community as brothers and

---

7. Benedict XVI, encyclical *Deus Caritas Est* (25 Dec. 2005), no. 3-8 http://www.vatican.va/holy_father/benedict_xvi/encyclicals/documents/hf_ben-xvi_enc_20051225_deus-caritas-est_en.html

sisters, members of the same family, is *caritas* incarnate.[8]

This is of course not to deny that human beings also have an inclination to avoid the uncertainty *caritas* brings them in. *Caritas* requires recognition of one's dependence on what others can only freely give: appreciation and commitment, compassion and care. To depend on the logic of the free gift is highly unsettling.[9] This unsettlement is what we tend to avoid, for instance by fantasizing that we our society is a matter of an enforceable contract. Therefore, the centrality of *caritas* to human societies is not self-evident. It has to not just be explained, but defended and preached.

'The relationship between God and man is reflected in the relational and social dimension of human nature', states the *Compendium of the Social Doctrine of the Church*.[10] (no. 110). This is in line with one of the major documents of the Second Vatican Council (1962-1965), were the then Roman Catholic bishops agreed on the statement that the human being is in fact not a solitary being, but 'a social being, and unless he relates himself to others he can neither live nor develop his potential'.[11] (Pastoral Constitution *Gaudium et Spes*, no. 12). This approach opens up the concept of *caritas* and makes it the foundation of being human. It clarifies how love for others, expressing itself in the desire that all will be well for them, is ultimately limitless. This comes to light, over and over again, but that often goes unnoticed. Take Jesus' famous parable of the Good Samaritan:

> A man was going down from Jerusalem to Jericho, and fell into the hands of robbers, who stripped him, beat him, and went away, leaving him half dead. Now by chance a priest was going down that road; and when he saw him, he passed by on the other side. So likewise a Levite, when he came to the place and saw him, passed by on the other side. But a Samaritan while travelling came near him and when he saw him, he was moved with pity. He went to him and bandaged his wounds, having poured oil and wine on them. Then he put him on his own animal, brought him to an inn, and took care of him. The next day he took out two denarii, gave them to the innkeeper, and said, 'Take care of him; and when I come back, I will repay you whatever more you spend.' […] Go and do likewise. (Luke 10:29-37)

---

8. Cf. Benedict XVI, encyclical *Caritas in Veritate* (29 June 2009), no. 19 http://www.vatican.va/holy_father/benedict_xvi/encyclicals/documents/hf_ben-xvi_enc_20090629_caritas-in-veritate_en.html
9. Ibid. 34.
10. *Compendium of the Social Doctrine of the Church* (2 Apr. 2004), no. 110 http://www.vatican.va/roman_curia/pontifical_councils/justpeace/documents/rc_pc_justpeace_doc_20060526_compendio-dott-soc_en.html
11. Pastoral Constitution on the Church in de Modern World *Gaudium et Spes* (7 Dec. 1965), no. 12 http://www.vatican.va/archive/hist_councils/ii_vatican_council/documents/vat-ii_const_19651207_gaudium-et-spes_en.html

Jesus does not so much instruct his disciples what to do, but he tells us what he sees happening and what should be valued and imitated. Connections are made via *caritas* between Samaritan and Jew, which is beyond the usual social boundaries, because the Samaritan recognizes the predicament of the other as concern of his own. In recognizing their fundamental dignity as threatened and violated, people who are habitually seen as standing outside one's own community, are spiritually and conceptually made participants of that community, are seen as family. From there, it is logical to help them to participate more fully, sharing the benefits and being seen as essential for the community. Through *caritas* we built communities and within these communities the members help one another to blossom.

In my view, this means *caritas* should not so much be seen as a principal to implement, something that is lacking if Christianity is lacking. The Mediaeval theologian Thomas Aquinas (1225-1274) considers *caritas* as not itself a virtue, but 'the form of the virtues' that are needed to maintain a decent and safe society.[12] This is scholastic language stating that our societal behaviour and social habits should not be replaced, but inspired by *caritas*. This brings us back to Hammarskjöld. In a world that exists in an unending plurality of connections uniting people in relations of mutual interest and responsibility, the point is not that what Hammarskjöld called the 'haves' should give something of their affluence to the poor and needy 'have-nots'. The point is that for us as a community of humans the quality of all our lives depends on our ability to make *caritas* the heart and soul of our connections. At the Second Vatican Council, the Roman Catholic Church made clear that this is at the heart of the Christian message: in Jesus Christ it is revealed that 'the new command of love was the basic law of human perfection and hence of the world's transformation'.[13] It is however not exclusive to Christians.

Ubuntu

Ultimately, *caritas* is the expression of the unobjectifiable conviction that it is fundamentally rewarding to have a committed relation to people who are different. Everybody has something unique and irreplaceable to offer and *caritas* is the attempt to enable others to really offer it. The idea that our society is not complete as long as not everybody has the opportunity to contribute to it in his or her own term is ultimately a matter of belief. The Christian tradition endorses this belief by insisting that every person is in his

---

12. *Summa Theologiae* II-II, questio 23, articulus 8 http://dhspriory.org/thomas/summa/SS/SS023.html#SSQ23A8THEP1; cf. *Compendium of the Social Doctrine of the Church,* no. 207).
13. Gaudium et Spes, no. 38.

or her special way an image of God and the outcome of history will be the full revelation of who is God. This clarifies that society is optimal when is brings everyone to his or her right, and vice versa, bringing everybody to his or her right is the way to optimise society.

Desmond Mpilo Tutu, the former Anglican archbishop of Cape Town, South Africa, has clearly explained why in his view 'God is definitely not a Christian'. It is impossible for God to exclude anything valuable and because there are clearly valuable elements in other religions, God's presence cannot be limited to Christianity (Tutu, 2011: 3-11)[14]. Tutu goes on to explain that the African concept of *ubuntu,* translated by him in the adage 'I am because I belong' as replacing the Cartesian principle 'I think, therefore I am', is for him definitely among the valuable inheritance that comes from outside Christianity. The concept, he thinks, is a necessary weapon against the Western culture of achievement that tends to make human beings expendable when they do not produce or contribute material things to the richness of society.

> In traditional African society, *ubuntu* [...] was seen as what ultimately distinguished people from animals – the quality of being human and also humane. Those who had *ubuntu* were compassionate and gentle, they used their strength on behalf of the weak, and they did not take advantage of others – in short, they *cared,* treating others as what they were: human beings.

Ubuntu is still highly valued in Africa, according to Tutu. Which is a good thing, in his view, for it makes it impossible, as he explains with a loose reference to the parable of the Good Samaritan, 'to pass by on the other side' simply because one does not want to become too involved. (Tutu, 2011: 22-23)[15]

Both the concept of *caritas* and the concept of *ubuntu* clarify how on a deep level commitment to society can never be limited to *my* society as *I* conceptualise it from *my* tradition, and to the people that contribute to it in ways *I* consider valuable. It requires involving those who are usually excluded, accepting what they bring as valuable for them and adding if possible what they may lack. We do not know where this will take us, but as Tutu makes clear, from a religious point of view this is exactly the uncertainty we should be able to face. The Parable of the Good Samaritan starts with the question of a Jewish scribe, who wants to know what it means

---

14. In 'God is clearly not a Christian: Pleas of Interfaith Tolerance', (Tutu, 2011)pp. 3-20
15. In '*Ubuntu:* On the Nature of Human Community' (Tutu, 2011) pp. 21-24

to love one's neighbour. Tutu understands Jesus' answer to mean:

> 'Hey, life is more exhilarating as you try to work out the implications of your fate rather than living by rote, with ready-made second-hand answers. fitting an unchanging paradigm to a shifting, changing, perplexing, and yet fascinating world.' Our faith, our knowledge that God is in charge, must make us ready to take risks, to be venturesome and innovative; yes, to dare to walk where angels might fear to tread.

This is not a plea to take risk for risk's sake, like some kind of spiritual bungee jumping. It is taking risks for the sake of humanity, finding a way forward by bringing into the community the best we have in our different traditions, because only that will take us to where we belong: a community in which the God who is *caritas* will be all in all. In that sense, from a Christian perspective, it is taking risks for God's sake. As God himself in Jesus Christ took the risk of becoming vulnerable unto death, in order to restore community with our human vulnerability.

Conclusion

As human beings, we are vulnerable beings. Dealing with our vulnerability means first of all to accept it and to realise that as vulnerable beings, we need one another so stay alive and to build a common world that enables us to sustain one another. In almost all of the current understanding of development and aid, this is forgotten. Already in 1958 the Jewish-American philosopher Hannah Arendt (1906-1975) saw the danger. She asked:

> Should the emancipation and secularization of the modern age, which began with a turning-away, not necessarily from God, but from a god who was the Father of man in heaven, end with the even more fateful repudiation of the earth who was the Mother of all living creatures under the sky?

For Arendt, this question was related to the launch of a Sputnik on 4 October 1957 and the successful attempt by the Russians to bring it into an orbit around the earth. The *New York Times* saw this as the first step of man to break free from the Earth and Arendt quotes a statement from the Russian space theoretician Konstantin Tsiolkovsky-Kaluga (1857-1935) who had inspired the Sputnik programme: 'Mankind will not remain bound to the earth forever.' For Arendt, the connection to the earth is the essence of human condition. The desire of mankind to escape the earth is a denial of its own existence (Ardent, 1958: 1-2). We need Mother earth to sustain us and as human beings, male and female, we are called to embody the grace she incarnates, thus showing our gratitude for that grace.

"This is my commandment", says Jesus according to the Gospel of John, "that you love one another as I have loved you" (John 15:12). Jesus led a life of grace and gratitude, we are told. This is the kind of life that can save.

References

Arendt, H (1958) *The Human Condition,* University of Chicago Press, Chicago.

Catherine of Siena (1980), *The Dialogue,* SPCK, London.

Hammarskjöld, D. (1954) 'The United Nations – It's Ideology and Activities' in A. Cordier, & W. Foote, (eds.) Public Paper of the Secretaries General of the United Nations. Volume 2. *Dag Hammarskjöld 1953-1956*, (1972) Columbia University Press, New York pp. 658-673.

Hammarskjöld, D. (1956) 'Old Creeds in a New World' in A. Cordier, & W. Foote, (eds.) Public Paper of the Secretaries General of the United Nations. Volume 2. Dag Hammarskjöld 1953-1956, (1972) Columbia University Press, New York pp. 195-196.

Hammarskjöld, D. (1957) 'A Room of Quiet (The United Nations Meditation Room)' in A. Cordier, & W. Foote, (eds.) Public Paper of the Secretaries General of the United Nations. Volume 3. *Dag Hammarskjöld 1956-1957*, (1973) Columbia University Press, New York pp. 710-711.

Hammarskjöld, D. (1974) 'Asia, Africa, and the West' in A. Cordier, & W. Foote, (eds.) Public Paper of the Secretaries General of the United Nations. Volume 5. *Dag Hammarskjöld 1958-1960*, Columbia University Press, New York pp. 380-387.

Hammarskjöld, D. (1974) *Markings,* Knopf 76, New York.

Lipsey, R. (2013) *Hammarskjöld: A Life,* University of Michigan Press, Ann Arbor.

Tutu, D. (2011) *God Is Not a Christian: Speaking Truth in Times of Crisis,* Rider, London.

Williams, S. (2011) *Who Killed Hammarskjold? The UN, the Cold War and White Supremacy in Africa,* C. Hurst & Co., London.

CHAPTER 16. DIGNITY AS A BASIS FOR THE POST-2015 DEVELOPMENT AGENDA: THE RELEVANCE OF THE LEGACY OF MARGA KLOMPÉ FOR A UNIVERSAL POVERTY ERADICATION PROGRAMME

Mirjam van Reisen

In the first place we are the inheritors of the unfulfilled aspirations of our ancestors posits the German philosopher Walter Benjamin (1991). He suggests that perhaps it is not our forefathers' (or foremothers') achievements that determine us, but the dreams they left behind. We become the caretakers of those dreams that were not realized and of the ambitions that were not completed by previous generations.

Marga Klompé, an icon of Dutch society, dreamt of a world governed by "loving care and justice", in which dignity for all was the basis of its organization, its governing structures and its laws. She was a leader in the resistance in the Second World War, a founding parliamentarian of the European Union, a negotiator of the Universal Declaration of Human Rights and Minister of Social Affairs; the first female minister of The Netherlands. This article takes her ambitions for a just global social society as a point of departure for a reflection on the post-2015 Development Agenda. How do her aspirations reflect in the Agenda for a future better world for all? Does this agenda sufficiently well reflect the ambitions that are carried over to us from past generations?

Connecting the future with the past

The post-2015 Development Agenda process encompasses the entirety of global negotiations for establishing a new global vision on the global eradication of poverty and sustainable development, a vision to replace the Millennium Development Goals (MDGs). The MDGs have set targets for 2015. The process has a distinct orientation on the future, but we can only think this future in today's present. Hence, this future is the future as we imagine it today. This present imagination of a future agenda is much influenced by our past.

Rothberg (2009) looks at how the present is produced from our memories of the past. He analyses remembrance of the Holocaust in the Age of Decolonization. In contrast to a theoretical approach of competing memories he proposes that "memories interact productively in unexpected ways". This theory provides an interesting conceptual framework for the analysis of the post-2015 Development Agenda. Rothberg's analysis reminds us that the post-2015 Development Agenda is a reflection of how society and members of society therein collectively produce aspirations that build on memories about the past. These evolve from our understanding of the past; from the normative and ethical ideals derived from this understanding.

This article sets out to reflect on this, based on the life of one person: Marga Klompé. She was the first female Minister of The Netherlands, a very concerned parliamentarian when the government was overseeing the brutal decolonization-process of The Netherlands with Indonesia. She was a leader in the resistance in the Second World War, which had a strong impact on her life. Marga Klompé was a negotiator in the Dutch delegation on the negotiations of the Universal Declaration of Human Rights. As a Minister of Social Welfare she laid the foundation of the social welfare legislation in The Netherlands. And importantly, she had experienced poverty in her own life, as a young person, which deeply affected her understanding of poverty, vulnerability and marginalization.

Defining Poverty

Marga Klompé was born in 1912 as the second in a family of five children. Her father was the owner of a small company. Unfortunately the family was thrown in poverty after he became mentally ill, a disorder from which he would never recover. Marga's mother, who was from German descent, refused to accept the charity offered by the churches, mainly because she (proudly) resisted what she experienced as condescending patronage that would accompany such support. In those inter-bellum years, churches prescribed over most aspects of family life: a persons marriage, reproduction, school, church-going and political affiliation were closely monitored. Instead of accepting the aid offered, the Klompé-women (mother and daughters) worked in all kinds of ways to try and make a living. Marga, who had a good intellectual brain, was sent to school and would teach to help provide income for the family.

The experience of poverty and dependency on aid very much define Klompé's understanding of it. She saw poverty as something that could happen to anyone. She refused to see poverty as something specific for a particular pre-defined group. She defined poverty as contextual, a condition that was the result of situational circumstances, as opposed to resulting from innate factors. She defined poverty as temporary – as something that could be overcome once the situations leading to poverty had been addressed. Her concept of poverty was deeply universal: everyone could one day become poor and anyone could come out of poverty under the right circumstances. She also identified an inalienable link between poverty and social protection; poverty resulted from the inadequacy of society to organize and provide social protection for its vulnerable members.

Her negative experience with dominant prescriptive church-based charity resulted in a clear vision to prioritize the protection of dignity of people living in poverty. To protect integrity and dignity, Klompé legislated by strictly separating material support, social support and spiritual matters. She did not accept that support to poverty-relief should be linked to conditionality in any way, and identified the respect of human dignity as the central principle to guide any support. Klompé reversed the relationship: social protection became a right enshrined in law that entitled any one without exception to live in dignity.

Marga Klompé went through a religious crisis before finding a deep spiritual foundation that would inspire her understanding of human dignity. She found herself eventually within the tradition of catholic social thought, and the responsibility to contribute in life to the social quality of family, community and society. In her later years she would actively engage with the churches, finding that a spiritual underpinning helped society in defining its social value orientation.

Her understanding of responsibility and society would underpin these convictions, which would form the basis of the social protection legislation put in place by subsequent governments after her appointment in 1956 as Minister of Social Welfare. She initiated the Law on Social Protection.

In Klompé's understanding the modern structuring of economic and social life progressively increased dependence between people as well as a dependency on circumstances beyond their control. A common shared responsibility for social risks was therefore a natural development (Borgman et al., 2012). This was the rationale for Klompé to start legislation for establishing universal social protection in The Netherlands (1965) and to replace the Law on the Poor of 1912. These efforts began with legislation on elderly care, recognising that during the Post Second World War period elderly care homes had insufficient financial means, which lead to residents living in extreme poverty, as well as abuse and maltreatment.

In Klompé's view, the government acceptance of an overall role of responsibility did not imply that it should provide and organize everything; the role of the state was to ensure that this responsibility could and was fulfilled. She left a lot of room for civil organizations and local governments to be in the lead for implementation, arguing that those closest to the people in need of support were in the best position to decide what they needed. In her view 'care' was a fundamental aspect to create a healthy social fabric in society and therefore should remain within the communities, but with support from the government to ensure equal and universal access to such support.

Klompé's view that dignity was central to any support informed her thinking that support could never be a 'one-fit-for-all' and she rejected standarised levels. She argued that needs could differ in different parts of society and that they would also change over time and therefore could not be legislated. She decided to add a complaints procedure to the legislation. This would allow for people to be treated within boundaries set by society itself through the complaints mechanism and within changing boundaries over time, in response to changing social perceptions of what constitutes the basis for a life in dignity.

A famous expression of Klompé was that people deserved 'a bouquet of flowers' on the table. In the Netherlands the offering of flowers symbolizes the celebration of life and they are offered at special occasions to welcome people, greet them and to express gratitude. Flowers have a deep connection to economic livelihoods of the past. In this way Klompé expressed her belief that dignity is not just a matter of survival and basic needs, but is associated with the meaningful existence of human beings as capable of celebrating life, participating in a social environment and contributing to the economic foundation of a society. Social protection programmes aimed at eradicate poverty should allow people to make such meaningful contributions to society.

In the post war period in the Netherlands, as elsewhere in Europe, severe poverty existed. The legislation Klompé initiated was predominantly national in character, but she had equally strong views on the need for European and global dimensions of such policies. The experiences of the war showed that inequality and marginalization leads to conflict, and therefore a universal global framework to guarantee dignity for all was needed.

Rights and International Responsibility

"Whereas recognition of the inherent dignity and of the equal and inalienable rights of all members of the human family is the foundation of freedom, justice and peace in the world." This is the first sentence of the Universal Declaration of Human Rights. Marga Klompé was a delegate of the Dutch Government to the United Nations. She was representing the Dutch Women Society when the Declaration was adopted, in 1948, according to her diary "three minutes before 12." (Borgman et al, 2012).

The Universal Declaration is the result of a deep-felt ambition to revert the violence of two world wars, which had destroyed Europe and pulled many overseas territories and their peoples into European hegemonic conflicts. It is important to note that the Declaration is entitled a Universal Declaration and not an International Declaration, emphasizing, as the first sentence of the Declaration does, the centrality of the dignity of each and every human being. The basis of these rights as natural and universal is a strong statement of the rejection of the Holocaust, slavery and colonial imperialism and carries the aspiration to create an alternative basis for global society based on mutual respect rather than domination. Klompé found the inspiration for the often difficult negotiations on a universal Human Rights framework in Archbishop Emmanuel Suhard. In 1948 the Archbishop of Paris wrote a pastoral letter entitled "le sens de Dieu" in which he advocated how care through love might provide a principle basis for the organization of societies. A meeting in Paris in September that year with the Archbishop gave support for her engagement in the negotiations, especially strengthening her understanding of the need to be tolerant in view of respect for diversity so that a universal Declaration could be adopted. Klompé was very much aware of the consequence of creating international (and West-European) standards – which she saw as the basis for increasing international collaboration based on shared values, and necessarily leading to decreasing national power.

The Universal Declaration of Human Rights provides a framework for the right of people to live in dignity and to not be poor and assigns global responsibility to protect this within the context of a broader framework of a dignified life. The legal framework recognizes social, economic and cultural rights on the one hand and political and economic rights on the other. However, in the context of the Cold War, emerging soon after the adoption of the Declaration, the ideological definition of the two blocks strived over the priority of freedom (the West) or food (the East), an ideological divide that trapped thinking on poverty and on ways to achieve its eradication. The divide locked the new independent post colonial countries into a new form of political, economic and military patronage in which they played second fiddler both in the West and in the East Block. The aspirations for independence made way for a battlefield between newly independent post-colonial countries that were extensions of the larger East-West Cold War. The development aid policies established in both camps were mostly an extension of the East-West battle and a means to protect influence in various parts of the world.

After the Fall of the Berlin Wall in 1989 the indivisibility of Human Rights (giving equal status to economic, social, cultural rights on the one hand and political and civil rights on the other hand) was proclaimed at the 1993 Vienna UN International Conference. The UN Summit on Social Development (1995) held in Copenhagen, provided a space for new agency for developing countries of the Global South in the new Post Cold war world order. For the first time ever, the Summit's Declaration included the recognition that poverty could be eradicated. In a logical extension of this observation emerged the need to accept responsibility as an international community to effectively eradicate poverty. The language 'eradication of poverty' is derived from this understanding and has replaced language of 'poverty alleviation' or 'poverty reduction' as goals falling short of the notion that poverty can and should be eradicated. In the latest revision of the EU's Treaty the objective of poverty eradication was introduced as the objective of its development policy (Mekonnen & van Reisen, 2012).

The Social Summit identified external factors as contributing to and exacerbating poverty. Poverty was defined as a condition caused by circumstances. Consequentially the text of the UN Social Summit does not include any reference to 'the poor' as this terminology was considered as degrading and thought to wrongly give poverty an innate presence in individuals. This language should be seen as a critique of the colonial language that linked the poor to people of colour, slaves or other marginalized people. The language of 'people living in poverty' was introduced to emphasise the understanding that poverty results from an inadequate environment. An action programme was agreed which put emphasis on the need to create enabling environments for social development.

Placing emphasis on the ethical imperative of linking action to the responsibility as identified, the Social Summit set concrete targets for the implementation of concrete policies geared towards the attainment of poverty eradication. These were concrete, identified where responsibility lay for implementation and set clear targets for their achievement. They were also time-bound. It was the first time that the Bretton Woods institutions, the International Monetary Fund and the World Bank, were identified in this way in such a programme. Drawn in rather reluctantly, the international financial institutions initially refused to accept the connection between finance, monetary and economic policy on the one hand and social policy and poverty eradication on the other. However due to strong public pressure pointing to the international debt crisis and the adverse impact of structural adjustment on social policies and the exacerbation of poverty resulting from these policies, the multilateral institutions accepted responsibility in linking their areas of policy to poverty. The UN Summit for Social Development identified areas of the 'enabling environment' where particular responsibility was given at the multilateral level to ensure a conducive global setting for national development. This was balanced with responsibilities accorded to national states in implementing the action plan. National states responsibilities related to all countries, both in East, West and the Global South.

From 1995 onwards the international financial institutions would increasingly include new language in their policy instruments: poverty – social dimensions – inequality, publicly accepting the responsibility for the impact of global policies in finance and economy for these areas. In parallel to this, they pushed the responsibility for these policies to the national level. In 1996 the Organisation of Economic Cooperation and Development (OECD), a club of western industrialized countries, elaborated a simplified set of time-bound goals and targets in a development policy context. This constituted an important reframing of the original goals, as their application was reduced to governments of developing countries and the framework no longer identified responsibilities of non developing countries and international financial institutions. In 2000, in preparation for the Millennium Summit, the OECD, IMF and the World Bank and the UN Secretary General presented a Document "A Better World for All" (2012), in which they presented seven goals, within a similar development framework, exclusively focused on targets for developing countries only.

Civic outrage demanded that the UN would adopt a document that reflected the original universal basis of the UN Summit for Social Development in its attempt to create an internationally agreed framework for poverty eradication. This outreach eventually led to the inclusion of an eighth goal, which expressed, rather inadequately, the dimension of international policy cooperation but the protest failed to redress the goals being applicable to developing countries only. Given that the seven or eighth goals were not presented for approval to the UN General Assembly, they were never officially adopted.

The Goals remained controversial in developing countries, where critics argued that the spirit of a universal global commitment was no longer respected and poverty was linked to developing countries only (Social Watch Report, 2001). The language that the agenda "could not be imposed, but had to be embraced" (A better World for All, 2000: 2), was confusing as the United Nations had already provided the basis for international consensus and hence the agenda was an imposed agenda. Developing countries had not been party to the negotiations of the reductionist Millennium Development

Goals but were now nevertheless asked to 'embrace' these 'imposed' Goals. Whether intentionally or not, the result was that international responsibility was essentially reduced to a (policing) task by the West to monitor the performance of poor countries towards the achievement of the goals. To confuse matters further, the subsequent process under the Aid Efficiency Agenda promoted the language of 'partnership' and 'ownership'. However, at the same time international donors began to use the Millennium Development Goals as a basis for new conditionalities, to which they linked both aid and trade interests and often pursued self-interests in market liberalization. For instance the so-called 'EU MDG contracts' linked support to governments to MDG priorities, but also to trade liberalization. In this way, financial support was usually accompanied by various donor-driven demands. It is only obvious that such aid was increasingly refused by developing countries, if they were in a position to do so.

From a women's leadership perspective, the Millennium Development Goals were a complete failure. The Beijing Declaration and Platform of Action (1995), and the extensive gender-relevant commitments included in the UN Summit for Social Development were reduced to one Goal on Maternal Health Care. This approach reflected a perspective on women that fails to recognize women's agency in society. The problem for women was to decide whether to engage with the Millennium Development Goals, even though they did not find themselves reflected in these, or to 'embrace' them. The 'embracing' of the Millennium Development Goals was for many women activists a reluctant and difficult decision.

The Millennium Development Goals were tied to a world order that still strongly reflected the colonial map of the world and one could hypothesize that the agenda was implicitly testing the performance of the former colonies based on criteria defined by the West. Mirroring this colonial map, the agenda of the Millennium Development Goals reads as a symbol of remembrance of imperialism. The agenda shows this history as an obstacle to the development of a new universal vision of responsibility for poverty eradication at global level that is based on equality and mutual respect.

Oat the same time, and more positively, it can be argued that the agenda of the Millennium Development Goals did provide a first policy platform that expresses a universal set of values expressing global intent to eradicate poverty, linked to an international agenda of concrete action. In that sense, the Millennium Development Goals can be read as a programme that translates universal global values in tangible and measurable results. This development agenda has also provided a strong recognition of the relevance of a social agenda. In 2010 the United Nations adopted the Social Protection Floor, based on extensive work by the International Labour Organization, examining the viability in terms of costs and implementation. Policies of social protection receive more attention generally, as an alternative and more holistic approach than the fragmentation of the narrow Millennium Development Goals. This could potentially provide a basis for more international attention for social protection legislation, whilst the UN's goal-setting of a social protection floor transfers the ambition to support universal protection to an international level. This certainly reflects the spirit of the Universal Declaration of Human Rights, which Marga Klompé so full heartedly embraced in 1948.

Peace and Women's leadership

The need to overcome colonial injustice was central to promote universal dignity – this was clear to Klompé, who as a parliamentarian closely followed the violent and complex process of the Indonesian independence from The Netherlands. As Minister, she was subsequently responsible for organizing the support for the many refugees and migrants from Indonesia, which would arrive in The Netherlands. During the following decades Klompé supported the ANC and its armed struggle, criticizing the apartheid regime and those, including companies, who supported it through investment and trade. She also as a Minister met with Palestinian delegations. Klompé hoped that international instruments would provide mechanisms to negotiate conflict and avoid war. The Holocaust had affected Klompé deeply and the question of how to avoid such genocide in the future was a serious and constant preoccupation during her life. In her view, the Universal Declaration of Human Rights formed the basis to build a world in which war could be avoided, with the dignity of human being as the central universal value. She saw the UN Security Council, United Nations and the European Union as important structures to maintain and negotiate peace.

The Second World War had deeply influenced Marga Klompé in a direct and personal way. She had to stop her studies of medicine in 1942 when the university was closed. She joined the resistance and was active as a messenger under the code name Dr. Meerbergen. She also played a role in the evacuation of Arnhem in 1944, after which she went underground with the name Truus van Aken. There is a story that she was in charge of several enemies soldiers who had been captured and she was asked to approve that they would be killed. However Klompé refused to authorize this and suggested that there were plenty of old castles in The Netherlands where these prisoners of war could be held so that justice could take its course once the war was over. Also telling is that, as a Parliamentarian, Klompé voted against a proposed expulsion of Dutch citizens, who had been found guilty of treason and collaboration with the Nazis, stating the principle that every citizen was entitled to their community and belonging therein.

She greatly valued personal responsibility based on individual conscience, which guided her brave role and leadership in the Dutch resistance. She also attached great value for the access of each individual to independent justice. Transitional justice based on dignity meant to Klompé that individual members of communities should not be excluded from the communities to which they belonged but that an active process of justice, reconciliation and reparation would help communities come to terms with the history of the war and move forward.

It can be argued that the leadership of Klompé in the resistance was the stepping stone to her political career. She built a large network of women volunteers and of political underground activists. The women's network was well connected, and also connected to the Dutch queen Wilhelmina. The Dutch Women Society would send Klompé as a representative to the UN after the war and through her participation in the UN her political competence was recognized. This resulted in the offer for her to join Parliament, which would eventually result in her Ministerial posts. It was the war, which had shown the competence of women in serving the public good, but which had also brought women together in the public sphere, and Marga Klompé would be a symbol of the political power for women that resulted from this.

The norms of society were not yet ready for women's participation in the public sphere. Marga Klompé would never marry as the Dutch law was still such that women had to resign from work outside the home once they married and had children. To avoid such a clash, Klompé did not marry and she would say, she never met the right person at the right time. But despite being much affected by the restrictive gender-prescriptions of that time in The Netherlands, Klompé refused to be defined by these. When a press conference was called with the announcement of her being inaugurated at the first female Minister of The Netherlands, she refused to answer question on the gender issue, stating that there was no difference between male or female Ministers ("other than that she had a make-up box in her drawer" – she would eventually sigh as journalists persisted on the question). The reason was clear, Klompé wanted to be Minister of social affairs for all Dutch people, and more importantly, believed that peace and social integration required wholeness of communities, rather than divisions. In this sense, she believed that focusing exclusively on the gender issue, did not help women or the communities of which they were part.

In the publication Women, War and Peace (2002), Sirleaf and Rehn, identify the many different ways in which women contribute to peace-building and conflict resolution through their engagement in and between communities, the knowledge of communities that they have and the role they play as communicators and messengers, giving guidance and moral authority to family and wider community members. The combination of skills and capacities that women bring to the table are valuable in (preventive) diplomacy (Isike and Uzodike, 2011). The organization of such skills may be different in different societies and at different times; but a deeper appreciation of what both genders can bring to the table of peace building and conflict resolution enlarges the scope of effective response mechanisms.

Based on a literature analysis of the role of women in pre-colonial societies in peacekeeping, Isike and Uzodike (2011) define women's participation in the caring side of society as an ongoing capacity that, if nurtured, would strengthen resilience of today's societies against violence. The contribution of Marga Klompé was to combine the ethics of a care society as a crucial foundation for peaceful societies. According to Klompé, the responsibility to strengthen care-based societies should be taken by governments and international institutions, recogising that communities themselves have the indigenous and intrinsic knowledge of how to organize that and that women have much to contribute to this. The agenda for peace building was therefore intrinsically connected to the agenda for poverty eradication and justice, based on a universal recognition of the need to care for each person in society. This inclusive conception related not just to the receivers of care, but also to the caregivers, especially women, recognizing the relevance and importance of this contribution to society. While for Isike and Uzodike such ethics of care refers back to pre-colonial traditional Ubuntu based African societies, and has the desire to restore the unbalanced society resulting from a patriarchal colonial intervention, for Klompé a ethical care society was a response to prevent the horrors of the holocaust ever occurring again.

UN Security Council Resolution 1325 moves the responsibility for involving women in peace and conflict matters to the highest international level. It recognizes the agency of women in prevention of conflict, protection in conflict and participation in peace building and peacekeeping. Subsequent resolutions have drawn attention to the desirability of inclusive community approaches to strengthen cultures of peace. A human rights culture and justice promoting active agency of all members of society are relevant to peace building and conflict resolution.

Activating traditional justice as one form of transitional justice promotes an inclusive community approach to assist communities to deal with wrongdoing and provide alternatives to a vicious circle of revenge "to activiate systems for truth-finding, resolving conflict, reparation, reconciliation and healing and can lead to forgiveness" (Mekonnen and van Reisen, 2011). "Memory attaches itself to sites, whereas history attaches itself to events" claims Nora (1989: 22); traditional justice focuses on memory, dealing with the actual place of violence as the place of interrogation and as a source for future conflict if not healed. This analysis links traditional justice to conflict prevention marking the importance of in-situ processes that enhance the agency of communities and their members to actively engage in local justice and healing processes.

The interrogating discourse on the need to have a greater involvement of women in peace building and conflict resolution has given focus to the importance of active and inclusive social relations at all levels, and especially at community level. It identifies the agency of women to promote inclusive social participation as a key component to peace building, in all its different forms, including the protection of vulnerable people, the creation of an inclusive social culture, education of values, norms and understanding of justice, and activating support mechanisms and care for people who are in need of assistance. In their combination the discourse on the need of women to be recognized in their capacity to contribute to peace building, has raised the question of the quality of the ethical and moral basis of society within the domain of peace building and conflict resolution.

"A life of dignity for all"

This article looks at the negotiation of the post-2015 Development Agenda as the productive realization of aspirations present today in our society, which result from the unfinished achievements of previous generation. A long-term historical background is provided by the combined and distinct processes of colonialism and holocaust, which produce collective memory from which senses of responsibilities in society are still being derived.

In a recent historical perspective deeper understanding of the realization of the Millennium Development Goals itself remains instructive for an understanding of the post-2015 Development Agenda. In the context of the post 1989 era, it was the first global universal proposition for the eradication of poverty after the end of the Cold War, even though it failed to fully overcome the heritage of a colonial world order in its design. The reworking of the Millennium Development stigmatized developing countries and in doing so carried the reminiscence of the colonial past. The post-2015 Development Agenda may be a chance to overcome this if becomes a global agenda that carries as a universal agenda the ideal of social societies where people are not poor. The social protection legislation, which was put in place in Europe in the post Second World War era can serve as a model to sustain societies that fight inequality and promote dignity for all.

The post Second World War period provides a basis for understanding the need of strong multilateral and international safeguards and the UN Security Council Resolutions provide a basis of strengthening the role of women in conflict resolution and peace building, and strengthen the community basis for societies that are built on relationships, care and (preventive) diplomacy. Whilst both genders are needed for this, greater participation of women in governance and leadership should enable this transition.

"A life of Dignity for All", is the title of the UN Secretary General Report on the post-2015 Development Agenda, linking its ambition to the opening sentence of the Universal Declaration of Human Rights. There is increasing consensus that the ideals for the future agenda should focus on the interlinkage of poverty eradication and social protection (especially health), inclusive and sustainable economic growth with a view to reduce inequalities, care for the environment, a rights based governance framework, the promotion of women's leadership and protecting societies from violence to promote peace.

The Joint Declaration of the group of African Caribbean and Pacific countries, (the ACP Group) and the European Union, who together make up a majority of 108 countries in the United Nations, emphasize the following five priorities (ACP-EU Council of Minister, 2014):

a. Basic living standards and a life of dignity for all, with a view to eradicating poverty in all its dimensions and to ensure sustainable well being. This would include, inter alia, improved health outcomes including through universal health coverage;
b. Inclusive and sustainable economic growth. The framework should be a key driver to reduce inequalities, create decent and productive jobs, and improve the sustainability of consumption and production patterns and promote structural economic transformation;
c. The sustainable use, management and protection of natural resources and the ecosystems services they provide;
d. Good governance, equality and equity, with a strong focus on vulnerable and marginalized groups and the empowerment and rights of women and girls;
e. Peaceful and stable societies and freedom from violence.

This agenda affirms that the ideals of today, projected in the future, carry forward the unfinished projects of the past. The agenda setting of the joint ACP and EU suggests that the post-2015 Development Agenda will comprehensively address a global programme and no longer just focus on developing countries alone. From the priorities that have now been set, it would appear that the promotion of women's participation will be identified as a priority, so enhancing the agency of women in fostering inclusive societies and communities. It expresses the desire that the dimensions of conflict and peace are fully integrated in this agenda, as a precondition for poverty eradication and dynamic, healthy and caring societies.

The Millennium Development Goals were never fully endorsed by the United Nations and this undermined their capacity to produce shared global commitments. It is important that the post-2015 Development Agenda will be adopted by the United Nations, so that all countries can fully participate. It will be in this act of global endorsement that the post-2015 Development Agenda will engage with the histories of colonial past and the Holocaust by seeking a common platform of negotiation to enhance global collaboration between countries at the highest possible level. In achieving endorsement of such an Agenda, the post-2015 Development Agenda could have the capacity to become a representation of a collective memory that carries the aspiration of a better world, which is based on the dignity for all.

References

A Better World for All (2000) *Progress towards the International Development Goals.* IMF, OECD, UN and World Bank Group.

ACP – EU Council of Ministers (2014), *Joint ACP-EU Declaration on the Post-2015 Development Agenda,* 39th meeting, Nairobi, 19-20 June 2014.

Benjamin, W. (1991) 'Thesen über den Begriff der Geschichte', in id., *Gesammelte Werke,* I/2, Frankfurt a.M. 1991, 690-708.

Borgman, E. and Reisen, van, M. (2012) *De Verbeelding van Marga Klompé. Perspectieven op de Toekomst.* Klement, Zoetermeer.

Borgman, E., Plessius, I. and Reisen, van, M. (2012), *In Liefde en Rechtvaardigheid. Het Dagboek van Marga Klompé 1948-1949,* Verloren, Hilversum.

Isike, C. and Usodike, U. (2011) Towards and indigenous model of conflict resolution: Reinventing women's roles as traditional peacebuilders in neo-colonial Africa. *ACJR,* Volume 11, No. 2.

Johnson – Sirleaf, E. and Rehn, E. (2002) *Women War and Peace.* Unifem, New York.

Mekonnen, D. and Reisen, van, M. (2012) The EU Lisbon Treaty and EU Development Cooperation: Consideration for a Revised EU Strategy on Development cooperation in Eritrea. *Law and Politics in Africa, Asia, Latin America.* 45. Jahrgang, Seite 269-380.

Moster, G. (2011) *Marga Klompé 1912 – 1986: Een biografie,* Boom, Amsterdam.

Nora, P. (1989) Between Memory and History: Les lieux de Mémoire. *Representations.* No 26. Special Issue: Memory and Counter-Memory. (Spring 1989) 7-24.

Reisen, van, M. & Mekonnen, D. (2011) Exploring New Spaces for Women in Transitional Justice in Eritrea and Zimbabwe, *Temperanter,* Vol. II – N.1/2.

Rothberg, M. (2009) *Multidirectional Memory. Remembering the Holocaust in the Age of Decolonization.* Stanford University press, Stanford.

United Nations General Assembly (1995) Report of the World Summit for Social Development (also includes the Copenhagen Declaration and Programme of Action). A/CONF.166/9, UN, NY.

United Nations General Assembly (2013) A life of dignity for all: accelerating progress towards the Millennium Development Goals and advancing the United Nations development agenda beyond 2015, *Secretary General Report,* UN, New York.

United Nations General Assembly (2000) United Nations Millennium Declaration. *Resolution adopted by the General Assembly*. UN, New York.

PART V - WOMEN'S LEADERSHIP IN GLOBALISED COMMUNITIES AS PEACE-BUILDERS

CHAPTER 17. REDEMPTION IN SINAI: A STORY OF SLAVERY TODAY[1]

Mirjam van Reisen

The Birth of 'Redemption'

This is the true story of the birth of a child in Sinai.[2] The name in Tigrinya given by his Eritrean mother is: Ra'ee. Ra'ee means Redemption.

The birth of Ra'ee was not a happy one. On the day she went into labour, Ra'ee's mother was tortured, as she was each morning. Chained to the other prisoners, she was electrocuted and beaten. Several hours later Ra'ee was born. When she delivered the baby she could not free her hands to pick him up as she was chained to the other prisoners. She had no cloth with which to cover him and to keep him warm. She could not hold him to feed him. She had no water to wash him. But despite all the odds, Ra'ee was there and he was alive.

Ra'ee's mother, HT, is a young Eritrean woman who escaped her

---

1. This article is based on interviews carried out by mobile phone and skype by Meron Estefanos, a journalist and activist for justice in Sinai. The stories of HT and Berhane were earlier published in: Reisen, van, M., Estefanos, M., and Rijken, C. (2013) The Human Trafficking Cycle: Sinai and Beyond. Wolf Publishers. For the security of the Sinai survivors mentioned in the article the full names are not provided.
2. The story is reconstructed from the interviews of HT with journalist Meron Estefanos and HT in 2012.

country a few months earlier to join her husband in a refugee camp in Sudan. She joined the 5,000 monthly stream of refugees who attempt to escape the open air prison which is her home-country. Eritrea enforces an unlimited 'military service', which is in reality a forced labour camp for young people, children and under aged minors. The conditions are harsh, poverty is rampant, there is no rule of law and prison conditions are unbearable. Detainees are held in ship containers placed under the hot desert sun and in holes dug under the ground. In Eritrea young people have no future, and they will risk an (effective) shoot-to-kill policy at the border to escape. HT fled to Sudan.

Her husband had left earlier and had arrived in a very large refugee camp in Kassala, called Shegarab. There he was waiting for HT to join him. HT, who was carrying his child, was able to cross the border. Unfortunately she never made it to Shegarab as an armed criminal gang abducted her. They took her to the Sinai instead. There she was chained to the other prisoners and tortured daily. She was asked to speak to relatives to collect ransom for her release. Now held in slavery, she was forced to beg and was tortured to make her do as they wished.

When HT's husband heard that she was imprisoned in Sinai he left the refugee camp and went to try and find her. Worried about her condition, he fearlessly put himself in danger to try and help her release or escape. However, he failed to find her and decided to go to Israel instead, so that he could collect the money needed to release his wife. Unfortunately in Israel he was detained under the so-called Anti-infiltrators Law[3], a law that allows the Israeli authorities to detain people, mostly Africans, who have entered the country 'irregularly' under the law. No exception is made for asylum-seekers, refugees or humanitarian circumstances.

Panicking about the fate of HT who was now very pregnant, and worrying about the need to help her release, HT's husband begged to be taken to court and in court explained to the judge the situation of his wife. The Israeli judge who heard his case took an extraordinary decision. He ordered that HT's husband would be temporarily released so that he could beg for money to collect the sum needed to pay the ransom for his wife.

Meanwhile HT delivered Ra'ee and was trying to keep her son alive under the most difficult of circumstances, begging her husband to collect the

---

3. This law was amended in 2012 to include irregular border crossings by Africans. The law has been successfully challenged in the Supreme Court but a new law was introduced by the government allowing the detention of African refugees in an isolated camp in the desert. The circumstances are so bad that in recent months demonstrations and hunger strikes have taken place to draw attention to the situation. The refugees have not been charged with any wrongdoing other than that they crossed the border looking for safety and asylum.

ransom for the release of herself and her son. Having given birth, the ransom had now doubled, HT had to pay for the release of herself and for her son.

HT's husband begged and collected money in Tel Aviv among the other refugees, among members of the Eritrean diaspora in Europe and from (poor) family members at home. He succeeded to collect the ransom and paid it to an intermediary in Tel Aviv. HT was finally released together with Ra'ee.

For HT it was now no longer possible to try and find safety in Israel and join her husband there. A large high tech protected fence was constructed by Israel to block African refugees from entry into Israel. HT was released close to the fence and begged to the Israeli military for water and food for her child. She was not allowed to enter. She was now so worried that her child would die from thirst and lack of food.

She was taken by the Egyptian military to a prison, as are most other survivors of Sinai trafficking, who are released in the desert. Why a prison? What was her crime?

In the prison she found no medical support, no access to a lawyer, no access to a court. HT learned that, in order for her to be released, she had to collect money for a plane ticket for her and her son so that she could be deported by the Egyptian authorities to the country she had fled: Eritrea.

HT's husband continued to collect money in Israel by begging, as he was not allowed to work. He collected the sum needed for the deportation of his wife and his son to the country to which he would never be able to return, Eritrea. A few months later, HT and Ra'ee arrived in Eritrea and live there now. Meanwhile HT's husband is still in Israel, trying to stay out of the hands of the authorities who could legally detain him indefinitely, as is the case for so many other Eritrean refugees; men, women and children. Why are they detained? Why should he be detained? What is his crime?

Ra'ee has never seen his father who, at great personal risk and fearless of the consequences enabled Ra'ee and his mother to leave Sinai torture camp. HT's husband is waiting for the day he will first set eyes on his eldest son. This is a family where two parents support each other and their young child across borders despite the injustices and tragedies inflicted on them. Ra'ee is their Redemption as they have shown courage, resilience and above all: love.

Slavery today: interrogating our responsibility

The aggression of the crimes committed in the Sinai is beyond comprehension. These are crimes against life itself. Babies are beaten. A child suffering from epilepsy is electrocuted. A human trafficker refuses to negotiate the ransom for four young siblings. A young man loses two healthy hands, because he is suspended from the ceiling. A mother gives birth while in chains. Women and men are raped and ripped of their dignity in front of children and loved ones. (Reisen, van, Estefanos, M. & Rijken 2012, 2013, Amnesty International, 2013, Human Rights Watch, 2014)

While being burnt, electrocuted and tortured the victims shout into mobile phones for help to their relatives: "please pay so that I can be released!" Those who cannot pay ransom fear being killed. Does this world exist? Is this the biblical land of Sinai where Moses received his ten commandments?

What is worse? The pain of knowing what is happening or the realization that it is easier for us to turn our head and look the other way?

Thousands of refugees, mostly from Eritrea, have been abducted, held captive in slavery in Sinai. The torture serves as a way to pressure the refugees to collect ransoms for their release. They phone parents, relatives, friends, and beg for money. The ransoms are high, very high. They have increased in the last five years as family members have paid these ransoms for the release of their loved ones. The torture is part of a new model of doing business – to make profit, lots of profit.

Who is right? He who refuses to pay for the release of a loved one so as not to promote the 'trade' in human beings, or he who pays (ever higher) ransoms to release his mother, his son, his child?

The Sinai Trafficking started in 2009 when Italy began to return Eritrean refugees to Libya. Libya deported these refugees to Eritrea and the refugees feared the punishment awaiting them on the forced deportation to the country they had tried to flee. Looking for a safe route and destination they attempted to try and go to Israel through the Sinai. The Eritreans that were kidnapped were able to collect the ransom, which quickly went up. Realizing that Eritreans were 'profitable' the organized criminal networks started to look for Eritreans and began abducting them from the refugee camps in Sudan and their surroundings.

Who is to blame? The country where refugees are tortured and extorted? The country that should have been a home, but turned its back on its own people? The country that refuses entry to refugees? The country that deports the refugees?

Israel built the big high-tech fence to stop the refugees. The survivors of Sinai Trafficking can no longer find security in Israel. Those who entered Israel prior to the building of the fence are labelled 'infiltrators'. Under a law amended in 2012 to allow the Israeli government to detain anyone who entered the state 'irregularly', the survivors of the trafficking can be detained for three years. They may even be held in detention indefinitely if they cannot return to their home country – as is the case for the Eritrean refugees. Despairing, traumatized, wounded, without any support, men, women and children, are held in prisons and detention facilities. They have not committed a single crime. Why are they in detention?

What is more questionable? To prevent survivors of torture and slavery to enter a country, or to put them in detention?

Little has been done to stop the international criminals that organize the Sinai trafficking and that works in collusion with the military, police and security officials in Eritrea, Sudan, Egypt and Israel. Those who organize such crimes and are responsible for its continuation enjoy impunity. The anti-terrorism actions in the Sinai have focused on the military security objectives and ignored the human dimension of the enslavement of Eritrean refugees.

Egypt detains the Sinai survivors and forces them to collect money by begging for the purchase of flight tickets. They are deported to Eritrea or Ethiopia. Deportation to Eritrea means an unsure future. The returning refugees have illegally left the country under the draconian Eritrean laws and can therefore be charged with treason. This can result in detention or even in the death penalty. They can be recommitted to the army and its forced labour camps where they will serve as slave labour to serve self-improvement programmes for Eritrean generals: to build their houses, work as slave labour on agricultural fields, in the mines or to provide sexual services.

How can the Sinai survivors be delivered from this vicious circle that holds them in slavery?

Churches have spoken up. As early as December 2010, Pope Benedict called for prayer for "the victims of traffickers and criminals, such as the drama of the hostages, Eritreans and of other nationalities, in the Sinai desert" (The Guardian, 2012). Pope Benedict and Pope Francis have continued to do so. In July 2014 The World Council of Churches adopted a communiqué, which "calls on member churches of the World Council of Churches in neighbouring countries and beyond to cooperate in dealing with issues of human trafficking in the Sinai desert that is costing the lives of many innocent persons daily." The statement followed a pastoral letter issued by four Eritrean Bishops in June 2014.[4] The letter asked

> "On top of the crisis of people leaving their country (..) the family unit is fragmented because members are scattered in national service, army, rehabilitation centres, prisons, whereas the aged parents are left with no one to care for them and have been spiritually damaged. And all that combined is making the country desolate."[5]

The four Eritrean Bishops have been commended for their courage to speak up in a country where the right to freedom of speech and freedom of

---

4. The four bishops are Mengsteab Tesfamariam, eparch of the capital Asmara; Tomas Osman, Eparch of Barentu; Kidane Yeabio, Eparch of Keren; and Feqremariam Hagos, Eparch of Segeneti.
5. Pastoral Letter, printed on awate: http://awate.com/eritrean-catholic-bishops-ask-where-is-your-brother/

religion mean little (Mekonnen and Reisen, van, 2014).

Sinai survivors reaching Europe

On 3 October 2013 a boat sank off the coast of Lampedusa. It carried some 600 Eritrean refugees. Many of them died. Among the survivors was Berhane. Berhane fled Eritrea when he was fifteen, to avoid the slave labour camp of the military service. He was kidnapped and taken to Sinai where he spent long months in harsh circumstances, being tortured severely. He collected a ransom of $ 38,000 for his release. He was then detained in prison by the Egyptian authorities and he collected the money for a ticket for his release. He was flown to Ethiopia, and ordered to go in one of the refugee camps. Seeing the lack of future in these camps, he decided to go through Libya and try to reach Europe. Berhane was on this boat that sank resulting in the deaths of almost 400 people. He was 17 when he reached the European shore in Italy. His name, Berhane, means Light.

Many unaccompanied minors from Eritrea have now reached Europe. As the age of the military service, de facto slave labour camps, in Eritrea decreases and consequently refugees are leaving Eritrea at an ever-younger age. Support workers find that these young people behave differently from any other young asylum seeker. It has been reported that many say that they are older than they are. They do this, despite knowing that as minors they would have access to asylum in the country in which they have arrived. Their priority is not their own safety, but their responsibility towards their family. They want to work and they want to help their families and those trapped in the situation of slavery in their country, in Sinai and elsewhere. They are impatient to enter the labour market and take their responsibility to contribute to the survival of other family members. As HT and her husband have also demonstrated, despite living in different places and unable to meet, they were able to join in carrying responsibility for Ra'ee and for each other.

The unsafe situation for legitimate asylum-seekers from Eritrea in neighbouring countries is a serious challenge for Europe. The European Union and its member states have an important role to play in resolving this situation, in identifying what can be done to change and improve the situation in Eritrea and enforce this; to help ensure safety for the refugees and asylum-seekers in neighbouring countries in Ethiopia, Sudan and Egypt and ensure that in these countries proper asylum procedures are in place; to stop the slavery and trafficking in the Sinai, stop the torture and forced begging and stop the impunity of the international organized crime networks that are involved in the abduction of people into slavery; to ensure that Israel carries out its responsibility to give a save haven to refugees and carry out its responsibilities under international law and to stop all deportations of refugees to Eritrea where they are punishable as traitors.

A Place of Evil

Ellen Johnson-Sirleaf and Elisabeth Rehn drew attention in their book "Women, War and Peace" (2002) on the increasing victimization of women, represented in increased human trafficking, slavery, sexual violence and killing of women. In Sinai all of these crimes against women come together. The Eritrean women come from a country where the war against a neighbouring country has taken over the entire social fabric (Selassie, 2011). Refugees fleeing national service become vulnerable victims of trafficking. Sinai stands as a place of memory of this evil. It demonstrates that a society that is driven by a patriarchal, authoritarian and colonially inspired military governance machine ultimately looses its capacity to care. Women are no longer capable to carry out that age-long function of bearing children, looking after family, including the elderly. Such a society, thirsty of love and care, becomes a desert of loneliness and pain, where everyone fights for survival.

The interrogation of the absence of women's leadership in the context of conflict resolution and peace building is not that it should replace the participation of men in such leadership (Isike & Usodike, 2011). The discourse points to the need for a leadership that is inclusive and above all which cares. A leadership that cares about families and that sustains the links between parents, elders, youth and children. A leadership that helps communities to look after those in need. A leadership that is engaged with the important matters of life and death, of giving birth and mourning. A leadership that allows mothers and fathers to raise their children in communities that gives a foundation of harmony. A society that no longer has the capacity to care, becomes a society of slaves.

The sexual violence associated with the Sinai trafficking cycle points to the embodiment of the suppression of women. The violent gang rapes, the sadistic sexual aggression, the forced childbirth resulting from rape, embody the quest of a total submission of women into slavery that has a strong sexual dimension. The body itself has become the subject of complete ownership of the slave owner. We can only begin to imagine how women can heal from this, how families can recuperate a sense of dignity and how society will come to terms with its total breakdown.

HT is now in Sudan, to receive treatment for the torture inflicted on her. The story of HT is also a story of resilience, of courage, of a man and a woman, trying to be a family, against the odds, being worlds apart, but caring for their child and each other. The story of Berhane, light, shows the power of hope, the power of the young who will move ahead to find a place where they belong and where they can contribute. Where they can work, and support their families. Where they can care for themselves and heir families. Against all odds, life stubbornly continues and refuses to give up.

None of the problems that relate to the tragedy of the stories of HT in Sudan, her husband in Israel, her son Ra'ee in Eritrea or Berhane in Sweden have easy solutions. But what is needed is the recognition that our world of today needs redemption from modern day slavery and that we all carry a responsibility for this to happen. This is the promise of the birth of Ra'ee: no matter where we are, we all carry the promise that we can deliver ourselves from slavery. This is the modern message from the Sinai: the responsibility to free mankind from slavery is still relevant today.

References

Amnesty International, (2013) Egypt/Sudan. Refugees face Brutal Treatment, Kidnappping for Ransom and Human Trafficking. Amnesty International, London.

Everyone Group (2010) Benedict XVI recalls the drama of the hostages in the Sinai desert [online] Available at: http://www.everyone-group.com/EveryOne/MainPage/Entries/2010/12/5_Benedict_XVI_recalls_the_drama_of_the_hostages_in_the_Sinai_desert.html (accessed 14 August 2014).

Ghondwe, K. (2012) The pope lifts the lid on Sinai's tortured Eritrean refugees. *The Guardian.* [online] Available at: http://www.theguardian.com/commentisfree/belief/2010/dec/09/pope-sinai-torture-african-refugees (accessed 14 August 2014).

Human Rights Watch. (2014) *"I Wanted to Lie Down and Die". Trafficking and Torture of Eritreans in Sudan and Egypt.* Human Rights Watch, New York. Available at: http://www.hrw.org/reports/2014/02/11/i-wanted-lie-down-and-die-0 (accessed 14 August 2014)

Isike, C.& Usodike, U.O., (2011), Towards and indigenous model of conflict resolution: Reinventing women's roles as traditional peacebuilders in neo-colonial Africa. *ACJR*, Volume 11, No. 2.

Johnson – Sirleaf, E., & Rehn, E., (2002) *Women War and Peace.* Unifem, New York.

Mekonnen, D.R. & Reisen, van, M. (2014) Religious Persecution in Eritrea and the Role of the European Union in Tackling the Challenge. In: *Religion, Gender and the Public Space.* (eds. Reilly, N. & Scriver, S.). Routledge, New York & London.

Reisen, van, M. & Mekonnen, D. (2011), Exploring New Spaces for Women in Transitional Justice in Eritrea and Zimbabwe, *Temperanter*, Vol. II – N.1/2.

Reisen, van, M., Estefanos, M. and Rijken, C. (2012) *Human Trafficking in the Sinai. Refugees between Life and Death.* Wolf Legal Publishers, Oisterwijk.

Reisen, van, M., Estefanos, M. and Rijken, C. (2013) *The Human Trafficking Cycle: Sinai and Beyond*. Wolf Legal Publishers, Oisterwijk.

Selassie, B. (2011) Wounded Nation. How a Once Promising Eritrea was Betrayed and its Future Compromised. Africa World Press, Trenton.

World Council of Churches (2014 07 08) *Statement on the State of Human Rights in Eritrea*. WCC, Geneva. (online) Available at http://www.oikoumene.org/en/resources/documents/central-committee/geneva-2014/statement-on-the-state-of-human-rights-in-eritrea. (accessed 14 August 2014).

CHAPTER 18. DESERTS, HIGH SEAS AND HOPE

Selame Kidane

Hope is the thing with feathers that perches in the soul - and sings the tunes without the words - and never stops at all.

Emily Dickinson

Introduction: from Tel Aviv to Via Tel Aviv

In the town of Adi keyih, in southern of Eritrea, there is an area colloquially known as Via Tel Aviv. The set of gleaming brand new housing developments are all too evident of the new influx of surplus income that has been received by the inhabitants of those homes.

It is so named because invariably each family that owns such a house, has been able to build and maintain their new found life of relative comfort because one or more offspring has made it across the Eritrean borders, across the harsh Sahara desert and survived human trafficking to land in Tel Aviv. With a job as part of the humongous workforce made up of Eritrean refugees, they are legally defined as 'illegal infiltrators'.

I have many friends who live a life on the margins of society in Tel Aviv; they queue for hours every month to renew a piece of paper that tells them, and everyone who comes across them, that they are illegal residents and do not belong. In this precarious status they remain, and there is absolutely nothing anyone is going to do any day soon to rectify the situation and make it possible for them to enjoy their rights as refugees.

Earlier this year protesting their treatment and particularly a new set of measures designed to make it even harsher on refugees and would be refugees, the inhabitants of underground Tel Aviv staged a series of walkouts. Men, women and children simply refused to go to work and sat at the park which has become a bit of a community hub in the derelict district of South Tel Aviv, which is a home to some 40,000 undocumented Eritrean refugees.

The response from Israeli employers couldn't have been more dramatic! They wanted them back and some even staged solidarity rallies of their own; there was no one to wash the dishes, the farms were deserted and fruit lay rotting. The streets were ridden with litter and assembly lines couldn't assemble anything. Like the inhabitants of Via Tel Aviv in Southern Eritrea, the businesses and hotels have also gained rather handsomely from the addition of an exceptionally amenable and hardworking workforce whose members are grateful for the opportunity to work all hours and demand nothing but the minimum wages that are turned down by everyone else in the country.

If one was to do a word association exercise about current day Eritrean refugees few would probably find positive attributes of strength and determination to associate with them. Poor, destitute and desperate would probably be top of the list. This is a stark contrast to even the previous generation of refugees who were considered highly educated and resourceful as well as committed to their national cause.

Eritrean refugees: the other 'push' factor

I once had a conversation with a remarkable young Eritrean man who told me of his absolutely harrowing story of 'survival', where out of a group of thirty-two friends and relatives who set out together only three survived the journey and made it to Europe via Malta. He is a final year engineering student in a London university, his story deserves Hollywood style rendition, and yet when I asked him if his family or his friends knew the odds he beat to get here, he told me: "who cares? Who wants to know? All my family are interested in is that I survived and I am in Europe, I made it!"

In Tel Aviv almost every single person has such a story to tell or not tell as is more likely to be the case actually. Often the story tells itself in the rare reports of violent domestic abuse perpetrated against the women who are trying to strand an unlikely reality together. Or the tragedy of a young mother who committed suicide leaving a newborn and a toddler behind, but the stories of indomitable spirit and undying resourcefulness never get noticed.

My friend Zebib, used to run a Women's centre in Tel Aviv, helping her fellow refugee women and their children in the process of piecing together the realities of such fragmented existence, and through my involvement at the centre I came to know many of these women and their stories.

Senait (not her real name), was an A student back in Eritrea and comes from a middle class family who are committed to educating their children. Her father's only dream was to see her progress with her studies. She too had a dream: to become a journalist, but in Eritrea both their dreams were unlikely to be realised. Senait couldn't face the reality of having to go to national service and becoming whatever the government intended for her, so she crossed the borders, crossed the Sahara and through Sinai she came into Israel, where she was detained for several months and unbeknown to her the conditions of her release was such that she had work as a fruit picker for several months. Still she didn't give up on her dreams of good education and a career. She never told her family what she did for a living and how she lived; she got on with her life as a farm hand. And it was only when she had an accident and damaged her legs that she actually almost gave in to the desperation of her situation and how far she was from her dream and that of her father. Today she is married and has a beautiful little girl, who probably has everything a girl of her age would want: two adoring parents who spend every last penny they earn not in Via Tel Aviv like many of their peers but on her. Because they both know that stuck as they are here in Tel Aviv they would never be able to give her the future that they would like for her without the amount of hard work and the commitment they put into raising their daughter. I dared to ask Senait about her own dream, and her response still rings in my ear:

> look at me... I work all hours to earn the basics, I haven't read a single book in so many years, no one knows how big my dream used to be. All they see is the refugee I have become. Sometimes I too feel that is all I am, all I have become. The only thing that keeps me going is my responsibilities to my little girl. She deserves a future that is not limited by the status of her parents, she is a brilliant little girl, she deserves the best of futures, and that is what I am going to give her.

That conversation gave me an insight into the real purpose of the villas in Via Tel Aviv and the many weddings, christenings, birthdays, etc that are celebrated in South Tel Aviv every week. They are actually physical representations of the glimmer of hope that persists despite traumatic past experiences and harrowing present reality. The villas and the children and the elderly parents being looked after, the endless 'celebrations' are what, many women at the centre are using to give meaning to an otherwise totally fragmented reality where nothing that they have become fits in with what they dreamt of becoming before leaving Eritrea.

Meanwhile back at the centre myself, Zebib and others were trying to put together potential programmes for the women's centre; an advise session, language classes, child care facilities. For me something was missing something that is essential in my own life, entertainment, pass time activity, a bit of fun. I desperately tried to interest the women in some such activity. 'A movie night perhaps?' I suggested only to be met with blank faces.

"Ok maybe something else; what do you ladies do in your spare time?" Manna (not her real name) was the first to respond. Everything about Manna including her tall slender body and her practical attire and footwear, tell of her resilience. Manna tells me she works endless hours, as a chambermaid, so she can earn enough money to buy her way out of Israel. Already she had been cheated out of her hard earned money a couple of times by people who promised her a way out. Given how hard Manna works for hours on end, one would expect her to be devastated at the loss of such large amounts of cash and also expect her to be very weary of anyone trying to sell her a way out of Israel. Not Manna. To her planning her exit is the only way of keeping hope alive; it is in fact the stuff that her hopefulness is built upon.

Three years after that planning evening in Tel Aviv and no doubt several failed attempts later, a few months ago I saw a picture of Manna on Facebook. In the background the unmistakable grey sky of Northern Europe and enough snow to tell me this wasn't an exceptional day in Tel Aviv. I was so excited for her and finally I could stop being sad about her statement from many moons ago:

> …sometimes even in my dreams I am folding sheets and making beds, if I wasn't working at a hotel on the seafront I wouldn't even have known I lived near a sea side, everything I do is centred on my dream of getting out of here. Our lives don't have room for movie nights or seaside outings.

Titi was about the only one in that group of women at the centre coordinating group who had a suggestion on what at first sounded like a great pass time activity – excursion trips into Jerusalem and all the other historical sites. I thought it was brilliant; here were a group of women who come from a very religious society and living with all the Biblical sites a very short bus ride away! Yet Titi's suggestion was received with the same polite but lukewarm reception as my frivolous suggestions of movie nights and seaside outings.

It was Easter season and Titi, who is a domestic home help for a middle class Tel Aviv family, had just come back from an evening prayer at one of the monasteries in Jerusalem. She has become more committed in her Coptic faith since arriving in Tel Aviv and spends all her spare time in church activities. She sings in the choir, she coordinates visits to religious sites for her fellow churchgoers and supports the priests in any way she can. Titi is happy and always smiling, but more importantly perhaps, she is content with her life in Tel Aviv. She puts due commitment to her job with the family, she earns enough to support her own family back in Eritrea, and has managed to strike a balance between her spiritual and physical needs. Her days are centred on her work and weekends with her church family. Her year is punctuated by colourful and vibrant celebrations of events on the religious calendar and satisfaction for her comes from knowing she is doing the right thing for her. Her friends respect her serenity even as they recognise that her way isn't necessarily the way for everyone and they tolerate her occasional sermons in return for her ever so supportive presence in the group.

That night, and every other night I spent in Tel Aviv, my biggest preoccupation keeping me awake was the worry that I would never ever be able to tell these stories (and many more) and tell of the resilience of these women and their resolve to keep going. Their ability to find something to hold on to, something to begin stranding their lives back together even after it has been shattered by traumatic experiences that many of us are not even able to imagine.

Of course not all of the women have stories of resilience; the surprise is that not many of them are actually like Hanna (not her real name), who left Eritrea as a teenager. The eldest of a family of several younger siblings and cousins looked after and supported by her lone mother who worked as a cleaner in Asmara. Hanna thought she was now old enough to find a way of supporting her mother and her siblings. Little did she know that her 'chosen' route would land her into the hands of traffickers who would sell her several times over, gang rape her mercilessly and beat her until she lost the use of several muscles in one leg. The story of her escape and arrival in Tel Aviv is a story that could fill volumes. Sadly her physical scars were nothing compared to the emotional scars that lay deeper and beyond the reach of her various attempts to strand her life back together again. She couldn't keep a job, for the demands of such long hours and hard labour were beyond what her weakened muscles could cope with. She was too emotionally fragile to cope with friendships and the many sexual advances from men who were simply unable to see what lay just underneath her youthful appearances and urbanite demeanour. And finally her search for solace led her into the hands of a religious cult leader who abused her vulnerability and inexperience and isolated her from the little support that she would have gotten from her fellow refugee women. All Hanna ever sought from him (and what he promised her) was that he exorcise the demons of Sinai out of her tormented soul. A few months after our last meeting a common friend reported to me that the 'priest' claimed to have exorcised the Sinai demons and was working on the Tel Aviv ones, Hanna was never the same again. My friend was asking "what hope is there for her if the demons are even here in Tel Aviv?" Hanna must have felt the same sense of hopelessness in the face of so many demons too.

At about that time I started thinking about the difference that is making a difference between those that are able to adjust to the harsh realities of life as an 'illegal infiltrator' in Tel Aviv and those that are not coping at all (the perpetrators of domestic violence and victims of alcohol abuse as well as those who have succumbed to over reliance on other avoidance tactics). I also started wondering if there is a scope for us to think of these hazardous journeys out of Eritrea as acts of positive hopefulness rather than the desperate measures of a generation unable to realise the aspirations of a once hopeful nation.

Perhaps it is the hopefulness instilled into this generation of Eritreans, a residual trait from the legacy of the independence struggle and its near miracle achievements that drives young Eritreans to be ever so hopeful and willing to overcome endless obstacles in the realisation of the goal of getting out of the country.

Although I do not have concrete empirical data, a majority of those leaving Eritrea are under 30 years of age; in Tel Aviv I would say about 26. Twenty-three years ago, at Eritrea's victorious independence, our 'illegal infiltrators' were mere toddlers. The oldest were probably carrying palm branches and dancing on the streets and the youngest would have been on their mother's backs as they danced. During the euphoric post-independence years many would have had their psychological births, the age at which a baby realises that she is separate from other entities (including the caregiver) and from this point on the village that is raising the child (in Eritrea it still takes a village), will be invested in teaching its young hopeful thinking. For this generation of Eritreans recent events would have made that lesson extra strong (potent). Eritreans across the globe and particularly inside the country would have been high on hopefulness following the attainment of the goal that took three generations of Eritreans.

Where previous generation of Eritreans were taught bitter perseverance and sacrifice, this generation of Eritreans will have been brought up on a staple diet of sweet victory flowing from a direct link of the experience of making a move towards a goal (an important element of hopeful thinking). If this hypothesis is true then hopefulness is somewhat a double-edged sword for Eritrean young people. It is both the force that is making it possible for them to choose exile as a pathway to goal attainment and it is perhaps the trait that is making it possible for them to survive even in the most unlikeliest of circumstances, such as in the case of my friends at the women's centre in Tel Aviv. Making it possible for them to work all hours and still manage to turn up at weddings looking ever so elegant and with immaculately turned out children on tow, on their only free day of the week.

Propelled by hope

Hope theorists define hope as the perceived capability to derive pathways to desired goals, and motivate oneself via agency thinking to use those pathways (Snyder, 2002). Here hope is conceptualised as an individual deference variable reflecting relatively enduring, cross-situational subjective appraisals of goal related capabilities made up of three major components: goals, agency and pathway.

Goals can be short-term or long-term, and inevitably they will vary significantly in terms of their importance or probability of attainment. When a goal is appraised and if it is of high enough importance to warrant continued mental attention then the person moves along the sequence to a phase where they consider the pathway and the agency.

Pathways represent a person's perceived ability to devise workable routes to goals, the resolve that makes people say: "I will find a way to get this done." (Snyder, 1998) People with high hope are more often than not able to imagine multiple routes and herein lies the difference that actually is the difference. When the individual encounters barriers to the goals (and particularly to goals with high outcome value) their ability to access other pathways becomes crucial.

Agency is the motivational component that propels people along their imagined pathway towards their goal. It reflects the individual's perception that she can begin to move along the pathway. It is the mental will power characterised by the internal speech such as "I am not going to be stopped." (Snyder, 2002) Like the ability to devise alternative routes, agentic thinking is also crucial as it provides the necessary motivation that ought to be channelled to alternative routes.

Thus hope can be defined as a positive motivational state based on a goal directed energy (agency), channelled through a considered pathway towards a chosen goal. When a particular goal pursuit has been completed (and a goal attained) emotions would cycle back to influencing subsequent pathway and agentic thinking, embedding hopeful thinking. When barriers are experienced those who are able to think of more pathways and muster enough motivation to pursue these would be at an advantage.

Thinking back to my many conversations with my friends at the Eritrean Community Women's Centre in Tel Aviv and their indomitable strength of spirit despite it all, and reflecting against the above theory (and similar others), some of what I have observed over the last few years begins to tell a story that is often untold about this generation of Eritreans. Of course no one has yet done any research into the phenomena that makes young people pay thousands of dollars for a space on a rickety boat or even a dinghy that is going to sail into the darkness literally and figuratively. However, could the fact that they were raised by a generation that actually fought against all odds and won their independence have programmed them to believe that there are near infinitive pathways to achieving their goal? Could they have developed an exceptionally high agentic thinking, a belief in their ability to 'finding a way' under any circumstances?

On my second or third visit to Tel Aviv Manna was recovering (only financially) from her latest setback on her quest to get out of Israel, and with a smile she told me that the "setback" was a lesson on human nature to all involved and that next time she would be more astute. I didn't think of it like that then but Manna's logic was actually no different to Zebib's when organisation after organisation were telling us that a Women's centre run by

Eritrean refugees in the heart of South Tel Aviv was simply impossible. Unperturbed Zebib just went about finding new ways to deliver services starting with an idea that actually generated the income required and provided much needed services (a child care facility for working mothers). Today the Centre runs numerous flagship programmes and doesn't even need the income from the crèche to sustain it.

Could the over dependence on alcohol and violence, that is more common in the young Eritrean men (anecdotal evidence) be ascribed to gender based differences measurable on the Hope Scales available to researchers? And more importantly would understanding all this facilitate the development of approaches that would enable us to support the psychological adjustment for those that are finding it hard to cope?

Of course not all the men have resorted to avoidance through alcohol and violence as a way of coping with their traumatic experience. In fact just as many women might also be finding adjustment difficult but their avoidance might be hidden beneath eating disorders or self harm.

I have also come across men that have shown tremendous strength and managed to come through such difficult experiences. Solomon (not his real name) is among the oldest Tel Aviv inhabitants I have met, through his currently frail body frame you can still see the tremendous physical strength that has carried him through a life of so much hardship. He was a young soldier during the independence struggle, but rather than be celebrated as a victorious hero he spent much of his life in independent Eritrea in and out of prisons for his vocal opposition against government policies and particularly the fate of his fellow former fighters. When he finally managed to escape from prison he took himself and his teenage daughters through the mountains he fought so hard to liberate and arrived in Sudan. Unfortunately all three were abducted and Solomon suffered horrendously at the hands of his abductors and their choice of torment for him was to rape his daughters before his eyes. When some ransom was paid by the family Solomon wanted one of the girls to be freed but the captors figured they would gain more by keeping the girls so they let him go instead, it took months before he recovered enough presence of mind to realise where he was. At the time I met him he had mobilised the community to collect enough money to free both his girls from the hands of captors, it was really clear that all he lived for was to see his children freed. Few weeks ago I heard both girls were now free from traffickers but still in limbo in Egypt.

Within hope theory any stressor can be conceptualised as that which interferes with the attainment of goal (starting with the most basic) and coping is the ability to effectively respond to a stressor so as to reduce psychological (and physical) pain. (Houston, 1988) High hope individuals will find more pathways to overcome the stressor and will also be more motivated to utilise those strategies. Higher hope people will also be more likely to find benefits (strength) in their on-going dealing with stressors (Tennen & Affleck, 1999) and less likely to use avoidance; a coping style linked to distress and decreased psychological adjustment when overused. (Suls & Fletcher, 1985)

Researchers have also found a link between higher hope and successful coping with unforeseen stressors (barriers to goal), (Snyder & Pulvers, 2001) enabling them to think effectively about the future, with full appreciation of the fact that at times they will face major life stressors. By contrast low hope individuals are more likely to catastrophise the future.

Successful adjustment is dependent on the ability to prevent major stressors by reducing, eliminating or containing them. High hope individuals are more likely to be flexible enough to find alternative goals in the face of immutable goal blockages. My friends building houses and supporting their families in comparative comfort at via Tel Aviv back in Adi Qeyih have found a worthy alternative goal of making something out of the fact that they are stuck in Israel without the prospects of making the lives they envisaged for themselves. For Senait and her partner it was pouring everything into her little girl, for Zebib and colleagues it was helping as many of their fellow refugee women as possible find the support that they need. All of this is meeting a need far more significant for the giver, than what the recipient might ever appreciate.

In my work with many refugees (both from Eritrea and other places), I have come across many people who are all too willing to entertain fantasies about 'magically' escaping their particular entrapment; unfortunately it sounds like Hanna may have fallen for that when she agreed to go through abusive rituals as solution. Many others in Tel Aviv come and demand that we talk to the UNHCR and effect their resettlement out of Israel. All this is a form of disengaged (avoidant) coping behaviour, more akin to low hope individuals, and often results in an unhealthy consequence, as well as a missed opportunity for learning from the experience of overcoming goal blockages.

Bittersweet triumph

Clearly the capacity that some Eritrean Refugee Women have shown for coping with numerous adversities, and the fact that many may have even thrived as a result of this experience, is a bitter sweet triumph as we know that many others have simply not had the opportunity to even contemplate alternative pathways that may have been available to them.

It is difficult to estimate how many have perished in the hands of brutal human traffickers torturing them to death in an attempt to extort ransom from their families. Many have also not made the journeys across the Mediterranean. At the time of writing, two such boats carrying at least 400 Eritreans in total are said to be missing for several weeks, one is feared to have sank off the Libyan coast from where it set sail over a month ago. Unfortunately such circumstances are far too frequent and yet refugees continue to make the journey. I guess there can also be over-hopefulness too.

Building with hope

As well as helping us understand the mentality that maybe facilitating the psychological adjustment of Eritrean refugees in Tel Aviv (and other destinations), hope theory can also provide a framework for developing a process through which those who are not coping can be assisted too.

When people lose hope they have little else to live for. Similarly if people avoid stressors through poor coping mechanisms, they will soon become disconnected from their goals. Hope theory provides a framework for therapeutic interventions by tapping into cognitive constructs involving people's perceptions as related to their goals. First, through their abilities to initiate and maintain movement towards a goal (agency) and their goal-related behaviours; Secondly, using their abilities to generate viable strategies in the event of blockages (pathways). Self-reflection through therapeutic intervention can therefore provide opportunities for those not coping to examine their agency or pathway thinking and be helped to raise their hopefulness by learning more effective agentic and goal-directed pathways.

This has got significant potentials for working with Eritrean refugees across the globe. Many have been through traumatic experiences and could be suffering from PTSD. Getting people back in touch with their original goal and helping them build their repertoire of workable pathways could potentially be an extremely rewarding therapeutic engagement.

I particularly think of people like Solomon, who could be helped to reflect back about the various obstacles in their lives and how they (life as a soldier, adjusting back into civilian life, escaping prison and being able to raise tens of thousands of dollars in Tel Aviv) can rebuild life using these very building blocks.

Perhaps if one had the opportunity to get to Hanna before the religious cult leader, one would have been able to get her back in touch with her goal of helping her mother and her siblings, using the strength that she had to survive the horrendous experience she had been through at such a young age.

Conclusion: A hopeful agenda for Eritrea

Last October when a boat carrying Eritreans sank and 366 people died, Eritreans across the world grieved with the bitterest expression of anguish coming from a massive memorial service held in Levensky Park in South Tel Aviv. Young men and women, priests and lay people wailed their heartbreak out. The torment of unrealised hope had come to haunt them: even after you pursue every pathway available and pushed yourself to follow every last one to reach a goal, sometimes that goal which seemed close and attainable enough, proves to be just the opposite.

A few months later the same crowd gathered in the same park refusing to go back to work until the Israelis sorted out their refugee policies. The same men and women gathered and demonstrated their determination to dismantle every barrier to them attaining their goal of living their dream of stability and security. The women's centre was abuzz with activities, organising the women and children protest day, hosting information session for wives of diplomats, organising the food rota for the protestors and child care facilities for those who need one, a sign that Eritreans in Tel Aviv always find a way back to hope.

Watching the endless coverage of those rallies on social media, listening to the speeches that were being made by young Eritreans, I too was riding high on the tide of hope rising from Tel Aviv of all places in the universe. I figured that if the policies of two governments (the Eritrean and Israeli governments) with such low hope for Eritrean youth are unable to delete the hope coefficient programmed into their psyche by the villages that brought them up, and if hope is such a persistent feature of Eritreans, there really is a good chance that we would be able to reverse all that has gone against us.

It is the low hope policies of the regime in Eritrea that have become an immovable blockage preventing the goal of many Eritreans from being realised inside their country. The search for alternative pathways leads many frustrated young people into choosing exile to attain their goal of personal development and security. Therefore the task of those of us fighting for a better Eritrea should include a fight for a high hope government with policies that facilitate the removal of blockages to the attainment of the goals of its citizens. We should also fight for policies that facilitate the setting and achieving of collective goals that enables the entire society to gain from common benefits. And finally as my friends have fully demonstrated, where there is a will there is always a way.

References

Houston, B. (1988) Stress and coping. In C. Snyder & C. Ford (Eds.), *Coping with negative life events: Clinical and social psychological perspectives* (pp. 373– 399). Plenum, New York, NY.

Snyder, C., Lapointe, A., Crowson, J. Jr. & Early, S. (1998) Preferences of high and low hope people for self-referential input. *Cognition and Emotion*, 12, pp. 807– 823.

Snyder, C. (2002) Hope theory: Rainbows in the mind. *Psychological Inquiry*, 13, pp. 249-275.

Snyder, C. and Pulvers, K. (2001) Dr. Seuss, the coping machine, and "Oh, the places you will go." In C. Snyder (Ed.), *Coping with stress: Effective people and processes* (pp. 3–19). Oxford University Press, New York, NY.

Suls, J. and Fletcher, B. (1985) The relative efficacy of avoidant and non-avoidant coping strategies: A meta-analysis. *Health Psychology, 4*, pp. 249– 288.

Tennen, H. and Affleck, G. (1999) Finding benefits in adversity. In C. Snyder (Ed.), *Coping: The psychology of what works* (pp. 279–304). Oxford University Press, New York, NY.

CHAPTER 19. A PLACE CALLED HOME: THE MARGINALISATION OF ZIMBABWEAN WOMEN

Grace Kwinjeh

There is a generation of young Zimbabweans, who left the country with their mothers, when they were just babies, with vivid memories of what the place, they used to call home, is like.

One of these young women is my daughter, Charmaine. She left Zimbabwe when she was just seven years old. She will be turning twenty next October. She first stayed in Belgium, than had to relocate to the United Kingdom, with her younger brother Clive, after I had to go back home to Zimbabwe. When I returned to Belgium in 2009, Charmaine relocated again to stay with me.

She is a hard-working and determined girl. She enrolled in the French education system, but then had to leave again for the UK, as a result of both the difficult economic situation and the difficulty of adapting to the French school system.

In spite of all those difficulties, Charmaine did very well in her A-level exams. She has now been accepted to study law at University level.

Charmaine's story is testimony of the children from Zimbabwe's many single female political activists, who endured years of separation with their children. Some senior women in the MDC, had to let their adolescent children go to the UK while they remained in Zimbabwe, staying for long periods of time without seeing them. I am so proud of their strength and tenacity. They are such a potential asset for Zimbabwe.

But, then again, I avoid to ask her the question which is always on my mind, because I fear the answer: "which place do you call home?"

The Zimbabwe diaspora woman: "out of sight, out of mind"

This chapter interrogates the positioning of Zimbabwean women who left Zimbabwe over the past 15 years, as a result of the multifaceted and prolonged struggle. Some left voluntarily, others were forced to flee by circumstances, beyond their control. The definition of women leaders is not confined to those who were in national and visible leadership only, but rather, also takes into account, women who were involved in political organisations from grassroots level. Many were forced to flee the country as a result of their political convictions and activism. Political persecution was not directed to those in mainstream politics alone, but civil society too, especially those who participated in the constitutional and women's movements (Human Rights Watch, 2006). There are also reports of teachers, especially in the rural areas, who suffered much persecution at the hands of Zanu PF's youth militia, just for being suspected of belonging to a particular opposition group. This chapter, therefore, seeks to start a conversation, on the whereabouts of these unnamed she-heroes or 'sheroes' of the struggle for democracy, to acknowledge their presence and to draw from their Diaspora experiences, in order to explore how they may contribute meaningfully to the rebuilding of Zimbabwe.

The lack of information concerning this important group of women, creates a solid case for further research into this area, given that the Diaspora is estimated at four million Zimbabweans, half of whom are women. The question of where the migrant Zimbabwean women, who have been at the forefront of the struggle at different levels in society, disappeared to and what became of them has been overlooked. There are many unsung 'sheroes' of the struggle, some like award winning and celebrated journalist Violet Gonda, who has been barred from returning to Zimbabwe. Gonda is one of the founder members of the popular UK based radio station SWRADIO Africa, which has since closed down due to financial constraints. She is on a Zimbabwe sanctions list, which includes senior British politicians among others.

The chapter gives an account of the political situation in Zimbabwe identifying how patriarchal power continues to dominate and has led to cycles of violence associated with the political processes. The chapter identifies how women have been affected by the political violence and how this has increased women migration. The chapter then looks at life in the diaspora as a new site of struggle, with new challenges relating to change and loss of identity. This chapter finally looks at the experience of loss, of no longer belonging, no longer being at the centre of the place called home. I will conclude by looking at the way in which women in the diaspora have found new forms of expression and organisation to survive and counteract the negative impact of the experience of losses on their lives.

Election violence affecting women's political participation

In what seemed like a progressive, seamless flow of historic events, which started with the fall of the Berlin wall in 1989, immediately followed by the process that led to the collapse of the Apartheid South-Africa regime, a new era was ushered in, as winds of change blew over the Southern African Development Community (SADC) region. The political mood changed, to encompass language that had to do with the inclusion of the previously marginalised groups. An environment was created for the increased participation of women in the public and private domains. In particular their participation in political decision-making which had hitherto remained a male preserve and has influenced priorities of budgets. An example often given is how male Members of Parliament (MPs), have pushed for resource allocation to make roads in rural areas to ease their travel, at the expense of building clinics to alleviate the suffering of women and children who often have to walk long distances in search of medical care.

Women now occupy notable positions of power at national, regional and even continental levels. The African Union Commission, which had long been identified with being a bastion for patriarchy, is now headed by a woman, Dr Nkosazana Dlamini-Zuma, who was elected to the position in October 2012. Other examples of female performance in countries like Rwanda constitute an impressive 64%, the highest in the world. SADC has affirmed its commitment to promoting women to positions of decision-making and power, the SADC Protocol on Gender and Development was signed and adopted by 12 SADC Heads of State and Government on 17 August 2008 in Johannesburg, South Africa. In this Protocol a commitment was made by Member States to achieve 50% women representation and participation in political and decision-making positions in the public and private sectors by 2015.

In Zimbabwe, women at present constitute 35% of Zimbabwe's Parliament, a figure which doubled after the 2013 harmonised elections, from the previous 17% in the 2008 election. This is a result of a provision in the new constitution, which was adopted in May 2013. This provides for a quota of 60 seats to be reserved for women. Women are selected through a proportional representation system. The seats are awarded to each political party according to the number of votes it receives. However, given the overall controversial nature of Zimbabwe's elections, and, the patronage system within political parties, the provision to promote women to positions of decision-making, loses its meaning. To date the opposition has disputed the outcome of the 2013 election, in which ruling Zanu PF made a clean sweep in most constituencies. The overall outcome is that Zanu PF women are the beneficiaries of this quota, since Zanu PF has the majority in parliament. According to those who contest the elections, the women who have taken these seats are the beneficiaries of the deception by their party and of vote rigging.

Another problem is that the system of selection of women across the political divide, has not been based on merit, but has rather rewarded those women who toed the party line. These women, selected on this basis remain hamstrung in parliament, as they don't have their independent support in a constituency. Therefore they have a limited possibility to push for policies that do not gain the support of the male leadership. The increased numbers of women in the current Parliament has not translated to any robust debate for policy changes that could benefit women.

So, despite the progress made at regional level to enhance women's participation in elections, there are major challenges in Zimbabwe. In 2009 the Research and Advocacy Unit (RAU) did research on the interest Zimbabwean women have in the politics of their country and found that women come out in large numbers to vote but that the voting patterns are affected by political violence, which has characterised elections since 2000. Reasons for not voting are associated with insecurity and fear because of the operating environment of intimidation and harassment. The report further indicates that the figures of women feeling unsafe during election periods has been rising steadily since 2002, with 70% reporting to be unsafe in 2008.

Violence during election time is a major issue that has tainted the credibility of Zimbabwe's elections, with the main opposition Movement for Democratic Change, (MDC) and other smaller parties still contesting the outcome of previous elections. Increased human rights violations are also reported around election time, these take the form of abductions, assaults, torture, rape and murder. AidsFreeWorld examined 70 alleged survivors, detailing 380 total acts of rape by 241 perpetrators. According to the report, many of these rapes were by multiple perpetrators, mostly identified as supporters of ZANU PF, and, in many instances, the perpetrators could be clearly identified by the victims. These women were interviewed in South Africa and Botswana, where they had fled into exile. Forty of the 70 women also reported that they had been severely assaulted, either before or after the rape, with sticks, electric cords, logs or metal rods (AidsFreeWorld, 2008). Failure to deal with violence in national politics and at political party levels has been the biggest stumbling block to Zimbabwean women fully benefiting from the protocols and declarations made at SADC level.

I together with three other female opposition leaders, including about 30 men, were brutally tortured on the 11 March 2007, while on our way to a prayer meeting for peace. I sustained injuries to my head and was unconscious for several hours after being beaten non-stop by several riot police, at a time. They only stopped to change hands after they were tired. I left Zimbabwe, in my pyjamas in an ambulance for South Africa where I received medical care. This is the case with many victims of political violence, who out of safety precautions have to leave the country abruptly to save their live.

Women leadership within the pro-democracy movement

In 1997 Robert Mugabe had been in power for 17 years after the white Smith regime had been overturned. The exposure of widespread corruption and misappropriation of public funds, popular disenchantment with the Lancaster House constitution (which gave President Robert Mugabe sweeping powers), and the desire by Zimbabweans for a 'home-grown' constitution, led to the formation of the broad alliance, the National Constitutional Assembly (NCA). It was composed of a wide array of civil society organisations, which ranged from the women's movement, trade union, student organisations, churches and professional bodies. It became a popular platform for mobilisation and organisation around issues of governance. This led to discussions around the formation of an alternative political movement, which would challenge Robert Mugabe's Zanu PF through elections. Thus the Movement for Democratic Changed (MDC) was formed, led by trade unionists Gibson Sibanda and Morgan Tsvangirai, and was launched in 1999. This was a watershed in Zimbabwe's history and the role women played in their individual capacities and as a movement is also key to understanding the overall successes especially in the constitutional movement. I was among the founders of the new party.

The way Zimbabwe's liberation narrative has been framed, often discounts the important and pivotal role that the women's movement played in both the constitutional movement, and later in the formation of the MDC. 'Her story' is often missing in spite of the heroic roles played by the women. One can mention for instance, Thoko Matshe, who was chairperson of the NCA, during the historic 'No Vote' campaign, in 2001, against a government sponsored constitution, which was meant to dilute and counter what civil society was suggesting, after mobilising views of Zimbabweans from all walks of life. Matshe, who is now based in South Africa, offered outstanding leadership to the broad alliance because of her integrity. Her meticulous leadership navigated around contentious issues on the constitutional reform agenda, and she kept the NCA together. Matshe led the NCA to victory, in a historic 'NO-VOTE'-campaign. This changed Zimbabwe's political face. More importantly, it dismantled the myth of the invincibility of the ruling party Zanu PF.

Other women leaders, who are now in the diaspora, are women's rights advocates, Lydia Zigomo-Nyatsanza and Yvonne Mahlunge-Gwashawanhu. Both are lawyers by profession and they both sat on the national Task Force of the NCA. Gwashawanhu is a practising law and at present plays a key role in educating women migrants of their rights.

The MDC under Tsvangira's leadership lost the plot altogether in terms of supporting and recognising the women in its ranks. The party, which has split into several formations in the 15 years of its existence, is now identified through a suffix to the name. The MDC led by Tsvangirai is now identified as MDC-T. The party has failed to deal decisively with issues of internal party cohesion among the different interest groups, which include women, as well as those to do with accountability and upholding the original founding principles of the party, which distinguished it from Zanu PF. Recent internal party violence has also badly tainted the image of the liberation movement, with the most recent case being the assault of former party, deputy Treasurer General, Elton Mangoma at the party head-quarters, Harvest House.

There are significant cases of victimisation of women within the ranks of MDC-T. Trudy Stevenson was assaulted at Harvest House after falling out with the party President. Lucia Matibenga, a party founder member, was removed from her post as Women's Assembly chairperson after falling out of favour with the party leadership. The failure by the MDC-T to dismantle the exhausted patriarchal model of power, premised on violence, has been its main undoing. The party is being torn apart by factional wars which pit Tsvangirai against his erstwhile right hand man, Secretary General Tendai Biti. Women in the party have also been torn apart, opting to support either of the two men. The MDC failed to build a formidable women's wing or movement, which would advocate and push for the interests of women not just within the party but at national level too.

Marginalisation of the diaspora in Zimbabwean politics

Zimbabwe benefits a great deal from remittances from those in the diaspora. According to Finance Minister, Patrick Chinamsa, just between January to November 2013, the country received $1.6 billion in remittances from the diaspora. While presenting the 2014 budget, Chinamasa went further to explain that the government would aim to harness the diaspora potential, by formalising a platform for dialogue through engaging the Zimbabwe Diaspora Home Interface Programme (ZDHIP), an entity through which the government aims to articulate its policies for engagement and investment with the Zimbabwe diaspora.

Despite the hardship of Zimbabweans living abroad and the benefits for the country of their contributions, the Zimbabwean leadership in general, across the political divide hold a rather condescending view towards those who have left the country - both male and female. This is the case irrespective of the motive behind their move, even if the departure was not politically motivated. The tenuous relation between the diaspora and the leadership became clear when MDC President, Tsvangirai, the then Prime Minister of Zimbabwe, visited London in 2009 and suggested that the Zimbabweans living in the diaspora ought to consider going back home, suggesting that they were wasting time. He was shocked to find that the Zimbabwean audience heckled and booed him (Mbiba, 2012).

The problem with the Zimbabwe political leadership is the general assumption that to participate fully in the affairs of the nation, one has to be inside the country. Zimbabweans in the Diaspora cannot vote, an issue on which both Zanu PF and the MDC-T seem to be in agreement. The Zanu PF dominated parliament of Zimbabwe, passed on 1 August 2014 the Electoral Amendment Bill, which takes away the right for those in the Diaspora to vote, contrary to section 67 of the constitution which protects the rights of adult citizens to vote. There have been no protestations from the opposition.

Women in the Zimbabwe diaspora

While the majority of the women fled violence in all its forms in Zimbabwe, violence remains a major issue that has resurfaced in their lives. Women in the Diaspora face the double jeopardy of being women and of also being in a foreign land.

The estimated 3-4 million Zimbabweans left especially to South Africa (2 million) and the UK (400.000) as well as Botswana (UNDP, 2010). The consequences are enormous. Families have been ripped apart. For instance, if the mother suddenly got an opportunity to practice nursing in the UK or the father had a chance to leave for Australia to teach. Other unmarried women with children had to make career choices and leave their children in Zimbabwe with relatives while they went out in search of work. Male and female migrants have suffered significant losses, not only in terms of what they owned at home, but even in terms of their careers. In the UK for instance nurses have been hired in the nursing and elderly care service industries, while many were qualified for other professions. As JoAnn McGregor (2006) pointed out: "Deskilling and a loss of status were problems for many of the qualified nurses who had relocated to the UK, and also for some of the older trainees in Britain, who had experience as professionals outside the health sector, or had run their own businesses." Some Zimbabweans in the Diaspora and especially those on asylum have not seen their families for over a decade.

In the United Kingdom and the United States there have been increased reports of domestic violence as a result of reversed roles. Women may find it easier to find work in social services, mostly as care workers while their husbands remain at home to look after the children. They hope for professional work as they would at home, to preserve what they traditionally see as their dignity and standing in society. Women have been more able to adapt, becoming breadwinners. This may result in a cultural shock and the men may feel emasculated and disrespected by their wives. This seems to be a cause of domestic violence in the Zimbabwean diaspora. The men have found it hard to understand the change in gender-roles. Their coping mechanisms include drug abuse, violence, sometimes femicide or suicide.[1]

In a report on *Zimbabwean Nurses and Teachers Negotiating Work and Family in Britain,* men interviewed often described nursing as a negative career choice. A former teacher recalled: "I trained as a nurse due to my immigration status - that was back in 2000, it was the only way to be stable" (McGregor, 2006: 9). Another male teacher who retrained elaborated:

> I didn't take the nursing job willingly, I just found myself without other opportunities, so I'm not motivated to go further through with the training, I felt I wouldn't last long, so I almost quit. I'm still undecided, I did a diploma not a degree in nursing – I chose not to go on because I didn't think I'd last long... I still feel a teacher, I decided to go into nursing because of a lack of opportunities for teachers, I thought of nursing as a job for females (McGregor, 2006: 9).

Now these two citations are interesting for an analysis of gender relations in the Zimbabwe diaspora and the reversal of roles. Women are

---

[1] From reports in social media: "Distraught mum kills self, two daughters in US", newzimbabwe.com, 02.07.2014; "Mum may have killed son before starting fire", Thurrock Gazette, 5.12.2014; "What's pushing Diaspora spousal killings?" Creed Mushimbo, Newzimbabwe.com, 12.10.2013. There is the reported case of 47 year old, Angela Mtambu, who killed herself and her two daughters, using suffocating nitrogen gas, at their upstate home in New York. Press reports indicate that Mtambu had to be admitted to Pennsylvania mental institution after being overcome with grief. There is the case reported in December 2013, of 45 year old, Cathy Mhlaba of Shoebury, in the United Kingdom, who is reported to have killed her son after which she took her own life, by starting a fire in her black Vauxhall Vectra. Mhlaba was in the leadership of the local MDC structures in Southend, were she was well respected. Many cannot fathom what led to her tragic end. Another heart breaking diaspora experience is of domestic violence. You have the case of the late Canada based Professor Otilia Chareka, who was bludgeoned by her husband, Patrick Chareka, in front of their young children. It is reported Chareka will spend at least thirteen years of his life in jail. In washington, USA is another case f Mary Mushapaidze was killed by her husband Mthulisi Ndlovhu, during a row over dirty dishes.

facing a huge backlash as a result if this.

The problem associated with the reversal of gender-roles has resulted in lengthy discussions on the popular news-site for Zimbabwean diaspora members: Newzimbabwe.com. Zimbabwean women in the UK are starting to organise themselves, mobilise support and build awareness for women caught in domestic traps of violence. Several organisations mobilise and raise awareness around this issue of domestic violence, such as the Zimbabwe Women's Network in the UK, (ZIWNUK) and P.H.O.E.B.E (Promotion of Health, Opportunity, Equality, Benevolence and Empowerment) which promotes greater inclusivity, encouraging a greater number of black and ethnic minority women and children to receive domestic violence support and counselling services across Suffolk.

The issue of domestic violence is intimately linked up with the overall sense of insecurity of the migrant communities. The situation for migrants and asylum-seeker remains insecure. In South Africa for instance the recent Documentation of Zimbabweans Project (DZP) permits for Zimbabweans living in South Africa, will be renewed under a new dispensation and will be called Zimbabwe Special Permit. But generally the situation of undocumented Zimbabwean migrants remains tenuous.

Despite these challenges women have found ways of organising and supporting themselves, their families and their communities. The Zimbabwe Women Achievers Awards (ZWAA), provides a platform in which women recognise their achievements and express their hope. Based in the UK, the ZWAA attracts Zimbabweans from all walks of life, and once a year at an event characterised by glitz and glamour, the women celebrate their successes.

Nora Chengeto Tapiwa – Tribute to a leader of women in the diaspora

(The source of this story is: Sofia Javed (undated) Nora Chengeto Tapiwa of Zimbabwe. Biography.)

A person who has very much inspired me is Nora Chengeto Tapiwa. She was a well-known leader of Zimbabwean exiled activists in South Africa. She was one of the founder members of the Zimbabwe Diaspora Development Chamber, (ZDDC). This organisation aims at creating cohesion and unity among the Zimbabwean diaspora, in South Africa, and beyond.

Tapiwa grew up in rural Zimbabwe during the liberation war. She became the organising secretary of the Zimbabwe Congress of Trade (ZCTU) union and hence became targeted by the government's suppression of political opposition. She was threatened and in 2003 Tapiwa decided to leave Zimbabwe with her two children. She fled to South Africa. Two years later the Zimbabwean authorities destroyed her house in Harare as part of a demolition programme called Operation Murambatsvina. This operation would result in an estimated 700,000 members of the Zimbabwe's working class community becoming homeless (Tibaijuka, 2005).

In South Africa, Tapiwa began to organise the refugee community and she formed the Global Zimbabwe Forum (GZF) with a group of more than 2,000 refugees, which grew to a large umbrella of 40 Zimbabwean organizations in exile. Advocacy towards the South African government to acknowledge the plight of Zimbabwean migrants and recognize them as refugees, succeeded in a waiver of visa requirements for Zimbabweans seeking asylum in South Africa.

The experience of women who fled has been like jumping out of the frying pan into the fire. In 2008 xenophobic riots broke out in South Africa against Zimbabwean refugees. This resulted in over 50 deaths among them Zimbabweans, and women were also targeted for rape and other forms of abuse (Romey, 2008).

Tapiwa worked at the Johannesburg Mayor's Migrant Desk and the South African Red Cross Society to coordinate humanitarian aid to migrants, and provide shelter and food to the victims of such attacks. She established the Tapiwa Institute of Leadership, specifically aiming at women; She motivated this:

> I want to encourage women to have confidence in themselves and believe they are no different from their male counterparts. Women, as mothers, are more passionate in making peace. They can keep nations together, the way they keep their families together. (Javed, undated)

Tapiwa received the Award of Woman PeaceMaker in 2010. Sadly, she passed away on 18 March 2014.

Conclusion

In Zimbabwe, women at all levels have given leadership to, and played an important role in, transformational politics. With President Mugabe in power for nearly 35 years, the country badly needs a more inclusive form of leadership. However, the patriarchal power structure, inherited from the colonial domination, has not been deconstructed, despite the efforts of women and social movements to establish alternatives. The cyclical violence associated with political elections has specifically targeted women. Women in politics are routinely suffering from violence and abuse and removal from positions if they fail to please the party leadership. The patronage system has silenced women politically, despite the new law promoting women's political leadership and guaranteeing women parliamentary seats, in conformity with the SADC protocol.

The 2 million women living in the diaspora face many challenges. Adapting to new circumstances, they find work (often in the care industry) below their training or capacities. Having work, while their husbands have difficulty in finding jobs, creates tensions within the home and the changing gender roles lead to domestic violence. The insecurity of many migrants, especially those who don't have documents, compounds the intra-household tension. While the Zimbabwe government recognises the contribution of the diaspora in monetary terms, it has failed to recognise the diaspora in terms of its political participation. Generally there is a sense that Zimbabweans in the diaspora are marginalised. A new generation of young adults has grown up in the diaspora. These young adults are Zimbabweans, but the question is, will they call Zimbabwe home?

References

Aids-Free World (2009) *Electing to Rape. Sexual Terror in Mugabe's Zimbabwe*. Aids Free World, New York. (p. 18).

Human Rights Watch (2006) *"You Will Be Thoroughly Beaten". The Brutal Suppression of Dissent in Zimbabwe*. Human Rights Watch, New York.

Javed, S. (undated) Nora Chengeto Tapiwa of Zimbabwe. Biography, available at: http://www.sandiego.edu/peacestudies/institutes/ipj/programs/women-peacemakers/about/nora-chengeto-tapiwa.php (accessed 4 August 2014).

Mbiba, B. (2012) Zimbabwean Diaspora politics in Britain: insights from the Cathedral moment 2009, *Commonwealth & Comparative Politics*, 50:2, 226-252.

McGregor, J. (2006) Professionals Relocating: Zimbabwean Nurses and Teachers Negotiating Work and Family in Britain, *Geographical Paper* No. 178.

Reeler, A. (2011) Zimbabwe women and their participation in elections, *Briefing Note*. RAU.

Romey, F. (2008) Double Jeopardy for women migrants, *Pambazuka news*, 2008-06-05, Issue 378.

Tibaijuka, A. (2006) *Report of the Fact-Finding Mission to Zimbabwe to assess the Scope and Impact of Operation Murambatsvina by the UN Special Envoy on Human Settlements Issues in Zimbabwe*, UN, New York.

UNDP (2010) The Potential Contribution of the Zimbabwe Diaspora to Economic Recovery, Comprehensive Economic Recovery in Zimbabwe. *Working Paper Series*, UNDP-Zimbabwe office.

CHAPTER 20. "GIRLS MAKE MUSIC, WOMEN CREATE CHANGE": ALTERNATIVE APPROACHES TO FIGHTING FOR A LIVING WAGE IN LONDON

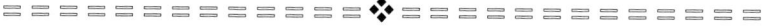

Robyn Stocker

The Scene

"What do we want? A Living Wage! When do we want it? NOW!" These familiar words echo across Brixton town as strikers make their voices heard, loud and clear. Most of these voices are female who believe they deserve respect and value in the workplace. I wish I could say they believe this without a shadow of a doubt, but the reality is that women have been conditioned to feel more uncertain about their decisions and to question themselves. Of course men do also, but it seems to be a more common theme for their female counterparts. A woman's value and position in society has been underrated for far too long.

The fact that these bold female campaigners have chosen to participate in such a movement demonstrates the underlying spirit of strength and determination. And one of the things that fortify this willingness to stand up is the support offered through the collective voice.

I am one of these women. We work in the service industry for a successful branch of a company with 21 branches across the UK. In 2013, the company was taken over by a larger national company. To protect the identity and reputation of these organisations, I will refer to the branch I work for as the Branch, the company as the Company and the current parent company (with interest in different countries) as the Parent.

The strikers add up to 69 members of the recognised trade union, of which a good majority is female. On the union's current six-person committee, there are an equal number of male and female representatives.

For the strikers, the last five months has been an intense emotional rollercoaster experience encompassing feelings of passion, unity, solidarity, progression, disappointment, frustration, breakthrough, tension, renewal and victory. But the fight is far from over.

The Cause and the Community

In 2007, staff balloted for industrial action and won a staggered agreement that took them above the poverty line. But this wage has since proven to be inadequate as a living rate and in early April this year, the Branch union members balloted to go on strike following negotiations that started in October 2013. The Greater London Authority recommends a London Living Wage, as it is the minimum prescribed amount necessary for living a sustainable life in London. The same applies to the Living Wage, which is the rate set to apply for the rest of the UK. Several organisations are already proud Living Wage employers: Lush Hand Made Cosmetics, Transport For London, The National Portrait Gallery, ABTA Travel Association and KPMG, to name a few.

A unit with a strong female presence, the strikers currently challenge the system, demanding the Living Wage as a basic human right.

Brixton is fast becoming a haven for wealthier residents, yet the community bonds remain strong and there is a reluctance to let go of the original grit and integrity of the old community. Some of the longstanding local residents know the story all too well. The Branch is a well-known landmark in the heart of a vibrant community. People either use the space to meet, work or unwind. Or people gather outside on the renowned Windrush Square, named after the Empire Windrush. This was a ship that hailed from Jamaica in 1948, carrying 492 immigrants many of whom then settled in Brixton where the nearest Labour Exchange was situated at the time. This historical setting is a poignant reminder of the spirit of strength of the working classes. The Brixton riots, sparked in the 1980's also offer a rich tale of historic significance to this local community, based on rebellion against institutional racism and oppression against minorities. Despite widespread regeneration, in places you can still feel a sense of struggle, riot and revolution that linger in the air. So it's not surprising that alongside the steady rise in power for the underdog, women are joining the uprising. And constituting at least half (if not more) of the world's population, they form a major cog in the overall works.

Women are key to the process of peace building within communities.

Because of their nature and alternative perspective, they provide the balance in the human equation. Throughout history, women have been at the centre point of the home, family and as such, the community. By nature, women also bring a range of approaches to the table; non-violent methods of protest, creative approaches and nurture over aggressive resistance. These characteristics complement women's ability to also stand strong, be assertive, use logic and strategize. These traits are typically associated with masculinity but strong female leaders express both aspects, just as well-rounded male leaders express a good balance of masculine and feminine traits also. The bottom line is that a balance of energy is needed and this can only happen where all aspects of healthy human traits are present.

The Challenge and the Secret

During the original negotiations prior to strike at the Advisory, Conciliation, and Arbitration Service (ACAS) in December 2013, the Company made an offer that would provide an increase in wages and work towards reaching the current living wage within approximately two years (£8.80 per hour). However, with no seeming further opportunity to negotiate, staff would always be lagging behind by two years with no commitment to ever reaching a rate that would match a current Living Wage.

Over the last four months, we have taken to the streets of Brixton and London to promote our message. During this period, we have been on strike thirteen times, protesting loudly outside our workplace and at strategically selected locations to raise our profile across local, national, and interest specific media. We were so passionate and inspired by the cause that we created our own brand "Living Staff, Living Wage", to represent our message: "All living staff deserve a Living Wage." We also enlisted the support of a number of celebrities who have been willing to endorse our campaign.

With our range of creative abilities, we pooled together and came up with engaging and entertaining ideas of how we could build a marketable brand to front our campaign and we have used everyone's strengths and the rich range of skills to create dynamism and liveliness to drive the movement forwards. Using music, art, drama, design, film and photography, amongst other talents, combined with productivity, efficiency and smart management and marketing skills, we recognise that by creating engaging processes, morale stays high and in turn fuels members and the community to keep going without which we would sure as hell crash and burn.

More recently (this July), following the three-month strike period, we returned to the negotiating table. The Company made an improved offer. The premise of which, £9.10 per hour would be reached by September 2016 and that we would have the opportunity to renegotiate in June 2016. A rough calculation suggests that by this time, the Living Wage will be estimated to have risen to about £9.70 per hour. Although the gap is much smaller, we still feel reluctant to accept an offer which means we are still lagging behind by a fair amount and there were also additional terms in the offer that did not sit well (for the purpose of this piece, I won't go into the details). Ultimately, we recognise the need to be practical in the application of the requested increase yet we are reluctant to settle for a situation whereby we still feel regarded as exploitable. The Company's overall stance, and certainly the Parent's attitude towards us still do not provide us with the reassurance that we are valued. At the time of writing, the results of the vote are yet to be released.

Through this work, we drew a lot of attention from the community and the media. The BBC, Channel 4, ITV, Evening Standard and The Guardian to name a few, covered our story. Our Facebook "likes" and Twitter followers rose into the thousands. We have repeatedly been approached to speak at conferences, rallies, marches and events to share hints and tips for other groups and to inspire people to stand up for what they believe in. We are regularly approached by people who ask us if we have achieved what we want. When we respond "no", the general response is one of disgust at the company and praise to us for our tenacity. People admire our spirit and want to learn our secret. The Branch is the only recognised Union of all of the Company's branches. Yet staff from four other branches have now been in touch and have told us that our campaign has encouraged them to unionise. How did we draw such attention and what sets us apart from other campaigns?

I believe the key element to our success is the innovative and youthful spirit of our campaigners. Not only do we have a large presence of women, but we also draw people who tune into their brilliant and creative minds. A huge proportion of the workers at the Branch are freelancers, others are students and a small minority work full time. It is a truly special place, and many of the staff choose to stay for a number of years owing to the sense of mutual respect, support, openness and community created by the type of employee that the Branch attracts. Through my own observations, I have found that the above-mentioned traits are often present in environments where there is a strong presence of women and "creative" workers.

As expressed by the branch secretary of the union and also one of the other female representatives, "I think there's so much loyalty at the Branch that you will find really difficult to find at other places and I think it's a fair thing for us to have, a Living Wage. I don't think it's asking the world."

They Exploit, We Create

One of the approaches we have been keen to employ as part of our campaign is to ensure that we take every given opportunity to keep lines of communication open with the Company. With so many different perspectives and skillsets, communication and maturity of approach has meant that there is something very real and genuine about the strikers. This in part is owing to the fact that there is a healthy blend of female and male leaders driving the campaign. And when I refer to leaders, I consider every single person actively involved in driving our campaign a leader. I believe that the hierarchical perspective of a leader can no longer apply. To me, a leader is any person who is respected by others, who inspires others and encourages positive growth.

As mentioned previously, another reason why the campaign is so successful is the high proportion of strikers developing careers in the creative industry. These are the people who bring life to the workplace and a main reason why the Branch is so popular within the community.

Ironically, the casual nature of the employment also seems to justify the lack of real value offered to employees. And the industry is filled with these. It has been proven that providing better conditions for staff and valuing their contribution encourages productivity and as such should be given priority. But the reality is that employers offer this flexibility of work under the false guise that they are "understanding" and "accommodating". In fact it suits them and allows them to manipulate staff to meet their own corporate agendas. Employees lose negotiating power and legal rights in the workplace owing to the lack of formal security and become objects for value extraction. What does that say about corporate perspective on the creative industry? And since the creative industry values the expression of qualities associated with femininity and not just masculinity, what does this say about corporate perspective on the feminine?

Outside of my job at the Branch, I work as a DJ, trainee music producer and manage a project called "Girls Make Music". The aim is to promote access for women to forge careers as music producers and sound engineers. I also teach young girls how to be a DJ and music production skills, encouraging more women to be an integral part of the music creation process and become leaders in this field.

The nature of my work and my situation requires a flexible working structure and this organisation is one of the rare companies that offers flexibility alongside some form of security. I truly appreciate this but it doesn't give the Company license to profit by paying an unfair wage. In contrast, the management style used by the strikers seeks to promote growth and inclusivity of members, giving them a voice and platform to develop as people, allowing them to own their experiences and take leadership in areas where they feel confident, willing and able.

To be continued...

The Company's response to our industrial action is to continually shut down the Branch on the days when we strike. As a paradox, the make-up of the

Company's management is also a marginal majority female. I must clarify that not all managers are effective leaders. As I stipulated earlier on in the chapter, my definition of a leader is not so much a person's position of authority but a person's ability to manage, inspire and lead others effectively to grow and develop. The traditional patriarchal style of leadership is still very much present in the actions of the Company's approach to management and no doubt within most corporate companies. And so I think a large part of moving forwards will be to encourage both women and men to use a supportive stance to women taking leadership. Sheryl Sandburg, the COO of Facebook, writes:

> Since there are so many more men at the top of every industry, the proverbial old-boy network continues to flourish. And since there are already a reduced number of women in leadership roles, it's not possible for the junior women to get enough support unless senior men jump in too. We need to make male leaders aware of this shortage and encourage them to widen their circle. (Sandburg, 2013, pp.71)

Good leaders are honest with themselves about who they are and what they want. One female striker who has worked at the Branch for several years, at the prospect of settling for a below par offer for which she would be entitled to backdated lump sum pay, proclaimed: "I may be broke but I'm not cheap".

Good women leaders are not trying to fit masculine stereotypes. It is very common for women who have taken on leadership roles to be shunned by both men and women for acting like men. But if both women and men were to embrace their feminine and masculine qualities and genuinely apply a balance of these traits to any given situation, the product would be organic. The male strikers are remarkable; they seem adept at also embracing their feminine qualities and are able to reach a real balance. This balance in society has been tipped way too far one way and it needs to swing back to settle at a happy medium. More women's leadership in decision-making is therefore necessary according to Sheryl Sandburg:

> Real change will come when powerful women are less of an exception. It is easy to dislike senior women because there are so few. If women held 50 percent of the top jobs, it would just not be possible to dislike that many people. (Sandburg, 2013, pp.50)

I realised very recently how touched I feel by the campaign. My participation has taken a lot out of me physically, mentally and especially emotionally. Many times, I have been on the verge of throwing in the towel. Leadership is a challenge and I have learnt day-by-day better ways of managing this role. I saw a glimmer of hope though, a sign that my work as a leader and our work as a team of representatives does pay off. Not necessarily in monetary terms or in terms of physical reward, but in terms of witnessing evidence of the rise in women's leadership.

One of the young female strikers spoke up at a recent meeting:

> All of those things [challenges with continued industrial action] I think can be tackled pragmatically, we need to do more fundraising, more of us need to step up and take responsibility... if we let [the Company] with everything they've been doing, grind us down, we'd be submitting to them and we'll have to go back to say oh you know, did we get the Living Wage? Well, almost. And that's what our campaign is, it's Living Staff, Living Wage. (Anonymous, 2014)

Picture a group of beautiful and inspiring women, sat conferring at a table in a bright and airy café. Some young, some older, but all with the type of determination and passion that cannot be stood in the way of. These female strikers took it upon themselves to gather together and draw up a detailed plan that would assist us all in the decision-making process of managing the ballot over current negotiations. This was the type of scene that I longed to see—a demonstration that women's work can be as much appreciated as a wonderful part of life as is the contribution of men.

I have repeatedly been told by male colleagues in my work as DJ and teacher that my presence is welcome. It "takes the edge off" and "brings a different energy to the group, we feel more settled". It is clear that developing a strong vision of women's leadership, representation and participation in peace building in communities is imperative.

Every single person living and breathing should by birthright be afforded a Living Wage. Women by birthright should be afforded respect. Recognition and value equates to fully functioning people and flourishing employees. Feminine traits such as compassion, sensitivity and tolerance add power to the human mix and effective female leaders are invaluable to progression in society. I believe that men and women alike would benefit greatly from supporting women to become positive leaders and promoting a more comprehensive leadership style in the workplace. Women should not and no longer need to comply with damaging standards from times past.

Laurel Thatcher Ulrich (2007), a famous historian and former professor at Harvard University, sums this up in one beautiful statement: "Well behaved women seldom make history."

References

Anonymous (2014) *Discussion during a union members' meeting.* [conversation] (Personal communication, 5 August 2014).

Sandberg, S. (2013) *Lean In: Women, Work And The Will To Lead.* Random House Company, New York.

Thatcher Ulrich, L. (2007) *Well-Behaved Women Seldom Make History.* Random House Company, New York.

CHAPTER 21. HOME-BASED CARE: THE POWER OF WOMEN TO CONNECT VULNERABLE MEMBERS OF THE COMMUNITY

Catherine Schook

For one person, it might be chicken noodle soup. For another, peeled grapes with missing pits. Whatever the comfort food craving or reassurance from a caring hand, our memories of sick days often have a glimmer of a woman's smiling touch. It seems no coincidence that in many countries women dominate the health workforce in over 75% of paid positions according to the World Health Organization (WHO) (2008). These care providers frequent our homes as well as our communities no matter their age, ethnicity, or availability.

As women have the ability to increase population growth courtesy of their reproductive organs, child bearing and rearing seems only the beginning. Bestowed upon her XX chromosomes comes a lifelong evolutionary characteristic of protection and nurturing. Our lineage has created an expanding chain throughout time, links labelled as "child" and one day perhaps as "parent". The roles within these links can interchange where a parent cares for a child and one day, a child for a parent. At the rate of population growth and differing age groups however, we'll have more "parent" links then ever before. In 2011, one in six European Union adults were over the age of 65. One in twenty were over 80 according to Eurostat (2013). The "child" links are looking a bit stressed.

An unbalanced chain is forming, especially for those that do not have a "child" link below them. For those families living in a rural setting with children nearby, as informal carers they are aware of the aging process and newly acquired responsibilities. Thanks to non-age specific technology, communication and nonphysical caring with a faraway aging family is common and scheduled weekly. Yet if none of the children are 50 steps away from their childhood front door at all times, responsibility can often fall to others, the non-familial others. Here enters the 75% female dominated health workforce in a variety of colourful positions.

One common example is of mom and dad growing old on the front porch in their rocking chairs with iPads and it will be the home care assistants, the health aides, "the help" that will come to their rescue when daughters and sons cannot. According to the WHO, home-care is roughly defined as satisfying people's health and social needs while residing in their home by providing appropriate and high quality home-based health care and services, by formal or informal caregivers, within a balanced and affordable continuum of care (WHO, 1999; WHO, 2002). An informal care giver, another keyword in this discussion about women's access to elderly care, is remarked as a carer that looks after family, partners, friends or neighbours in need because they are ill, frail or have a disability and the care they provide is unpaid (Eurocarers, 2007). Children fall into this category, along with aging spouses.

To place this topic in its historical context, let it be known that in the beginning of the 20th century, large-scale hospitals and medical institutions were built to care for the sick, the wounded and disabled, and the frail (Risse, 1999). Children's hospitals and mental institutions were also constructed during this time yet in the 1960s, a beginning replacement model started to take shape. So as to avoid long stays in medical institutions for both children and older people, new polices focused on improving nursing homes and elderly residential homes with such labels as integrated care, continuous care, deinstitutionalization, community care organizations and home-based care (WHO, 2008). Now in the 21st century, it is preferable to stay within one's home and maintain a routine with controlled customized care (Economic Policy Committee and the European Commission 2006). As alternatives become available to those favouring to age at home versus an institution, a selection process is now available for who will care for them, in what way and how often. Older children sometimes are not even a part of this equation.

The aim of this chapter is not only to discuss aging and its complexity in quality and care, but also to highlight unseen female informal care providers, a working force that has thinned out since urban sprawl and smaller family sizes became normalized. These women do not receive compensation in monetary form and their efforts are often coupled with paid care, which is highly demanded and globally short in supply. Several questionnaires and interviews were prepared for this chapter heading and the results are presented in a narrative format. The roles of the participating female caregivers range from daughter-in-law to granddaughter, from living 50 steps away, to living in another country. Within these stories, the interchangeability of the "child" to a "parent" link in the familial chain and the inheritance of caring can further be understood.

Tiny's granddaughter

Tiny is currently 93 years old. She is living at home in a small village in North Holland and she enjoys the comforts of egg salad on toast and has a history of spoiling her grandchildren with peeled pit-less grapes ("A few grapes were a luxury back then she says, now this is very common food"). She is nearly blind and she has four daily visits from home-care aids as organized by a home-based care organization. Thursday night is her scheduled shopping night and that is with one of her granddaughters. Tuesday is with the other granddaughter ("My sister also comes by once a week and does the same that I do").

This granddaughter, a questionnaire respondent, knew she wanted to work with people at a young age, especially when deciding her educational path: "I did always want to do something concerning people. That's what I like, having contact with the people around you that you work with and for." It was a trip to the dentist that sealed her fate: "I asked my own dentist if I could join him an afternoon in the office to see how everything works in a dental practice. I liked it so much and found it that interesting that I eventually made my career choice." Perhaps it came naturally to her, choosing a helping profession: "The care for your teeth and socializing with people were the two key features that interested me about my job."

This granddaughter joined the informal caregiving workforce in 2013 when her grandmother got sick and moved to be closer to her immediate family: "I would always visit her every other week, but now it's standard I visit her every Thursday night to help her and keep her company." When questioned about priorities and how this granddaughter decides what to do during these nightly visits, she answers: "Her priority is my priority then. She's cared for four times a day. My parents help out a lot too. So when it comes to getting her medication and meals ready, that is taken care of by the care people. I keep her company."

What this granddaughter does though is something more than just keeping Tiny company: "Whenever it's necessary I'll water the plants, clean the toilet, do the dishes and we visit the mall around the corner together. A real 'outing' for her." She even receives secret grandma compensation: "My grandma sometimes sneakily gives me 10 euro, because she thinks we deserve it. She's very happy when we visit and likes giving us a little something."

As someone that dedicates one evening a week to the needs of someone else, the question of why a young, career-oriented woman would give her time is asked. Her cool response: "She always took such good care of us and now she needs that care. I love doing it for her because I see her spirit is lifted. I'm a caring person at heart anyway. I think the people that need it most deserve it and I like doing it then." This granddaughter has a brother and a father, (Tiny is her father's mother) so when questioned about the qualities she brings to caring that her male counterparts don't, she replies: "It is because they are not as involved with my grandma as we are. The people that are there most for her are me, my sister, my parents and my aunt. Women cope with it differently than men do I think. Less patience and not such a strong bond I think. Women tend to care more than man do." Interesting that the list of individuals that are on the caring schedule (not including the paid help aides) are 80% female. Perhaps this "caring gene" has been hereditarily passed down to this granddaughter through her mother and the good care of her paternal grandmother. The combined family unit has reversed roles in providing care and is individually responding.

Karl and Irmgard's daughter

Originally from Germany, with parents still nestled in German farmland, Karl and Irmgard's daughter left for the big city early on, leaving behind two siblings living closely to their parents. Once the mother, 83, was stricken with dementia and the father, 88, was too exhausted to care for his wife, the immediate family was called into action. She recalls: "The total body care has to happen by someone else. But first my father wouldn't let anyone in. […] He takes her out walking and he can hardly walk and she is still very strong […] And he said to the family, 'Please come and live with us because I can't do all of this.'" Luckily a few steps away lived the older brother and his "saint-like" wife and she started to care for the mother: "My sister-in-law is the fall back scenario. I mean she has to do it everyday."

After two years of the sister-in-law caring for the mother, Karl and Irmgard's daughter addressed the next phase with her father considering the growing burden on one family member: "And he says, 'No no, nothing will be changed. I will take care of your mother until she dies and I hope you will help. That's the situation. And she's done everything for us and now we do everything for her.'" With baby steps, the daughter residing in the Netherlands hired a weekly cleaning lady. Soon a weekly aide was hired to help with bathing and cooking.

However while recently on holiday, a dreaded phone call came from her younger sister saying their father needed to go to the hospital considering complaints of exhaustion and heart problems. After his release with recommendations of rest, the father asked again for the daughter to stay. Her reply: "You have to be dying before I come more frequently. And then he says, 'Ah, [cough cough] I think I am going to die.'" In order to leave him and her mother in better hands, without placing more responsibly on the sister-in-law (who at the time had the mother living at her house from bedtime to 15.00 the next day), 24-hour care entered the conversation.

"You have that very often in Germany with farmers. If you bring a farmer to an elderly home, he'll just leave. So we have a lot of women from Poland and Slovakia, they come in and they live with the elderly people for a month, sometimes two months. And then they go back and someone else comes for a month." It took some getting used to, with a decrease in staff down to one person, and some behavior and control change with Papa, however Maria is currently living with Karl and Irmgard. She is an older Slovakian woman, as selected by the daughter from a home-based care organization, that will return home in a month and another will take her place. Already, the parents are taking to her and the sister-in-law only houses Maria. However the sister-in-law's perspective, as a care provider not even related by blood, stated eloquently why she gives her time: "It's part of life. You raise your children, your parents die, children don't need that much care anymore and then you start all over again. What more can you do?"

Eventually, nonphysical informal care can be achieved across national borders if there is a telephone and a home-care organization to call. With a family unit of three children however, two of which living nearby, the saving grace was the daughter-in-law. Not an instance of genetics but an example of a woman individually responding.

Mrs. VHVW's daughter-in-law

While the granddaughter gives her time every Thursday evening to Tiny, the daughter-in-law, her husband's mother, knows her as Mrs. VHVM. With a shift in perspective from one caregiver to another with the same elderly woman, including alternative roles and responsibilities, perhaps the richness of the informal caregiving in a family unit can be witnessed in this participant's responses.

From an early age, the daughter-in-law was raised in a close family: "Family life was important, communal meals, coffee in the evening and on weekends." Like her daughter, this daughter-in-law also found the helping professions and its education enticing: "I decided to go to nursing school, to have something to fall back on." With a nursing education, she now works as a healthcare assessor: "As a community care giver, I'm caring for physical tasks, coordinating the tasks and I support the client in their home situation."

Her caregiving roles are a bit more in-depth than her daughter's: "We do groceries, read her mail because she's almost blind, assist her going outside. We check the safety of her food, clean up her 'accidents', change medication, and check her clothing. Sometimes we help her get showered." When it comes to planning priorities, one is strikingly clear: "Our first priority is taking her outside. She thoroughly enjoys this but can't do it by herself any more. We shop together as much as possible at the local mall." As tradition repeats itself with the daughter-in-law, family meals are also occasionally organized: "Every so often I take her to our home on Wednesday to have a meal with us. However, because she has a strict diet, eats slowly and not in the tastiest way, I don't do this too often."

Lucky for Mrs. VHVM, she raised a son with connections: "Her son works at a organic grocery store, so he takes care of the groceries." However balancing of the care priorities has been difficult recently considering a decline in health: "We have spent the night with her over a period of time, because she couldn't get in or out of bed by herself. It's getting better now, but cognitively speaking she's gotten worse, which increased her dependence on care."

The daughter-in-law describes her role as a caregiver by saying: "I'm caring and love to make someone else happy. Actually it makes myself feel good if people appreciate what I do." When the conversation turns to the man's role in caregiving, her response mentions Mrs. VHVM's son: "My husband struggles with 'defecating accidents'. Helping with the physical needs, especially personal hygiene is hard for him. I myself don't really mind with this aspect of caring, probably because of my nursing background." When questioned why she believes it is women who provide care for others, she responds: "The wife was at home caring for the children, the man provided income. You still see this with the elderly. I myself think that care giving is closer to women then men, if this is genetic I don't know." Lastly, it was asked if she had any ideas how to make a community more elderly-focused. Her response: "An afternoon program, with a possible communal meal or coffee, could decrease social isolation. A long afternoon/evening with a program would be a welcome break."

The Golden Age

In these stories of women providing care for a blood relative or a family member related by marriage, no matter the relation, they give their time and physical and mental energy for years. As these narratives pinpoint, a person's specific caring role for an elderly family member differentiates and certain skill sets or "perks" are put to use. A granddaughter's Thursday evening is free, the son works for a grocery store, the daughter-in-law has a background in nursing to help with medications, a daughter finds and contacts the best services. If the family unit works together in utilizing their strengthens and schedules, the balance is more equal. If it falls to one person, as the example in Germany, the quality of care decreases in not just the recipients but also in the givers.

Another similarity between these narratives is the elderly person's desire to be outdoors. Being outdoors and socialization is a part of human behavior, no matter what age, so a trip to the mall or a walk with a balancing arm could make the difference. Even the daughter-in-law made the recommendation to include an afternoon elderly programme to decrease social isolation. Perhaps this topic is being examined too closely and the desired end result to achieve healthy aging is simply human interaction, preferably from informal family caregivers.

Women have an inherited attribute of nurturing as passed down the familial chain. The participants mentioned within this discussion strengthen that statement as witnessed in their monthly, weekly, if not daily commitment to caring for an older individual, whether blood related or not. The informal caregivers role has been decreasing with the growing presence and demand of non-familial care considering the family's move in being farther away. Globalization has allowed the spread of populations, however when someone turns that golden age, the vast spread and absence of people, especially family, is no longer desired. It's the comfort, the family connection, the trips outdoors, those interactions are the ones women can not only provide but also cherish. The woman's role in connecting the elderly population is of significant importance and without it the family unit is not complete. In order to face global aging, family responsibility needs to be re-prioritized where individual roles are formed to fill certain gaps for the benefit of the aging family member. The leaders of this change will lie within women, as it is their role within the family and the community to nurture, solve problems and provide comfort, even in the form of peeled grapes.

References

Eurostat (2011) The greying of the baby boomers: a century-long view of ageing in European populations. Luxemburg: European Union. Available at: http://epp.eurostat.ec.europa.eu/cache/ITY_OFFPUB/KS-SF-11-023/EN/KS-SF-11-023-EN.PDF (accessed 16 August 2014).

Economic Policy Committee and the European Commission (2006) The impact of ageing on public expenditure: projections for the EU-25 Member States on pension, healthcare, long-term care, education and unemployment transfers (2004–50). Brussels: Economic Policy Committee and the European Commission. Available at: http://ec.europa.eu/economy_finance/publications/publication 6662_en.pdf (accessed 16 August 2014).

Risse G. (1999) *Mending bodies, saving souls: a history of hospitals.* Oxford University Press, Oxford.

World Health Organization (1999) *Home-based and long-term care: home care issues and evidence.* Geneva: World Health Organization. Available at:

http://apps.who.int/iris/bitstream/10665/66096/1/WHO_HSC_L TH_99.2.pdf?ua=1 (Accessed 16 August 2014).

World Health Organization (2002) *Community home-based care in resource-limited settings: a framework for action.* Geneva: World Health Organization. Available at: http://www.who.int/hiv/pub/prev_care/isbn9241562137.pdf (accessed 16 August 2014).

World Health Organization (2008) *Spotlight on Statistics: Gender and health workforce statistics.* Geneva: Department of Human Resources for Health. Available at: http://www.who.int/hrh/statistics/spotlight_2.pdf?ua=1 (accessed 16 August 2014).

World Health Organization (2008) *The Solid Facts: Home Care in Europe.* Copenhagen: The WHO Regional Office of Europe. Available at: http://www.euro.who.int/__data/assets/pdf_file/0005/96467/E91884.pdf (accessed 16 August 2014).

PART-VI A REFLECTION ON THE CHALLENGES OF REBULDING POST-CONFLICT LIBERIA

CHAPTER 22. INTERNATIONAL SOCIAL RESPONSIBILITY

Lecture on the occasion of the celebration of the 85th Dies at Tilburg University, Tilburg, Netherlands on Friday, 9 November 2012

By H.E. Mrs. Ellen Johnson Sirleaf, President of the Republic of Liberia

Rector Magnificus, Professor Philip Eijlander;
The Executive Board of Tilburg University;
Faculty, Students;
Members of Parliament and Officials of Government;
Corporate Leaders and Leaders in Social Responsibility;
Former Prime Minister Lubbers;
My Fellow Liberians; Ladies and Gentlemen:

Let me say how delighted I am to be in the Netherlands once again, and to be here in Tilburg, a city that is growing in prominence economically, culturally and particularly in the field of education.

Thank you, Tilburg University, for the kind invitation to be your guest of honour and to address this esteemed Tilburg family as you celebrate the 85th Dies. It is an honour to be associated with an institution recognized for its research and as the best-specialized University in the Netherlands every year for the past five years.

I am especially honoured to have been selected this particular year, 2012, as you mark the 100th anniversary of the birth of an extraordinary woman,

Marga Klompé, the first female Minister of the Netherlands, whose life bore striking similarities to my own – an activist and an advocate for equal rights – and it is a pleasure to be able to speak on a topic that is her legacy and this year's special theme, "International Social Responsibility."

Marga Klompé's work in negotiating the Universal Declaration of Human Rights was inspired by the need to provide a life of dignity for everyone, irrespective of their culture, religion or ethnicity. She argued that societies were becoming more complex, and therefore society had a responsibility to care, so as to protect the dignity of every person. Her message was as relevant then, over sixty years ago, and it resonates even today.

I join in celebrating the life of this courageous woman, who went on to negotiate the Universal Social Security Bill, from which Dutch Society continues to benefit. Marga Klompé had a vision of a society based on institutional structures that promoted the protection and preservation of values, which in turn, created a healthy and tolerant society with a focus on assisting the unprivileged as an entitlement and not charity.

International Social Responsibility

On the topic of international social responsibility, we would need to speak of the inequities of our world, and what has to be done to mitigate or eliminate them. Inequities and variation in natural endowment are inherent constants in the human condition. Some of us are taller, stronger or smarter than the average person. Some regions encourage agriculture, horticulture and aquaculture much more than others. These differences occur naturally, and it would be unfair to begrudge any person or region for their naturally occurring advantages.

We know, however, that the moral strength of any society can be gauged on how it treats the most vulnerable – the children, the elderly, the disabled and the poor. On this scale, our global society has made strides, but is still wanting. There is so much more to do, and it is in this context that international social responsibility takes shape.

Over time, some of us are able to build on our advantage and become even stronger. Hard work, persistent effort, effective planning are all qualities that some possess much more than others. In societies where the individual's rights are protected, and stability and security maintained, people thrive. We must always respect and applaud such success.

We must also note that power seeks power, and history is replete with instances where advantages, whether naturally endowed, legally or illegally acquired, are wielded against the public interest, and short-term benefits accrue to but a few. Ultimately, however, this happens to the long-term detriment of the collective good.

The 2008 financial crisis is one example. The disproportionate influence and advantage of a small group of people threatened the entire global economy. Even in a country like Liberia, which is not directly connected to international finance, we felt the resulting credit crunch when investment and remittances declined. Another instance of the institutionalization of an advantage that works against the greater good is the role of women in society. One example that comes to mind is the stubborn discrimination against women across all societies: the obvious wage gap between men and women for performing the same job; the smaller number of women in positions of public trust; the absence of a choice of a career; and the wholesale obstruction of 50% of the world's population from equal participation in political, economic and social life.

With time these inequities become institutionalized to such an extent that its beneficiaries no longer even notice them. Only its victims see them and care, since they must live with the consequences daily. Your role – my role – is to work to end these disparities. Our responsibility is to reform our institutions, organizations and entities – local, regional, national and international – so they reflect the equality of persons for which we all strive.

At its most basic, international social responsibility is concerned with the development of the human person. A major thrust is to ensure human development and security through empowerment and sustainability, along with greater equity and productivity. The end result of international social responsibility must be to promote and preserve a peaceful world order, protect the environment, and bequeath to succeeding generations a more stable and a more humane international system.

International social responsibility is made necessary by multiple issues, the most important of which is the vast gap that exists between the rich and the poor within countries and We live in an unequal world that is increasingly becoming even more unequal. We live in a world where it is now possible for individuals to pay tens of millions of dollars for recreational trips to space when millions of school children still walk miles to unlit classrooms that do not even have enough chairs and desks, and some are forced to sit on the floor. That we are comfortable with such a world, that we will sit on the side-lines and let this continue, is blight on our collective conscience. Through international social responsibility, we move outside the margins of society to include those who have been excluded.

Let me highlight, though, some of the good news: between countries. Between 1990 and today, we have made tremendous progress in reducing some of the inequities within and between our societies. I can provide anecdotal evidence of how empowered women have become in my country.

When I travel in the countryside, and I see how women are far more assertive in taking part in discussions in their communities. They tell me that they no longer sit down and let the men decide. As I travel across Liberia and Africa, I am both amazed and humbled by the number of young women whose options for future aspirations have expanded. Today, they say boldly, we want to become President; we want to be a Prime Minister. To those young people we say, indeed, international social responsibility is beginning to take root.

The 2012 Millennium Development Goals (MDGs) Report also gives cause for hope. It notes that three important targets will be met well ahead of the 2015 end-date. Even more heartening is the observation that "while challenging," meeting the remaining targets is well within our reach, if governments do not waver from their commitments.

The Report notes that, for the first time since records on poverty began, the number of people living in extreme poverty has fallen in every developing region, including our own sub-Saharan Africa. Preliminary estimates indicate that the proportion of people living on less than US$1.25 a day fell in 2010 to less than half of the 1990 rate, and during the same period over two billion people gained access to improved drinking water sources; the share of slum dwellers in urban areas declined; and improving the lives of at least 100 million people.

In revising its poverty statistics, the World Bank observed that, when one takes into account increased population between 1981 and 2005, global poverty rates have fallen by about 25 percent. Unfortunately, this is not as encouraging as it sounds since these aggregate numbers do not account for differences between regions. China's large population and impressive progress over the period skews the aggregate number. During that period, China's poverty rate fell from 85% to 15.9%, or by over 600 million people, accounting for about 50% of the decrease in global poverty. We applaud this reduction, the lives of at least 100 million people having been improved, and those improvements keep mounting. Yet, I say, the numbers are disappointing, and the pace of improvement is still unacceptable.

Over 3 billion of our fellow human beings still subsist on less than US$2.50 daily. More than a billion children live in poverty, and tens of millions lack access to adequate shelter or safe drinking water. At this pace, it will be difficult to halve extreme poverty in some of our lifetimes.

Allow me to use my own country as an example of why and how such a pace is frustratingly slow. Liberia's current population is about 4 million. Our vulnerable employment rate exceeds 60%, as most of our labor force lacks the kinds of skills that would make them marketable. Our infrastructure is weak, making transactional cost prohibitively high for small businesses. The price of capital remains high, resulting in high interest rates, short lending periods and, consequently, high default rates, which in turn, further increase lending and transactional costs.

Most of the world's poor live in countries like Liberia. If we are to reduce poverty, then aid is not enough. It has never been enough.

When I came into office in 2006, the National Budget of our entire country was US$80 million – perhaps something equivalent to some of the budgets of your universities. Our Central Bank reserves were a mere US$5 million. It didn't take a rocket scientist to tell us that US$80 million would not meet all of the vast the needs of a collapsed economy and destroyed country.

We have made great progress, but even that must be seen in context. Our National Budget today has climbed to $687 million, a great leap from the 2006 figure. However, the cost of paving the road that links the center of our country to its southeast will cost US$405 million; and restoring our large hydro-electric generator will exceed US$250 million. Countries like ours – with high unemployment, little or no infrastructure and small resource envelopes – are host to the world's poor, and if we are to reduce the inequities that exist in our world, how we see these countries, and how we engage them, will have to change.

Please note that it is not for the lack of resources that these disparities exist. The aggregate unreported wealth of individuals in tax havens is equal to the combined size of the United States and Japanese economies. This is about US$21 trillion, all of which, according to the Tax Justice Network, is held by 100 million people. But just listen, of this $9.8 trillion is held by just 100,000 people.

This is not an attempt to criticize the success of those who have piled up the billions, but an opportunity to show the stark inequalities that still persist in our world – where a country with under 4 million people cannot afford paved roads and entire populations are cut off from the rains during six months, and 100,000 people are able to hold about $9.8 trillion dollars in unreported earnings. We have all heard the statistics, but they warrant repetition. It is important to keep in mind that every statistic represents a life – a child, a mother, a daughter, a father.

International social development must address human development. I believe that the UN System is correct when it observes that human development encompasses more than the rise and fall of incomes. We need to create a global environment that allows people not only to develop their potential but to also lead productive lives. I also believe that the UN membership is correct to move beyond the old policy of non-interference in the internal affairs of a sovereign State, to intervention in the interest of a repressed people, under the policy of the Responsibility to Protect.

According to the Overseas Development Institute (ODI), poverty reduction will occur as a result of the rate of growth and change in income distribution. This is within countries and between countries. We must also note that reduction in inequality and income differences will help spur poverty reduction. If we want to end acute poverty, if we want to improve opportunities for all of the world's people, countries and regions, international social responsibility must address these inequalities.

Conclusion

Let me close by saying the new dynamics of population growth, developed country stagflation and financial stress suggests that the world is at a crossroads. We must either adopt new policies and strategies to bring the world's poor nations into the competitive and contributive arenas of development through the exercise of international social responsibility, or we face the reversals of prosperity in the richer nations of the world.

The time to act is now.

The time to bring about women's equality is now.

The time to address poor education in children in poorer nations is now.

The time to bring international responsibility to all nations in an interdependent world, where everything you do, and say, also has ramifications for us, is now.

And every time we succeed or fail, you feel the consequences.

The new Global Development Agenda, now being formulated, the one in which I participate as co-Chair, in going beyond the Millennium Development Goals to formulate an agenda that, indeed, will be global, coming from rigorous global consultations, will reflect an agenda and an objective that says we cannot allow our people in the world to be poor.

Poverty must be eliminated. We must formulate this.

We must demand this.

We must insist on it.

And we must act on it. I thank you.

CHAPTER 23. LAUDATIO

On the occasion of awarding an Honorary Doctorate from the University of Tilburg at the 85th Dies to H.E. Mrs. Ellen Johnson Sirleaf, President of the Republic of Liberia

By Professor Dr. Mirjam van Reisen, Endowed Chair of Marga Klompé

Friday, 9 November 2012

Madam President,
Excellencies,
Distinguished guests,

"Our dream has the size of freedom" are the poetic lines with which you gave inspiration to the people of Liberia: Liberia, the country of freedom.

The country of hope, for so many who found refuge in it after the dark days of slavery. The connection of your country with the United States speaks for itself. But so does the connection with Europe. It was the Dutch East Indian company that was among those firms, trading slaves from West Africa to the Americas. It has deeply affected the realities in your country. You have described this in great detail in your book: "This Child Will Be Great."

Madam President, we warmly welcome you to European soil. This is your own continent in so many ways. I am reminded of your maternal grandfather, who was German, and who lived in Liberia where he met your grandmother.

Madam, on Wednesday you received the highest distinction of France at the Elysée Palace from President Hollande: la Grande Croix de la Légion d'Honneur. This well deserved honour is surely a sign of changing times. The entry of a new era, away from the days that European countries competed over colonial control and rule in Africa, and over access to its abundant natural resources. Away from competition between Dutch, French, British and German territories. Today Africa and Europe are finding each other in very new ways.

Our images are painted by the past. The destruction of the civil war in Liberia and in Sierra Leone shocked the world. We all remember the pictures of adults and children that were maimed, the pandemonium frightened us all. You had the courage to go back to your country, assemble the women, organise their participation in a constructive force to stop the conflict. Your influential report "Women, War and Peace" published by the UN in 2002 has helped in understanding the role that women play in conflict, not just as victims, but as agents, who have a choice, to accept, to participate, to resist, to mediate, to call their fathers, brothers, husbands and sons to account. In conflict we all carry responsibility. Women can choose to help end conflict. This is what you have shown. It has inspired women all over the world, and led to the groundbreaking UN Security Council Resolution 1325.

You have shown the power of imagining the future with fresh eyes. As the Flemish painter Permeke put it: "I don't paint what I see, but I paint what I think I have seen." While we paint we create a reality, we create our future. Our imagination is what we become. Therefore how we imagine the future is how we shape reality. I was in Monrovia at the invitation of your government this summer. I walked into one of the townships and a young boy of some 18 years old approached me to guide me around and finally brought me to his mother's place. His family had been destroyed by the civil war, his father, a government official, killed in front of his eyes, his mother, uneducated, fled with her children and in all those years of growing up, this kid had not once gone to school. What did he want, I asked. To go to school. To find a job. And his mother, sitting in front of a shack, was just grateful. Grateful for peace. Grateful for a quiet night. Grateful for the little freedom offered by a country in peace.

Madam President, the expectations upon you are immense. It is not enough that you were bold in firmly denouncing corruption, when western countries supported the corrupt leaders of your country during the Cold War. It is not enough that you suffered the pain of prison when you demanded democracy loud and clear, and we in the west continued to support the dictatorial regime. It is not enough that you climbed the ladder of a professional, first as Minister of Finance, then as World Bank Advisor, next as Under Secretary General of the UN, and gave all of this up to serve your country. It is not enough that you have heard the cries of your people and responded to it. We need you now to succeed to construct the future: to get the children to school, to create jobs, to build roads, to build homes, to bring democracy, to keep the peace. To realise the dreams created through the hope which you embody as President.

At this Dies we celebrate the 100th birthday of our first female Minister: Marga Klompé. She bears much resemblance with you. She also had German roots. She resisted Nazism and became a leader in the resistance. She served in the United Nations where she assisted in the negotiations of the Universal Declaration of Human Rights. She served in the European Assembly working for regional peace on this continent. She realised the first law on Universal Social Protection in the Netherlands.

As you have, Marga Klompé demanded respect for the human dignity of all, asked for all of us to carry responsibility for justice and peace, individuals, politicians, companies. We all have our role to play. As you are, she was a spiritual woman of faith. And like you, she was a pragmatic realist.

And as you, she was and is supported by a strong, supportive and loyal sister. Your achievements are no small feat. You have shown the world that women can lead. That African women can lead. That women can lead countries out of conflict. That women can play a pivotal role in bringing peace, in making peace, in keeping peace. That women are good economists, good financial analysts, good strategists. That women care, as daughters, mothers, wives, partners and as leaders.

In Europe we look at your achievements and wonder, is this the new Africa? The new Africa won the Nobel Prize for Peace in 2011. Europe won the Nobel Prize for Peace in 2012. This surely provides a basis for a partnership for peace and prosperity between our continents.

Madam, I congratulate you on your bold and courageous steps, which will remain to inspire the people of our continents to believe that peace is possible. 'Our dream has the size of freedom' - indeed, but reality needs exceptional people with your courage and inspiration."

PART VII – THE PRAXIS OF ENGAGING WITH WOMEN'S AGENCY IN PEACE BUILDING

CHAPTER 24. "SHOW ME YOUR FRIENDS, AND I WILL TELL YOU WHO YOU ARE": THE ROLE OF REHABILITATION PROGRAMMES IN REDUCING RECIDIVISM AMONG PRISON INMATES

Vickie Wambura

Benjamin Baraka, a young 21-year-old lad, was arrested and sentenced to Nairobi West Prison in 2005 for fraud. He was sentenced to three years in prison. In April 2007, he joined the existing prison primary education programme. At first, Benjamin's grades were very low but he was determined to turn that around. He worked hard, put in extra hours of learning and assignments, proving he was up to the task. At the end of that year, Benjamin was at the top of his class and his teacher and prison officials were proud of him. He had a bright future ahead of him and was full of so much potential. Prior to his release, Benjamin sat for the national exams and when asked his plans when released, he retorted that he would go back to his former ways of forging cheques. He went on to say that this is all he knew how to do and it put food on the table and a roof over his head.

This was almost seven years ago and this first hand encounter helped shape my thoughts about the challenges facing prison rehabilitation in the country. The presence of peace doesn't mean the absence of crime. In fact, crime violates personal peace. It constitutes an invasion of personal space, and is an assault to the peaceful state on the victims. While the whole nation may not be at war, the victims feel and live in a different reality irrespective of whether the crime caused them to suffer physical hurt and pain. When statistics and numbers are read out about declining or increasing crime rates it's important to take a step back amidst the applause or disproval and visualize the actual human faces on both ends of this tragedy. Both the victims and perpetrators are our brothers, sisters, mothers, fathers and relatives. The reduction of crime and the active effort towards reducing repeat offence is central to peace building in our society. My personal thesis is that if we get rehabilitation right then we will have better and safer communities. That is why I established the organization Nafisika Trust.

From the Beginning

It was just about Christmas in 2006 after spending my gap year in Belgium on a cultural exchange programme. I was back home in Nairobi and was in the process of applying for a student visa to return to Belgium. One evening I watched a TV news story that described the dilapidated state of prisons in Kenya. The first thought that crossed my mind was, "Who spends Christmas with prisoners?" I immediately got excited at the thought of doing something about the conditions during the Christmas season. However, it took me a while to gain access into prison as I didn't know how to go about it, but in January 2007, Pastor Simon Mbevi of Mavuno Church introduced me to Nairobi West Prison, a men's prison in the heart of the city.

Needless to say, I was excited to walk through the prison gates to offer my services. I had it all figured out, so I thought. I was going to paint the prison together with the inmates. This would enable us to bring a facelift to the prison as well as allow me to spend time with the inmates and to get to know them personally instead of as statistics. It seemed like a great plan until I met the officer in charge of the prison together with her staff officers. My brilliant idea was immediately turned down as they told me that they had just painted the prison and didn't need any more painting. My bubble burst. At 21 years old I was a little intimidated by all the officers in the room when I asked what else I could do. They looked at me blankly for what seemed like forever until one officer spoke out. She said that they had just started an education programme but lacked books and stationary. I jumped at it and offered to get the learning resources they needed.

So two weeks later, I returned with over 150 books and dozens of pens and pencils. I had managed to raise money, which was donated by my family who encouraged me to take on this crazy challenge. When dropping off the books, I requested to take a tour of the prison to see the conditions in which the inmates lived. I walked past their living quarters, rest area, common hall and kitchen when I saw a small dark room that acted like a classroom with eight students. One inmate acted as the teacher and they scribbled in their exercise books. This scenario moved me to look deeper at what they were learning. So I glanced through their books and I was moved to inquire more. I began to learn that there weren't any trained teachers commissioned by the prison service to teach at the prison, despite them directed to have a school programme. At the time they only had one class that would sit for the national exams but they were barely prepared to do so. So I offered to teach and they agreed! On that day, I taught English and it was an amazing experience.

I continued to frequent the prison on a daily basis as I taught English and Mathematics. It was the most fulfilling experience in my life and after a few weeks I began to think that I could do this for life. So in an attempt to discover my purpose, I postponed my education in Belgium to the next semester and continued to teach in prison. After a couple of months I completely discarded the idea of studying abroad and decided to pursue a road less travelled. I decided to dance to the tune that resonated in my heart; I dedicated my entire time to teach in prison. I had no clue where this would lead to but I had found something greater for which to live. It was something beyond me, something worth living for.

My encounter with Benjamin reshaped my thinking of social change. I began to understand that I was dealing with a systemic challenge that needed a different approach. I needed to understand the roots of the problem and begin to address them from different angles. I studied about rehabilitation globally and the different approaches from the East and the West. I analyzed the situation in our prisons deeper and formulated approaches that would address the causes of re-offence in Kenya.

The state of the Kenyan prisons and partnership with Nafisika Trust

The Kenya Prisons Service has its origins in the colonial era where its main role was to incarcerate and punish Africans as a means of pacifying them. Traditionally, the prisons service had been a department of the Ministry of Home Affairs under the Office of the Vice-President. Vice-Presidents were basically political appointees serving under the whims of the president and lacked the muscle to effect changes unless there was goodwill from the president. As a result the inherited legacy of the prison system was maintained. Largely ignored in the post-independence years by subsequent administrations, a radical shift was needed if we were to break away from having prisons as punishment centres towards becoming rehabilitation centres.

This journey began earnestly in 2001 when the then Vice-President and Minister of Home Affairs Moody Awori began to institute reforms to the service to address the years of rot and neglect. This shift meant that prisoner reformation would no longer be a by-product of imprisonment but rather a deliberate action taken by prison personnel. This was the birth of rehabilitation as a priority of the Kenya Prison Service. Over the years, the Kenya Prison Service has improved on its service delivery and approach in rehabilitation of prison inmates. It has been a herculean task to change the more than 40 years of neglect and change the established culture and attitude towards rehabilitation. Behind this reform has been the hard work and dedicated service of the prison service workers who have had support from the very top echelons of the service. Their dedication and determination to turn around prisons form centres of punishment to centres of reform deserves applause.

However given the demands of other sectors of the economy, substantial expenditure on prison programmes ranks low on the list of official priorities. It is because of this that the prison service created the Open Door Policy where they could partner with non-profits like Nafisika Trust to support their rehabilitation processes and programmes. This policy has enabled a flourishing partnership between Nafisika Trust and the Kenya Prison Service since 2007 when I first walked through the prison gates of Nairobi West Prison. Our work has not been without its set of challenges, such as fighting mind-sets, getting resources and establishing new cultures and norms, but it has been worthwhile. Today Nafisika Trust and the Prison Service can boast of our work and success stories from the hundreds of reformed inmates and a positive environment in prison. Through this work we have been able to fully understand our resource gaps that are needed to make our work more effective. Four key areas stand out for us in no particular order: finance, infrastructure, technical expertise and technology accelerators.

The vicious cycle of recidivism

While there was a form of industry and training built into the system, it did not have rehabilitation at the centre. Inmates could learn some skills such as carpentry. However built within the criminal justice system were sentences that included "hard labour", which usually entailed punitive and unproductive tasks such as crushing stones for hours on end. This in effect created "hardened" criminals bonded in camaraderie brought on by the suffering they endured together while in prison. This does not create safer communities upon release of these inmates when they complete their sentences as they quickly fall back into the same company and get back into crime again and therein lies the vicious cycle of recidivism. We have since established that understanding the causes of recidivism is key to successful rehabilitation and achieving peaceful neighbourhoods as a by-product.

Many reasons and factors have been put forward as causes of criminal behaviour. The interesting thing is that none of the reasons are unique to criminals. It's a complex issue that cannot be easily deciphered. If it was that simple then it would have been solved a long time ago. Every child is born with a lot of promise, and somewhere along the way, irrespective of social standing, they take different paths. Some choose crime. This occurs with families further complicating and blurring the different reasons. We have however noticed a few things that stick out among many inmates. Dysfunctional families are common among inmates. Research by the Texas Department of Criminal Justice show that 70% of children born of incarcerated parents end up in prison (2008). Absentee fathers, child neglect or negative home environments for children lead to increased crime in children. Low education standards, which then contributes to poor employment and poverty, has been shown by Marano to be a contributor to choices to get into crime as individuals try to make a living through illegal means (2003). There could be many other causes and this is a knowledge gap that should be addressed even if in a minimalist way.

Among the causes of recidivism is unemployment. After prison, the most crucial thing ex-inmates need to get back on their feet is a source of income. Many inmates leaving prison are at the bottom of the pyramid and do not have much financial support to start life over again. On the very day they are released many have no housing, food for the night or even the bus fare to get them anywhere. It's an "out of the frying pan, into the fire" scenario. The truth is crime has a "reward" of sorts or else no one would get into it, and many go back to crime.

Societal stigma is a major challenge that ex-inmates face in their bid to get reintegrated and accepted. Society has a very negative and warped view of prisoners and they extend this to them even after having paid doing time. Stigma is almost like a second prison for these individuals. They serve their time in prison but when they get out, society continues to punish them despite their best efforts to change. When society refuses to give a second chance to these men and women, they condemn them as second-rate citizens, which brings frustration and causes them to rebel into a life of crime once again.

In this fast changing world many inmates lack relevant skill sets to get into gainful employment. An IT professional jailed for five years will find him or herself hopelessly outdated upon release. The current model doesn't enable inmates to continually improve on their skills. While it may be argued that a prison is not a school, we believe that a balance can be struck to enable prisoners with some professional training to continually access updates or practice in a limited way in their profession. This way they will still have some relevance in society upon release. There is also the need to adopt ex-inmates into the right kind of networks when released. The Confucius quote says "Show me your friends and I will show you your character". No doubt we are a sum total of the people around us and with the right kind of people around us then we are almost assured of a successful future. Inmates do not have these kinds of networks and also their lack of exposure is a limiting factor in their life.

Nafisika Trust approach—the power of volunteers

The face of the Kenyan inmate is very youthful. According to Njono, earlier surveys published in the Kenya Youth Fact book using data from the Kenya economic survey showed that a significant number of offenders are between the ages of 18 and 25 (2010). The data shows that out of 96,726 convictions, 54.3% were of this age group. If the 26-50 age group is added to this number, it rises to 88.4%.

The majority of the volunteers that give their time and expertise are young too. It is part of our strategy to attract a pool of young volunteers who are of near similar age as the inmates. While all are generally welcome, we do have a preference for university students and young professionals who are eager to pass on the skills they have. Over the past year alone, these volunteers have given ten thousand hours of service. Every year Nafisika involves an average of 60 volunteers in its programmes and this is often a defining experience for both inmates and volunteers alike.

Working in partnership with the Kenyan Prison Service, Nafisika Trust runs programmes in Counselling, Education, Entrepreneurship and Re-entry. The reason we run these programmes is because the majority of inmates have not had adequate access to education, exposure and opportunities. This in turn sets them to be at the bottom of the pyramid in life. The economic gap grows wider and the cycle of crime continues. Our programmes are a strategic attempt to narrow the economic gap by providing skills that will enable individuals to have access to employment and break the cycle of crime in their lives and that of their children. These four key areas that I will expand on below are run mainly by volunteers and through partnerships forged with interested groups and the Kenya Prisons Service.

Counselling

Nafisika runs both psychosocial and substance abuse counselling that targets prison inmates that suffer from psychological issues or have a history of substance abuse. We have noted that many of the inmates come from unstable and broken families. The absence of role models at the family level leaves many of these young people vulnerable to anyone who wants to create a new reference point in their lives as appertains to education, attitude towards work and money, and social standing. The effects of these have been devastating. Many youth get caught up in the wrong company and acquire bad habits. Substance abuse is the most rampant amongst the youth and is a major barrier to employment. This challenge requires trained psychologists and counsellors to address it effectively. We have partnered with the psychology department of the United States International University, a private university in Kenya to enable us to deliver quality counselling and family therapy in the prisons.

Education

Literacy rates among prison inmates are quite low. Many of the inmates dropped out of school at an early age and lack the most basic writing and numeracy skills needed to get by. While poverty is a contributor to low education standards among inmates, there are those who quit school on their own volition and got into crime as a way to avoid parental control and guidance. It is challenging to deal with such inmates because of the years of "miseducation" they have and not many feel the need to get back into formal education since they have lived a life convinced that it has no real value. The persistence of our volunteers and that of the prison warders has however made steady headway in changing these perceptions. Through counselling sessions we have seen increasing numbers join the literacy classes and work on their reading and writing skills. They have been able to shed off the shame that comes with being illiterate and take steps towards taking charge of their lives. Having a goal to work towards has proved to be therapeutic to the inmates, allowing them time and space to accept the challenges they faced as part of what shaped their decisions, realize the consequences that similar choices would have and most importantly, overcome the effects of their past lives. A few of the inmates go on to take the national examination and some proceed to study for their "O" level examinations. This in turn improves the employability of these inmates. We also have a long-standing volunteer-run computer skills education programme in which we teach basic computer literacy skills to those who already have some proficiency in reading and writing.

Employment Programmes

Our Employment Programme consists of entrepreneurship training and business incubation projects. We have partnered with KCA University to deliver an entrepreneurship course that develops self-awareness, assists with career goal setting, and acquiring financial literacy, and sales and business plan development skills. These programmes equip inmates with skills to enable them either secure employment or start their own.

Re-entry Programmes

Prison service ends when an inmate is done serving his time. While this should be a joyful time, an ex-inmate quickly experiences the woes of life after prison. Many ex-inmates experience stigma and rejection from society and some find it hard to get jobs as they may not be adequately skilled or are not employed because they have a prison record. Nafisika walks with ex-inmates down this difficult path and helps them get on their feet as fast as possible. Before release, inmates go through interview sessions with Nafisika and prison staff to help them envision their lives after prison. We hold family therapy sessions so that the bond between them and their family is strengthened. Upon release we hold their hand through the tough times. We also link individuals with prospective employers, support them in starting a business or get them to college to pursue higher education.

Something to feel good about—The Entrepreneurship Programme

The Entrepreneurship Programme is the biggest and most impactful programme we run. The majority of the inmates are eager to take this class despite its intensive nature. This quarterly programme takes inmates through the ins and outs of how to start and run a successful business. Those who attend feel that it is most beneficial to them after being released, especially since their criminal record lowers their attractiveness in the formal employment market. The skills they gain in this programme give them a competitive advantage. The curriculum jointly developed by Nafisika and KCA University teaches the inmates to discover themselves and their potential away from crime. It also teaches them how to best position and brand themselves, how to write business plans, how to raise capital and to keep appropriate accounts for their business. We like to think of this as a discovery of who they are and what they can achieve. At the end of the programme, inmates graduate with a certificate in Business and Entrepreneurship from KCA University.

Two inmates released from Nairobi West Prison recently have put into practice what they learned in our Entrepreneurship Programme. Both former security guards arrested for assault but exonerated three years later. One of them now runs his own clothing business in downtown Nairobi and offers professional writing services for clients who need help with tender documents and related documentation. These skills were learned while in prison and are an example of how properly tailored rehabilitation programmes that resonate with the inmates can be transformative. The former inmate also volunteers his security skills, learned at his former job prior to incarceration, at his local church in the face of terror threats in the country. Another inmate has gone on to run a successful vegetable farm in his hometown of Gatundu. When asked about the impact of the Entrepreneurship Programme he had participated in while in prison, he stated that it helped him learn how to write a business plan, think through important steps in starting a business and keep proper records of accounts. He knew he couldn't get his former job back but he is now happy to have something of his own and is able to support his wife and two children.

References

Institute of Economic Affairs, (2010) *Youth Fact Book: Infinite Possibility of Definite Disaster.* [pdf] Nairobi: Institute of Economic Affairs and Friedrich-Ebert-Stiftung. Available at: http://library.fes.de/pdf-files/bueros/kenia/07889.pdf (accessed 30 June 2014).

Marano, L., (2003) Analysis: Prison Education Cuts Recidivism. *United Press International*, [online] (Last updated 1.42 PM on 10th September 2013). Available at: http://www.upi.com/Odd_News/2003/09/10/Analysis-Prison-education-cuts-recidivism/UPI-88041063215765/ (Accessed 14 March 2013).

Texas Department of Criminal Justice, 2008. *Incarcerated – Children of Parents in Prison Impacted.* [online article] Available at: http://www.tdcj.state.tx.us/gokids/gokids_articles_children_impacted.html (Accessed 11 July 2014).

CHAPTER 25. THE HAND THAT ROCKS THE CRADLE IS THE HAND THAT RULES THE WORLD: WOMEN´S ROLE IN IMPROVING COMMUNITY SECURITY

Agnes Dinkelman

In 2002 Liberian women, tired of war, wanted their men to arrange an agreement on the negotiating table. They followed the call of Leymah Gbowee to no longer have sex with their husbands. What was the strength of that intervention? They had a good view on the driver that in this case shaped reality: the hunger for power. They understood that the fight for power fails when women embarrass men by talking to the media about the "powerless" situation of their men in the bedrooms of their homes. The women also were aware of the possibilities of solidarity, because together one can achieve more. So, what in fact did these women do?

The Liberian women took the space they had to influence their world. Beyond that, they understood how to effectively address the issue from the position they were in, knowing what they stood for together and determined: to bring an end to violence and rape, to bring peace and to work on dignity from there. So what can we say about "their position", "their space" and about "understanding the drivers that shaped reality" to effectively address an issue?

The combination of danger and violence causes a strong increase of dopamine and adrenaline to the brain. It makes the archetype "warrior" feel strong and valuable, it helps him to move away from fear but also disconnects him from other human beings, according to Bourke (1999). Men who live in hostile situations are therefore dominantly led by gaining control and managing risks. The hunger for power as the dominant value decreases if the circumstances change: no more war, no more fights, decreasing hostility. I have observed this in my encounter with former DRC warriors and in my work with European policing officers who returned from Afghanistan. The change of circumstances did its work on the value level: there was mistrust and alertness before, back in a safer environment their base attitude towards the world around them changed. In the new situation we saw cooperativeness and openness for the rules and codes of the society in a calm and responsible way.

So how are women to cope with situations of violence? Women have the beautiful position to really make a difference in community security. They are married to the men, mothers of the children and sisters of each other, and have intimate relationships with all of them. From their position they can sense, pre-sense, see and foresee, interpret and monitor what is happening in their communities, and their interpretations are therefore insightful into the development of conflict. After all, given this position they are well positioned to give meaning to what they sense and see and so develop a deep understanding into the context of which they live.

Women can also use their space to become educated, to give impulses for change, and to take leadership in their communities. The space of women is often limited in comparison to the male position due to traditions, law, and determination of men, external family or religion. So what can women do given the position they have, acting within the space they have, to improve the situation of community security?

My writing is based on my experience as an analyst and practitioner on social dynamics, community security and women leadership. I will share observations from real cases without disclosing identities of actors for reasons of confidentiality. I would like to explore here examples of how women can use a limited space to leverage the situation in conflict. Such examples provide insight into the leadership of women to create community security on a personal, communal and national level.

Coping with hostility

Safe places hardly exist. I learned this by working with a diverse group of people around the globe, either in groups or with individuals, in villages, offices and institutions. I am always struck when people mention the hostility they meet in their lives. Mothers and daughters-in-law might fight over homework, power and privileges. In companies and institutions I have seen people fighting for the better-paid job, competing in a way that leaves no space for collaboration. In every environment there is insecurity.

So then what is a secure community? I consider a secure community a safe place which can have the size of a country or be as small as a family; where people can trust each other, where they know that no one will harm them, cheat on them or betray them. In a safe place there is dignity, respect and support. We have to face the truth; safe places hardly exist, so there is no other way than to purposefully deal with hostility. Hostility makes people cautious and withhold themselves from developing talents and sharing thoughts and ideas. In the end, an unsafe human environment is costing us what we so desperately need: trust and inclusiveness in an emotional, social, economic and spiritual way for peace and prosperity.

Some people confront unsafe places heads up and with stretched backs; ready to act, gain control and diminish risks that they feel can undermine their status. Others lay back and act cautiously because they don't want to get involved in any serious threats. Young girls living in communities where violence is common often behave this way. When I describe their behaviour as "as an attempt to be invisible" they laugh, recognizing it. Some people measure their position carefully, consider the situation, calculate, avoid hostility as much as possible, and at some point take their chances to avoid the next violent threat. These are all responses to cope with hostility. A child soldier from Sierra Leone, according to Mooy's work, shows this in a clear way by stating, "I ate from the human heart so the ones who saw me were frightened […] as everybody was aware that I was a bad person they wouldn't dare to hurt me" (Mooy, 2008, pp.19)

All warriors share the desire to come to grips with insecurity through power and control. But unguided warriors are dangerous warriors. Thomas Sankara, the murdered visionary president of Burkina Faso, stated that a warrior without education is a potential criminal, according to the video Thomas Sankara: The Upright Man (Pan AfricanMarkets, 2006). We therefore need to consider more carefully the coping mechanisms employed to address insecurity and hostility.

People are coping with hostility at all levels. World leaders avoid threats too and try to stay in control. Opponents of Stalin in Russia were executed and not allowed to become a threat. Later Brezhnev made his competitors retire while Khrushchev sent them to far away countries as ambassadors for Russia, as narrated by Yeltsin (1990). Gorbachev allowed his opponents to come back into politics to show the world that he was serious about the idea of "glasnost", meaning openness. In the same spirit, Obama asked his direct opponent within the Democratic Party, Hillary Clinton, to be his Secretary of State and overcame their antagonism by offering her a position next to him. World leaders act like all humans by having a personal view on the feeling of safety for themselves and their position. In geopolitical interaction, Gorbachev and Obama tried to let cooperation prevail. Their challenge was to cope with an environment that forced them to take position in a world shaped by hostility, control and power.

Identifying values as a basis for coping mechanisms

Coping with control, power and hostility can be done in different ways motivated by different values and according to prevailing circumstances. Mwenda put it this way:

> It is possible that a corrupt dictatorship in one country at a given time is what is necessary to achieve rapid change. But it can become dysfunctional in another country with different social and political dynamics. The building of a national identity and an effective state in homogenous Rwanda under a Tutsi president may demand honest government; but in heterogeneous Nigeria or DRC, corruption may be the glue to bring and hold diverse interests of powerful elites together. There is no one size that fits all." (Mwenda, 2014).

My argument is that in order to improve safety and security in communities it is crucial to understand that there is no standardised way to respond to violence. Circumstances differ, issues disputed over are not the same, cultures may differ and people respond in different ways. In trying to address hostility, a range of coping mechanisms can be used that are motivated by different values. Human behaviour originates in values. In order to increase the range of coping responses to hostility we need to review the values that underpin behaviour. In our attempt to understand a situation we should observe and assess the values of that community. This profile of values can provide us with the information needed to determine what kind of interventions may be effective.

Let me give you an example. I worked in the Netherlands with minority leaders that have an African or Asian background. These leaders perceived reality in a total new way once they understood how to use the perspective of values and worldviews, considering the circumstances they were in. The younger leaders longed for more influence. They wanted to lead their community towards more involvement in the Dutch postmodern society. The elderly leaders didn't let them and they withheld information from the next generation and prohibited their actions or ignored their requests. During our meetings it was identified that one of the crucial issues for the elderly leaders was the question of a dignified retirement. They felt responsible for the fact that they took their families to a new world and didn't succeed in their goals of pride, honour and prosperity. Without addressing these issues properly, the elders stayed unwavering in postmodern questions and attempted to stay in control and by doing so, they prevented the youngest generation fitting into society. The younger leaders in our sessions understood they had to earn their leadership position by gaining the trust of the elders by honouring them. They had to make clear that the experience and knowledge of the elderly would be part of their moral compass while navigating a new world. Only addressing the need for tradition and cherishing the culture and honouring the families would not be enough to change leadership positions. We also had to understand the need for dignity and respect so that the elders could retire in a honourable manner. It would help them to be proud of their offspring to take leadership and behave in ways they felt were correct.

In unsafe places the urge for power and control is a dominant value. To increase women's leadership in community safety, it is important that women can identify how values impact choices and behaviour, knowing that everybody is coping with power and control in their own interest.

Educating male 'heroes'

Unsafe places in the domestic domain are quite common. One third of women throughout the world will experience physical or sexual violence by a partner or sexual violence by a non-partner as the World Health Organization (WHO) concluded recently (2013). Domestic violence is power driven. The violator is in control, the victim is calculating. In domestic violence situations, the violator (often but not always male) does not postpone the satisfaction of his needs. This inability is a real threat for women.

Women can put domestic violence and rape on the agenda. The most effective way to do so is to reset or re-emphasise what constitutes a "code of conduct" for a man. This can be the impetus for an identity transition: from the archetype "warrior" to a "community man". Violence and rape no longer fit in this archetype. When men want to adapt to the new identity they have to leave the warrior archetype in which rape is common. The more men identify with the concept of "real men" the more they will reduce violence. Women therefore have to push male leaders to subscribe to the code against domestic violence and rape and to correct the men that are violating the code. Men's involvement in maintaining the code is also important. They should correct their peers so that the issue becomes a matter of honour, pride, embarrassment and shame. To maintain a new code, male involvement in correction and blaming is crucially important.

If we approach the violators in the archetypical role of "warriors", we can see that a key value is "to be in charge". Using violence is a very common way for them to achieve their goals. We need to change the circumstances in a way that can provide the men with new roles, in which they are in charge again but in a different and non-violent way. A transitional process of male identity starts with the question of "What is a real man?" And beyond that, "How could a real man become a hero?"

Women can use their feminine qualities to start a process of support for men to become more open for what the community needs them to be: to protect the women from other men; and to build houses, hospitals and schools; to create perspective for the children; and to allow women to be their partner in the development of the family and the community. Men working on items like these deserve to be perceived by the community as "real men".

Heroes could be described as real men (or women) who know how to empower the community and have an attitude of understanding and support. They are able to move away from hostility and find ways to cooperate and facilitate dignity and social, economic and spiritual growth. Heroes could be described as leaders who serve the interests of all living creatures in the community.

I propose that a possible intervention for addressing these questions is to organize regular gatherings. As this issue is important for the whole community, it is important to get everyone involved. An example of such gatherings is the community meetings at the grassroots level in both urban and rural Rwanda initiated by the government. About 50 families living in a neighbourhood or village called Umudugudu have formed the lowest administrative entity in Rwanda. The Umudugudu gatherings are used by the government as an information channel where citizens can be informed on policies. The gatherings also are used by the community to deliberate on safety issues, social behaviour, and about conflicts between neighbours and conflicts within the home. The citizens choose the leaders of these gatherings themselves. Such an existing framework would be an excellent basis for the development of "real men" in community security.

In our case as we explore an intervention on domestic violence and the transition of men from a "warrior" towards a "real man" who is of great value to the community, women leaders could start with gatherings in their village supported by the leading and respected "real men". At the start, women leaders have to explain the central issue and give information on legal or policy requirements. Male and female leaders have to make clear that the community cannot prosper without everybody being accepted as a member of the community and everybody taking their role. The question brought up is "what do we consider a real man?"

The next stage of the intervention could be the invitation to reflect on the question. It urges participants to avoid talking about "me and myself" but to externalize and speak about "the man that is doing the things real men do", or "a man who is behaving without hostility, taking responsibility by finding ways to build peace, like heroes do". The women of the community can sit around the group of men and reflect on the discussion when they get the floor. They can tell stories in which they express how they expect the men to contribute to the family and the community. This way the community can standardise the behaviour they think is useful to the group, for both women and men. Domestic violence is one of the issues on the agenda.

These are important post conflict tools and women leaders can make a start with this identity shifting process. They can organize and facilitate these intimate sessions where men and women work on the transition of the identity of men. In these meetings they can find ways to become "a real man" and a hero. Health and governmental institutes, policing forces and Non-Governmental Organizations (NGOs) can support the process by communicating information on behaviour that responds to a code for manhood that does not rely on violence.

Women's involvement in early warning in radicalization

Some regions, such as the Middle East, North Africa and Sub-Saharan Africa, are threatened by terrorist groups like ISIS, Boko Haram and Al Shabaab. According to Kwok's work, these groups are growing steadily and financed by wealthy sources in the Middle East or Indonesia (2014). The extremists receive funds from Southeast Asia through oil in the caliphate or kidnappings in Africa. This extremism threatens women and men with their liberty and independence.

The geographical playing fields of these groups transcend the borders of nations. The Islamic State (IS) caliphate creates a situation that leads to a new possibility for meeting, talking and collaboration between the West and the Arab world. African leaders also have to decide on a strategy and to overcome differences so that they may act jointly and quickly before the situation gets out of hand.

Looking at it from the perspective of values, the members of the terrorist organisations are motivated by a desire for more power and control. The urge for power and control leads to the law of the jungle that is full of concepts as "eat or be eaten", instant satisfaction, honour, pride, brotherhood and the idea of following leaders without questioning.

We have to understand the degree of attraction that these groups exert on young people. The attraction can lie in the idea of adventure, of being invincible, untouchable, unbeatable, and being a part of the winning team. These groups offer young people a way to make the world understand that they are fed up with what they see as humiliation through Western oppression.

They find the legitimacy of their actions in the Quran. The groups take the view that everyone must take the holy book literally without interpretation. This view gives them full control over what they want civilians to think and how they want civilians to act. The similarity with the Christian Inquisition is striking. In late medieval times the Inquisition had the exclusive right to setting the standards, judging and punishing people. Today we seeing in IS a new manifestation of the values and behaviour that fit with dominance, male superiority and the value of hunger for power. We need to deal with this trend. Women are crucial in this process.

Young people who are considering joining terrorist groups need counterforce. They need to be firmly corrected by the people around them to address and contradict both the defected logic and the urge for control. In these young people we have potential warriors that are falsely informed and who need proper firm guidance and adequate information that is well adjusted to their goals and values. Mothers should be encouraged to pick up on early signs and to observe and reflect on new ideas of their sons and daughters. Communities can contribute by organizing an early warning service for police forces and the military. Governments and donors could invest in television programming with debates that include experts on the issue as well as young people. This will help identify the defects in the logic of the jihadist movement, to prevent young people from becoming criminals.

As mothers and sisters, women have the best position to sense and pre-sense changes as their sons and brothers become attracted to the jihadi movement. The men in the family can become informed by the narratives that are spread by fundamentalists in real life or through the Internet. Mothers need to know (and should be informed) that they have the power to intervene. They have the position to help their children to see what is right and what is wrong. There are too many women who do not understand that this is within their power, especially when it comes to their sons. These mothers and sisters need to become the first responders. We could facilitate meetings where women can learn to read the first signs, how to respond and what to do. Community leaderships should support women so they can start to provide de-programming training and provide psychological and spiritual support.

The hand that rocks the cradle...

The challenges to community security are serious. They have to be addressed with an understanding that values drive behaviour. To diminish hostility, values need to be shaped or reshaped. Community processes that intervene at the level of values to shift identity are therefore key to promote long-lasting community security.

At the local level women can play a very important role in resetting the value systems that define boys and men and identify new male identities that allow men to be valuable for the community in a non-violent way. Using their space they can make an important contribution to improve community security, like the Liberian women who responded to the call of Leymah Gbowee in 2002. The examples of the identity shift for men after conflict and the undermining of the support of extremism show how women can address hostility in a constructive way. In early warning, which is increasingly relevant within the expansion of extremist terrorist organisations looking to recruit young people, women have an important role to play in education, identifying young people attracted to these organisations and addressing, as a community, effective responses. Men have an important role to play as peers, demanding non-violent behaviour that is valued and respected by the community as positive masculinity.

Unsafe places can become less unsafe over time, with leaders who respect their people and demand non-violent, constructive behaviour. The more secure society is, the more people can feel safe to work on social and economic perspectives. Women leaders can initiate this process and increase the number of women leaders leading communities, institutions and homes. Women can educate their children to become real men and strong heroes and heroines that understand how to intervene to the hunger for control and power. As the poet William Ross Wallace wrote (1890): "The hand that rocks the cradle is the hand that rules the world".

References

Bourke, J. (1999) *An intimate history of killing*. Basic Books, New York.

Conflicthantering (2013) Interview met Leymah Gbowee: "Morele kaders zijn kapot en verdwenen". *Tijdschrift Conflicthantering*. 5th ed. (2014-12-18).

Kwok, Y. (2014) The ISIS Extremists Causing Havoc in Iraq Are Getting Funds and Recruits from Southeast Asia. *TIME*, [online]. Available at: http://www.time.com/2888423/isis-islamist-state-in-iraq-and-syria-indonesia/ (Accessed 30 August 2014).

Mooy, G. (2008) *De wil om te doden*. Athenaeum, Amsterdam.

Mwenda, A. (2014) What produces success or failure of nations? *The Independent* [online]. Available at: http://www.independent.co.ug/the-last-word/the-last-word/9054 (Accessed 30 August 2014).

Pan AfricanMarkets (2006) *Thomas Sankara: The Upright Man*. Available at: https://www.youtube.com/watch?v=J5USbA701SI&feature=youtu.be (Accessed 30 August 2014).

Wallace, WR. (1890) *Beautiful Gems of Thought and Sentiment*. The Colins-Patten Co., Boston.

World Health Organization (2013) *Violence against women: Global Picture Health Response*. Geneva: World Health Organization. Available at: http://www.who.int/reproductivehealth/publications/violence/VAW_infographic.pdf?ua=1 (Accessed 30 August 2014).

Yeltsin, B. (1990) *Getuigenis van een opposant*. Anthos, Baarn.

CHAPTER 26. CHALLENGING THE STATUS QUO AND UNLEASHING THE HIDDEN POWER OF WOMEN: THE ZIMBABWEAN EXPERIENCE

Chikomborero Mafuriranwa

The story of Rose Mapango, age 38, Area Trainer Seke, Mashonaland East Province

I was deeply traumatised by the rape I experienced during the period of conflict. I was raped by a "good Samaritan" from the nearby village as I fled the violence in my home area. This man was a friend of my late father and I had known him from childhood. I went to his home so that I could board a bus to Harare from his village since it was safer there as the cadres had not yet occupied the area. My plan was to proceed to Harare to seek refuge at my brother and his wife's house. I decided to seek refuge in Harare as I was informed by my brother that the situation in urban areas was less tense. Cadres had attacked our village the night before but luckily, I had fled with my neighbour and my two-year-old son whom I strapped to my back and fled to a nearby mountain. The next day, I walked to the nearby village, at whose market I had planned to catch the next bus to Harare. It was not safe for me to board a bus from my village, as I was afraid of being followed by cadres who would be milling around at the market harassing people. Unfortunately for me, the "good Samaritan" I had affectionately addressed as "Uncle" all my life left his wife sleeping in their matrimonial bed, tip-toed into the room where my son and I were sleeping and sexually violated me during the night.

The next day, I left with my neighbour for Harare. On arrival in the city, I did not narrate the rape incident to my brother or his wife but simply kept it to myself, though I would cry myself to sleep every night for two months. After the Government of National Unity was formed and since a government arm for peace called the Organ for National Healing, Reconciliation and Integration was put in place, I decided to go back to the village since this new Ministry vowed to ensure that peace would be restored in communities. Well of course that was what I made myself believe yet the real reason was that I did not want to be judged for having yet another baby out of wedlock by my brother and his wife so I thought it best to leave their home before my pregnancy became visible. I put on a brave face and convinced my brother to let me go back to the village, yet deep down inside I was choking with fear—the fear of being alone in that hut and experiencing yet another attack.

On returning to the village, my neighbour invited me one hot Wednesday afternoon to a club meeting that took place 500 metres from our community fields where we had been tilling the land in preparation for our next maize planting season. We met with ten other women from the village and sat under a tree. I had no reason not to join this meeting since it was 12:00pm and the sun was at its peak, its rays burning my face, and we had decided to take a break. The meeting's agenda for that day was on how it was important for women to seek counselling for the trauma they experienced and how it was up to us to break the cycle of violence. Those words rang in my head and I then made the decision to visit the clinic the next day since I was now five months pregnant and had not registered for antenatal care. The nurse was not as friendly as I expected, however she attended to me and advised me on the steps to follow.

I was tested for HIV and tested positive, however I received post-test counselling and was advised to return to the clinic after a few months for more tests. I walked home feeling confused and angry—angry for letting that scumbag have his way with me. I was determined on revenge. I had a few sinister ideas in my head, like burning him to death in his hut in the middle of the night. "That wouldn't be so bad", I thought to myself and grinned.

The following Wednesday, my neighbour invited me for the club meeting under the tree. Again we sat down and discussed issues of peace as it was the topical issue of the time. After the meeting, I shared my experience with my neighbour and she referred me to an Area Trainer from the club who had been trained on counselling.

Over a period of three months, my personal healing process took place. I began to feel less and less bitter and became more hopeful for the future. I have forgiven my violator though I have not sought justice for this crime. I realized as we learned more on gender-based violence in the club that my case would probably be dismissed, as there was no adequate evidence left from the crime since several months had passed. However a year later, I now have a healthy baby girl who is free from the virus as I underwent successful anti-retroviral therapy.

I have also been leading a community-based intervention for approaching our traditional leaders advocating for punishment of perpetrators of violence against women. Our Chief openly supports us and I am on the lookout for cases of violence in the community and refer them to the Chief's Court that meets every Saturday. Our Chief's Court is an important part of our community structure and most people seek to have issues addressed under Customary Law rather than seeking Litigation which they view as tedious, complicated and above all, expensive. Due to us playing the watchdog role as women, men in the community are now afraid of abusing women in any form. I do not regret the day I joined that club meeting under the tree for it has given me a new outlook on life. I am also able to defend other women and girls and give them the power to protect themselves despite my not having received that opportunity myself.

The name of Rose Mapango is fictitious as to protect her identity.

The impact of the conflict on women

The conflict that took place in Zimbabwe prior, during, and after 2008 was highly gendered in nature and negatively affected women more than men due to the patriarchal nature of Zimbabwean society. The colonial era worsened this as colonial power solicited male labour and provided them with passes for the urban areas, while women were left behind in rural areas. In modern day, women resultantly have less educational opportunities than men and form the majority of people living in rural areas. Men on the other hand work in cities and surrounding towns, with those who are married only returning home to their spouses on weekends and public holidays.

Women were highly vulnerable to attack by cadres due to the geographical spacing in rural areas and lack of coordination where the violence took place. They were raped, tortured and some killed. A main characteristic of these violent political clashes was the use of the rape of women as a weapon of war meant to weaken the opposing force.

The problems of women are three fold: lack of economic opportunities, lack of political participation, and violence and sexual violence.

Women also have limited economic opportunities as they do not own the means of production such as the land and only provide labour on their father's or husband's land. They also benefit very little from commercial farming and grow only very few crops for subsistence. This lack of resources hinders their participation in socio-economic and political processes; hence they are not able to take up positions of power.

Although women form the majority of the population, they are not adequately represented in national political structures. In Zimbabwe, women therefore have limited representation in Parliament and other forms of local leadership. Therefore, policies and laws are not conducive towards the socio-economic growth of women as it is men who formulate policies against a patriarchal mind-set. Hence the political representation is lacking to defend women's interests, including the protection of women against violence as well as measures to increase women's participation in decision-making processes.

Training workshops for women across Zimbabwe revealed that the patriarchal nature of Zimbabwean society is the main cause of women's violation during periods of conflict. Gender-based violence is rife in many communities. The presence of gender-based violence in homes easily spirals to other women in the communities. This is because culturally, women are exposed to gender-based violence by their male partners and other male members of their families and these cases go unreported. As a result, these men who are accustomed to abusing women within the domestic sphere without any punishment easily extend this violence to other women in communities during periods of political conflict.

Women who experienced violence during 2008 were displaced from their homes and lost their sources of livelihood in the form of crops and livestock such as cattle, goats and chickens. Some had their homes burnt down and were left homeless. Other women also experienced sexual abuse in addition to being displaced and losing their homes. However, they did not have access to health services such as Post Exposure Prophylaxis and Counselling as well as justice due to weak institutional operations in health centres such as clinics and local Traditional Chief's Courts as well as Magistrates Courts. Women are in dire need of counselling, treatment for HIV and STIs as well as justice from local and/or legal courts.

National Healing mechanisms for Peace

> Peace Begins with Me! Peace Begins with You! Peace Begins with Us!
> Ukuthula kuqala ngami! Ukuthula kuqala ngawe! Ukuthula kuqala ngathi!
> Runyararo runotanga neni! Runyararo runotanga newe! Runyararo runotanga nesu!

These were the aspirations expressed by the Organ for National Healing, Reconciliation and Integration (ONHRI) which was established in 2009 as one of three transitional arrangements created during the period of the Global Political Agreement (GPA) that was intended to facilitate the peace building process. The GPA aims to lay the foundations of addressing Zimbabwe's history of the cyclical political violence over generations. From 2009, three Ministers (among whom the Vice-President), representing Zimbabwe African National Union- Patriotric Front (ZANU-PF),

Movement for Democratic Change- Tsvangirai (MDC-T) and Movement for Democratic Change- Mutambara (MDC-M), gave leadership to ONHRI. The three founding ONHRI co-principals, ONHRI Chairperson, Vice President Landa John Nkomo representing ZANU/PF, Minister Sekai Masikana Holland (MDCT) and the late Minister Gibson Jama Sibanda (MDC), succeeded by Minister Moses Mzila Ndlovu. ONHRI was established to achieve restoration of the dignity of all Zimbabweans regardless of age, gender or creed; to achieve peace, stability, unity and prosperity for individual Zimbabweans, their families, communities, organizations and the country as a whole.

The co-principles agreed to adopt a national, inclusive, grassroots-based consultative strategy to gather the views of Zimbabweans on their vision of establishment of sustainable peace in this country. For 18 months the ONHRI focus was on the following broad areas of engagement, with a view to restore the tenets and values of the Africanness, Ubuntu Bethu/Hunhu Hwedu, of Zimbabwe. Following this process, ONHRI proposed to the government to develop a bill for the enactment of an Act of Parliament on Peace and Reconciliation processes in Zimbabwe. The proposed infrastructure for peace with its four elements was adopted by the cabinet in April 2012.

The Policy Framework proposes the establishment of an independent operational institution to be called the National Peace and Reconciliation Commission (NPRC) where "reconciliation" is inclusive of healing and reparations, and "peace" suggests negotiated settlement of disputes and prevention of future violence. The NPRC shall provide policy advice, facilitate the development of programmes and supervise implementation of programmes and activities for the promotion of equality, national healing, cohesion and unity.

The Voluntary Code of Conduct for Political Parties is for intra and inter-political parties to deliberate commitment through moral suasion to regulate the behaviour and conduct of political parties' officials, members and supporters. This instrument is meant to embed zero tolerance to violence in all political engagements and processes where internal disciplinary mechanisms and procedures would have to be enforced. Resort to legal enforcement would be through prevailing enacted laws.

The voluntary Code of Conduct for Political Parties is part of the documentation of the Nomination Court to be signed by every person wishing to become a candidate in Parliamentary elections. All candidates signed this on the 31st of July 2013 at the harmonised elections. The Code of Conduct defines in clear terms and lays down the consequences of indulging in any form of violence as a candidate during the course of elections.

The History Programme is intended to bring Zimbabweans together to discover the common ground they share. The programme is to pursue for purposes of learning from the past epochs of historical experiences to inform our future. It is hoped the launch of this programme will take place soon. ONHRI's hope is that Zimbabweans through traditional leaders interacting with scholars and clans will assist the history researchers to carry out their research work when they visit various areas in the country. The History Programme is still in progress, coordinated by Midlands State University (MSU) as recommended by ONHRI. A team of academics has been working with communities, traditional leaders and others as an inclusive healing exercise by its agreed methodology. The project aims to encourage Zimbabweans to appreciate their common cultural values and that they are one family.

The three co-principals identified Midlands State University where the History Programme was already ongoing to host new Peace Institutions that would carry out Peace Programmes for sustainability of the achievements of the ONHRI recommendations. This fourth element was still being created but its main focus would be to respond to and aim to address the complex concerns of survivors of violence, both perpetrators and victims. The base for the effective and sustainable Promotion of Equality, National Healing, Cohesion and Unity translating into positive peace should be through empowering all Zimbabweans politically, culturally, socially and economically through programmes and projects to eliminate poverty by creating sustainable livelihoods thus catalysing development and a resilient national economy.

Self-organisation of women

The Association of Women's Clubs (AWC) is a community-based organization that was founded in 1938 by an 18 year old visionary school teacher, Helen Vera, who was married to a traditional Chief, Chief Mangwende of Murehwa, Mashonaland Province in Zimbabwe. Helen was moved by the plight of women when she observed how extremely impoverished they were when they came to the Chief's homestead. They wore tattered clothing and went to the Chief seeking assistance for basic provisions such as food. During the early years of her marriage, Helen grouped together women in various villages under the Chiefdom into clubs. It is at this point that the seed of a social movement for women empowerment to fight the poverty that patriarchy brought about for women was sown.

The club's aim as set up by Helen Mangwende née Vera was to improve basic living standards of women. Members were taught basic home economic skills such as cooking, sewing, knitting and crocheting. Young Farmers' Clubs were also started for young women whose aim was to enable young women to take part in farming, which is the main commercial activity to enable them to be financially independent and provide themselves and their children and not depend on men. To date, the organisation consists of roughly 100,000 rural-based members spread across five provinces of the country which include Matabeleland, Mashonaland East, Manicaland, Midlands and Masvingo.

AWC has responded to numerous needs of women over the decades since its formation. During the early 2000s, due to socio-economic challenges such as increasing food shortages, a decline in health service delivery and more recently, politically-motivated violence; AWC has played a pivotal role in addressing socio-political challenges in Zimbabwean communities after the 2008 elections, with women playing a crucial role.

Based on the problems that they faced, women in their clubs collectively made the decision to take action to address the injustices they experienced. The story of Rose Mapanga highlights the opportunities that exist for women for them to unleash their hidden power and make positive changes for themselves and others in their communities.

International and local legal frameworks have also provided the background against which promotion of women's participation in governance, peace building and security can take place. The UN Security Council Resolution 1325 has provided the framework for work around women-led peace building initiatives in Zimbabwe. Nationally, the Constitution Making Process has also aided this.

True to AWC's mandate of training and information-dissemination to rural women, training of women on conflict transformation, peace and healing has been carried out in a fruitful partnership with Oxfam Novib since 2011. The training carried out under the partnership has significantly contributed towards closing gaps in the low participation of women in peace building and leadership at local and national levels. This is due to the fact that information on gender equality and women's rights creates the consciousness of security as a right. Women's clubs also provide a safe space where women can share knowledge and ideas regarding peace building. The clubs are structured and this enables the members to think proactively and shape their thoughts and carry out actions in an organized manner.

Women's clubs, in addition to creating a hub of knowledge and information sharing, also create a platform where women are equipped with lobbying and advocacy skills. This work is carried out to close gaps that are created when women have adequate information yet there is no conducive local legal or policy environment that supports their participation. Women are stronger as a collective and can engage themselves in advocacy to community leaders and other authorities at the national level.

Due to advocacy work of the clubs, women have also taken up local positions of authority and women-led community initiatives have been adopted. They are also more proactive than men on issues of the promotion of peace and are more effective change-agents. They have merged information and the traditional cultural systems in existence. Women have led the formation of Peace Committees that have carried out advocacy work to traditional leaders so that they adopt a more positive system that promotes the participation of women. Women have also negotiated for central roles in mediation of cases amongst rival parties that clashed during election violence.

Despite having limited academic knowledge and resources, rural women have the power to make a difference if they realise the power they have and are given a slight push. The desire they have to see a better Zimbabwe for future generations is the driving force behind their passion for peace.

Conclusions

"An eye for an eye makes Zimbabwe blind", was the slogan promoted by the Organ for National Healing, Reconciliation and Integration. Peace and reconciliation includes all Zimbabweans in accordance with the philosophy of ubuntu bethu / hunhu hwedu and provides basis reparation, restitution, compensation, among others perceived entitlements, arising from violent historical epochs of Zimbabwe. In the future, the details of peace building will fall under the purview of the National Peace and Reconciliation Commission as an institution, once legally established, to deal with the past and future occurrences of violence.

The Infrastructure or Architecture for Peace through the Zimbabwe National Policy Framework for Peace and Reconciliation bestows a legacy of solving disputes through dialogue rather than violent conflict to succeeding generations enabling a break away from the culture of cyclical political violence inherited from the past epochs of our history. Such violence has affected women in deeply traumatic ways as a result of which women have been shunned. The Association of Women's Clubs has been one of the mechanisms through which women meet, support each other, deal with the consequences of violence, organising security and protection and demand their place in the community and even justice. When women organise, they can change their lives in positive directions and lead communities to peace.

CHAPTER 27. ONE HAND CANNOT TIE A BUNDLE: PEACE BUILDING IN SECULAR AND FAITH-BASED COMMUNITIES IN UGANDA

Angeline Nguedjeu-Momekam

Introduction

I am not a victim of a conflict or post conflict setting. I grew up in the relatively stable environment of Cameroon long after the independence years. Yes, the Biafra wars of the seventies still lingered in the background as it had spilt over into Western Cameroon. Through the tales of my grandparents I was confronted with issues of conflict or displacement, but I now realize that I had a caricatured idea of survivors of war and conflict.

I now work within the field of conflict transformation and have spoken with many survivors. Listening to their stories has been humbling and at times frustrating. I have also experienced this work as rewarding as the ability to understand and empathise with the experiences of survivors of war and conflict has transformed my view of the world. In my experience, addressing women and peace issues in post conflict communities cannot be done with a detached or "neutral" mind-set.

My role is to accompany the implementation process of the programme strategy through identified local partners. Partners are selected based on their suitability in relation to the targeted communities. We sit together and discuss how to fill the identified capacity gaps. It is my role to oversee the institutional capacity building process tailored to the demands in line with the joint terms and agreements.

I have been struck with the gender dimensions of conflict and the incredible resilience of women who have encountered conflict. In this contribution, I want to share my experience of supporting communities who have gone through conflict. In the case of faith-based communities, religion plays an integrative role and offers a thread of hope to the marginalised.

I am interested to share my thoughts on how religion can be an important aspect of strengthening a community approach to peace building. This contribution is intended to be a snapshot from practice and highlights the challenges of supporting such interventions aimed at peace building in communities. It builds on my work as a conflict transformation officer in the Dutch Protestant aid organisation, InterChurch Organization for Development Cooperation (ICCO). The conflict transformation programme supports efforts that are aimed at societies where poor and marginalised rights of men and women are respected and where the rule of law prevails. The programme facilitates community driven interventions through both faith-based and secular local partners.

Northern and North East Uganda

The programme I am supporting is in Northern and North East Uganda. The peace process and subsequent massive return of former Internally Displaced Persons (IDPs) created new challenges. This region is afflicted by the remnants of two decades of insurgence of the Lord Resistance Army (LRA). The civil war in Northern Uganda that lasted for 20 years has had devastating effects on the community support mechanisms. Despite the ongoing reconstruction processes (including the Peace Recovery and Development Plan and the Northern Uganda Social Action Fund (NUSAF)) thousands of people are still deprived of economic opportunities, resulting in widespread poverty and insecurity. Women bear the brunt of gender-based violence, including genital mutilation that is practiced by the Sabiny in the East and the Pokot in Northeastern Uganda.

The majority of the former 1.8 million IDPs have returned home or have identified new villages to settle, but reintegration is still a fragile process that will need time and support in order to consolidate. Most of those that return are women.

Post-war latent conflict in Northern Uganda was characterised by the spirit of revenge, land grabbing, war trauma, and lack of knowledge about rights or even intimidation to exercise them. There are laws for the protection of land rights but there is no clear way to implement them because access to the legal justice system is limited and difficult.

Uganda can be classified as a highly Christianised country. Most Ugandans are practicing or loyal members of a church.

The post-war trauma for women

The results of the war for women and girls according to the annual reports presented by TEWPA (2012), ISIS-WICCE (2013) and UOMU (2012) to the funding partner organisation were dramatic:

> Abduction
> Sex slavery
> Rape
> Cutting of facial parts
> Death through torture
> Permanent deformation including vaginal fistula after obstetric disorders
> HIV/AIDS
> Other sexually transmitted diseases

Many women were without shelter and sleeping under the trees with their children. They gave birth under trees. Many women had lost their husbands, sons and relatives. Taking care of young children after left behind by the deceased husband puts a heavy burden on women. Trauma and stigma from rape and torture resulted in women being shunned by their spouses and communities. A great number of the abducted young girls and women returned with children fathered by their abductors and on their return, the women and children were also shunned. They now live as outcasts in their communities. This poses yet another problem of identity. It may also result in new conflicts owing to property and land ownership. Women may also find it hard to love and take care of the children resulting from rape by soldiers or rebels.

Women's organisations in Northern and North Eastern Uganda

The Teso Women Peace Activists (TEWPA) is a rural woman's based organisation founded in 2001 to respond to the challenges of unrest as a result of armed conflicts manifested in different forms in the Teso and Karamoja regions. TEWPA has strengthened the capacity of rural women in conflict resolution and transformation processes and stimulates dialogue through active involvement and participation of women, youth and other strategic stakeholders.

Isis-Women's International Cross Cultural Exchange (WICCE) is a global women's rights organisation that utilises creative strategies to generate and share information and knowledge to enable women to enhance their leadership potential and participate in decision-making. A partnership between Isis-WICCE at a national level and TEWPA at a regional level resulted in a joint intervention aimed at trauma victims in the Teso sub-region. An integral part of this programme is the exchange visits between trauma victims from different post conflict parts of the world. TEWPA has journeyed with Isis-WICCE to Nepal, Ethiopia, Somali Land, Rwanda and others on peace missions to identify different coping mechanisms of trauma victims.

TEWPA further produces and disseminates documentation on women led peace, reconciliation and conflict transformation initiatives in the programme areas. Some of the activities of this programme facilitate a broad range of community activities such as: cleaning wells, planting trees, charity walks/work and easy writing. The data collected from the field also feeds into the documents on monitoring of the UN Security Council resolution 1325 Uganda National Action Plan.

The Lira Women's Peace Initiative (LIWEPI) and the Kitgum Women's Peace Initiatives (KIWEPI) support the reintegration and resettlement of communities in Northern Uganda. The Conflict Transformation programme also focused on the rehabilitation of formerly abducted girls. Fifteen formerly abducted women and girls in Aromo Sub County were provided with skills in tailoring and goat rearing to support their livelihood and ensure effective reintegration and resettlement.

The Uganda Orthodox Mothers Union (UOMU) is a faith-based organisation that was formed in 2003. UOMO is a member of the Ugandan Joint Christian Council. As a legally registered faith-based corporate_body it is supported by three churches: the Church of Uganda, the Roman Catholic Church, and the Uganda Orthodox Church.

UOMO has been recognised within the church and outside for their role in women empowerment. Their strength is especially in empowering women within and outside the church structure to become agents of change with a strong focus on peace building and conflict transformation. UOMU's mandate is to empower women to effectively participate both in the development of the church and communities to build on sustainable conditions for conflict transformation. Activities include: organisation of events like World Women's Day of Prayer; celebrating International Day of Peace to allow women to articulate issues that greatly affect them; working with communities on women rights and obligations including gender-based violence in the northern part of Uganda; organising participation in community dialogue meetings on marriage and divorce bill; and sensitisation on gender-based violence.

The programme of UOMO has allowed women to articulate concerns within the broader church community. Examples of concerns are for instance the corrupt judicial system. The UOMO members advocated for reforms using the church structures. UOMO works very closely with the Inter-religious Council of Uganda and the Anti-Corruption Coalition Uganda. At the community level, it is important to mention that UOMO women have developed links to the district programmes and this has improved their participation. The UOMO also rallied against a controversial marriage bill debated in Parliament during the year 2012. UOMO sensitised communities so that the law would protect women when their marriage was dissolved. The controversial bill failed in Parliament and was not enacted as a result of concerted national advocacy from religious and secular organisations.

Lessons learnt

Religious and traditional leaders and the government of Uganda have played a significant role in sensitising community members to use non-violent means to solve existing family and community conflicts. However, some of the dogmas, traditions and beliefs both in church and society are still disempowering women and limit women's active participation in peace building. The biggest challenge with faith-based organisations is their strong male dominated structures.

UOMU acts within the framework of ecumenical collaboration in Uganda. It presents a strong voice of women. Women feel supported by their faith. The structural challenges that women face within the churches have been addressed by supporting the strengthening of collaboration of UOMO with other church structures as well as with secular organisations. For instance, collaboration with the Joint Christian Council of Uganda has been interesting to bring women's issues higher up the agenda of the Ugandan churches. However, the limitation is the focus of such interventions at the macro level.

The connection of the churches to community-based support focused on faith and values provides a very important framework to support women but does not have an ecumenical presence. Secular organisations are also better placed to address the government's policy, although the advocacy of the women in the context of UOMO proved to be successful in challenging the recent marriage bill. The collaboration with secular organisation was especially important to achieve this success.

Livelihood oriented activities by secular organisations are also an important part of the peace building package. These provide women's communities with assets, skills and tools, which contribute to the improvement of their living conditions. Secular organisations, such as Isis-WICCE have also played a key role in the important area of trauma healing and in organising international exchange for locally rooted community organisations.

Critically, the faith-based and secular organisations are complementary in their approach and in combination they may provide an important support system for community women. The collaboration between faith-based and secular organisations should therefore be encouraged and supported. In their complementary strengths they may help women to overcome the trauma of war. As the saying goes, "One hand cannot tie a bundle."

References

Badaru, N. (2014) Interview with Nelly Badaru. Interviewed by Angeline Nguedje- Momekam [*in-person interview*]. (1 August 2014)

InterChurch Organization for Development Cooperation (2010) InterChurch Organization for Development Cooperation CEA- Regional Strategic Plan 2010-2015, ICCO, Utrecht.

Isis-Women's International Cross Cultural Exchange (2013) Evaluation report to InterChurch Organization for Development Cooperation, Isis-WICCE, Kampala.

Kitgum Women's Peace Initiatives (2013) Annual report to InterChurch Organization for Development Cooperation.

Lira Women's Peace Initiative (2013) Annual report to InterChurch Organization for Development Cooperation.

Nguedjeu-Nkwenkam, A. (2003) *Non-formal basic education and vocational training for women's empowerment: a case study of the Cameroonian grassfield.* Ph.D. Universität Heidelberg.

Teso Women Peace Activists (2012) Annual report.

Uganda Orthodox Mothers Union (2012) Activities report.

Wikipedia (2014) Community. [online] Available at: http://en.wikipedia.org/wiki/ Community (Accessed 15 September 2014).

CHAPTER 28. CONFLICT, CONTRADICTION AND CONSCIOUSNESS: AN ARTIST'S EVOLUTION

The art of Milly Buchanan

The Cover of this book depicts a painting by Milly Buchanan. Milly Buchanan was born in Monrovia, Liberia in 1944 to a German-Jamaican immigrant and a Liberian aristocrat of Americo-Liberian descent. Milly's artistry began in Vevey, Switzerland, where her talent was first noticed, at the age of 10, by a prominent Swiss artist, Guy Baer. In order to paint her portrait, Guy Baer gave her a sheet of paper and some charcoal-sticks and told her to draw the three eggs before her to keep her still--the portrait he painted of her, "Jeune Liberienne" was sold to the Jewish museum in Vevey. Thereafter, Guy Baer tutored a young Milly once a week for nearly a year, imparting his classical technique in oil painting, which still characterizes her work today.

Her early work, mostly still-life, landscapes, and portraits, clearly followed the great European Masters of 15th century, but Milly developed her personal style of Afro-Cubism in the late 70's. Reminiscent of Picasso, Braque and Modigliani --her favorite artists to date-- Afro-Cubism was her shattered-glass art expression of the social-political turmoil in Liberia.

Milly uses the African concept of "Self"--meaning oneself, within one's tribe, and one's culture and land--to express her observations as an artist. Her work became influenced and affected by the culturally uprooted society in Liberia, the practice of "converting the natives to democratization", and her internal conflict of Christianity versus pagan ancestral worship. Her paintings vibrate with five or six layers of colors, a representation of the overlay of educated behavior atop the raw inner artist. And much of her work includes an "eye", which represents witnessing the timeliness of art, a female breast indicating the progeny of art, and the "dove of spiritual peace" as the Holy Ghost.

The 27 oil paintings in her "Crying-out" series are Milly's purest afro-cubist expressions and reflected the social, political, and economic turmoil that engulfed the Americo-Liberian society. The tumult drove Milly to other African countries in search of a common-denominator to art forms, and found inspiration as an artist caught-up in conflict, contradiction, and consciousness.

Truly a renaissance woman, Milly is also an architect, a conference interpreter and translator speaking five languages (French, German, Italian, Spanish and English), and a former model (including September 1971 Ebony Fashion Fair poster-model, Essence Magazine). Milly's extensive sub-Saharan Africa life, coupled with her personal and professional relationships with Africans from all walks of life (the late President Sekou Toure of Guinea to recording artists Hugh Masekela and Miriam Makeba to uncelebrated market women, students, farmers, and fisherman) have produced a unique perspective from which to artistically represent the essence of the African struggle and spirit of resilience and hope. Milly is also a founding member of the Union of Liberian Artists an organization that creates a forum for the exchange of personal experiences in various refugee camps, motivates young self-taught artists to develop their skills, hosts art exhibits and promotes their works.

Retired since 1998 as Advisor on International Affairs to the former President of Liberia and mother of five adult children and twenty grandchildren, Milly now focuses all her time on painting. As she reflects on her artistic track record over some five decades, impressions of mindset redirection, national reconciliation, and reconstruction in her native Liberia can easily be seen in the vibrant colors of Afro-Cubism.

CHAPTER 29. COMPREHENSIVE COMMUNITY CARE IN RURAL REALITIES THROUGH THE LENS OF JANNEKE VAN DIJK

======================❖======================

Mirjam van Reisen

Janneke van Dijk is a Government Medical Officer at the HIV clinic at Parirenyatwa Hospital in Harare, Zimbabwe, focusing on the provision of paediatric HIV care.She worked as a resident medical doctor at Murambinda Hospital in rural Zimbabwe in 2000, experiencing the diversity of pathology seen at a rural African hospital, and the devastation of HIV when no treatment was available. In 2003, she settled in the rural village of Macha, Zambia and worked as a resident doctor and research associate, later becoming the Clinical Research Director of the Macha Research Trust. She has been a long-time member of the Triple C approach of Comprehensive Community Care. This approach integrated training and awareness with operational medical care in deep rural settings.

Janneke van Dijk holds a PhD from the Erasmus University in Rotterdam:*Rural Realities in Paediatric HIV Service Delivery* (2003).She is currently an advisor of the Tilburg University Globalisation, Ageing, Innovation and Care(GAIC) programme. She is married to Gertjan van Stam and practices photography as a hobby. She is originally from The Netherlands.

The pictures show rural women simultaneously as entrepreneurs, mothers and care-givers, all at the same time. It shows the integration of care, livelihoods, dialogue and negotiation – not as separate tasks or identities but as an amalgamation of what constitutes a healthy village community. Her pictures show women as assertive and – often – happy members of a society where care is explicitly part of public existence. In this sense her pictures can be seen as a commentary of current metropolitan life, where care-giving is removed from the public arena and separated from economic spaces. Caregiving is here portrayed as an integral part of all daily activities.

Van Dijk shows care without reservation as a major part of community life that blends in with leadership roles, governance and the economy. In so doing Van Dijk points to the centrality of women as community builders in Southern African rural villages.

Picture 1: Portia, who continued the Murambinda Foster Home, established by her mother – after her mother's death, Zimbabwe

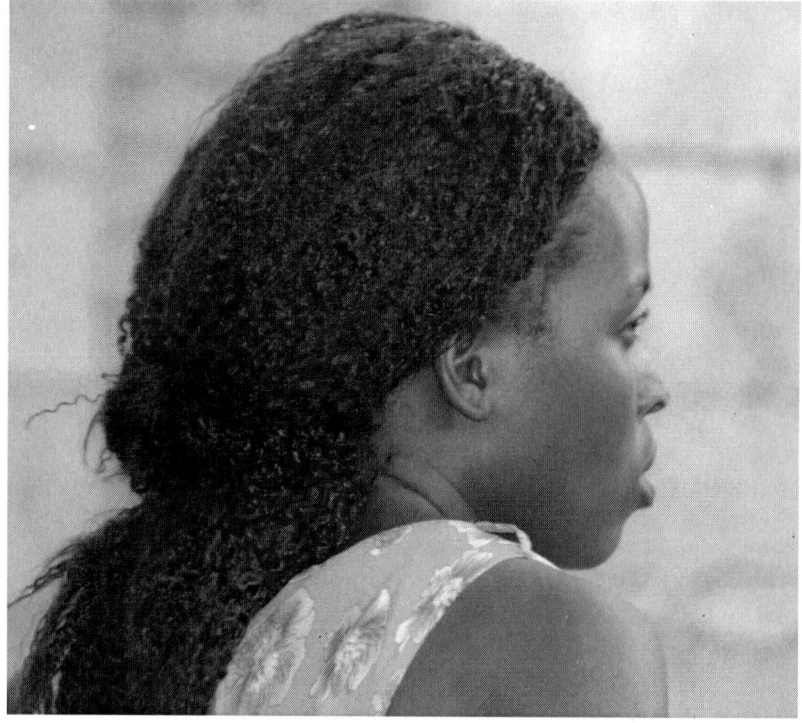

Picture 2: Women carrying baskets with baby in sling, Macha, Zambia

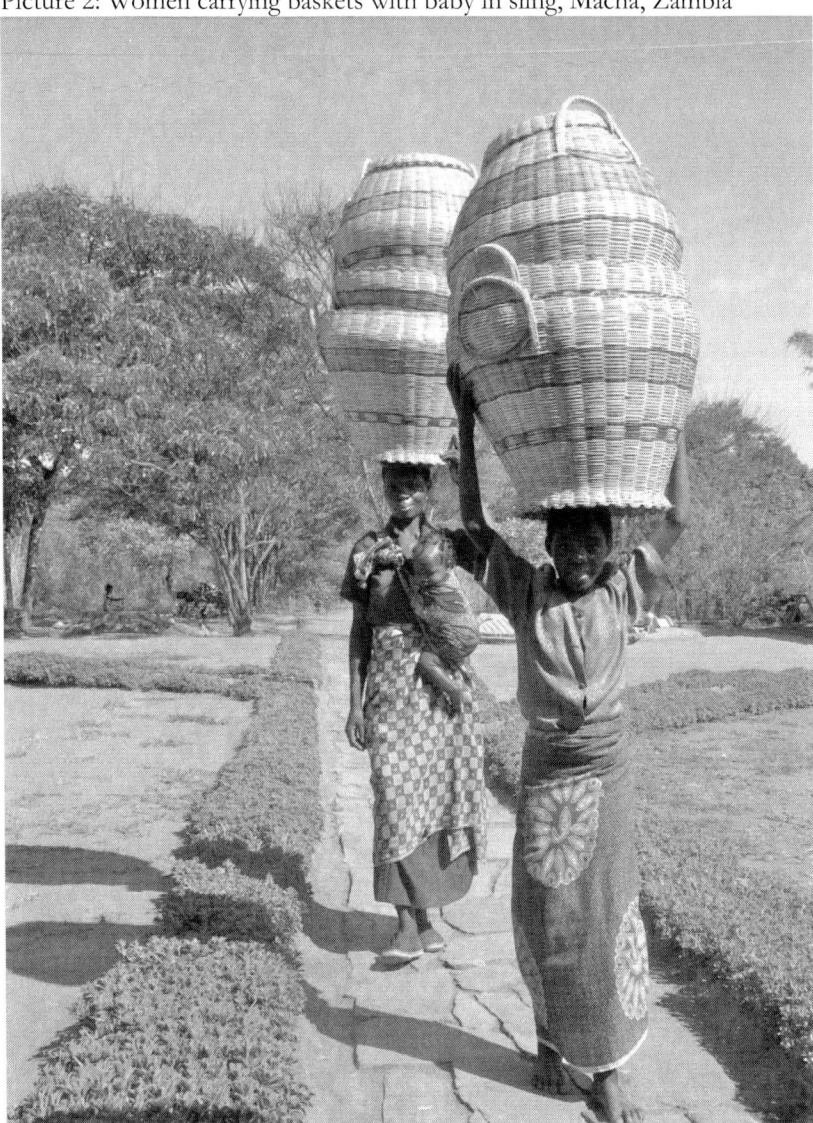

Picture 3: Opening of the Care House "Youth Day" in Macha, Zambia

Picture 4: Traditional Birth Attendant examining a pregnant woman during antenatal clinic at a local Rural Health Post in Zambia.

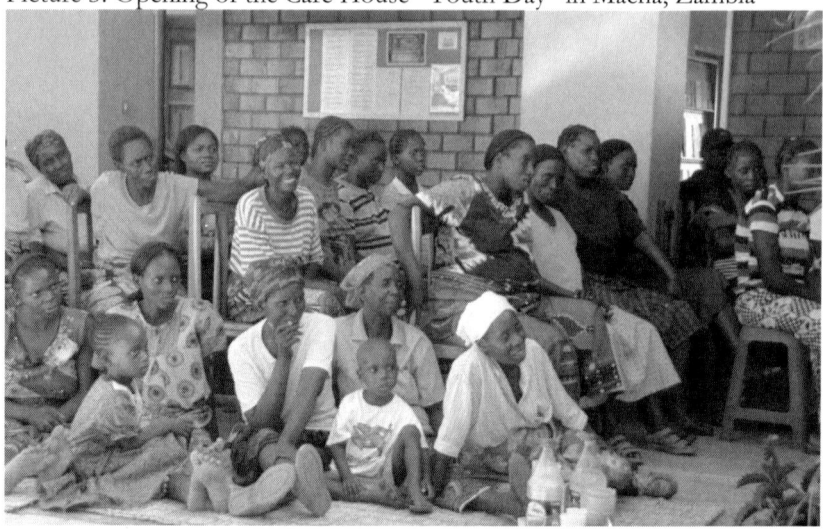

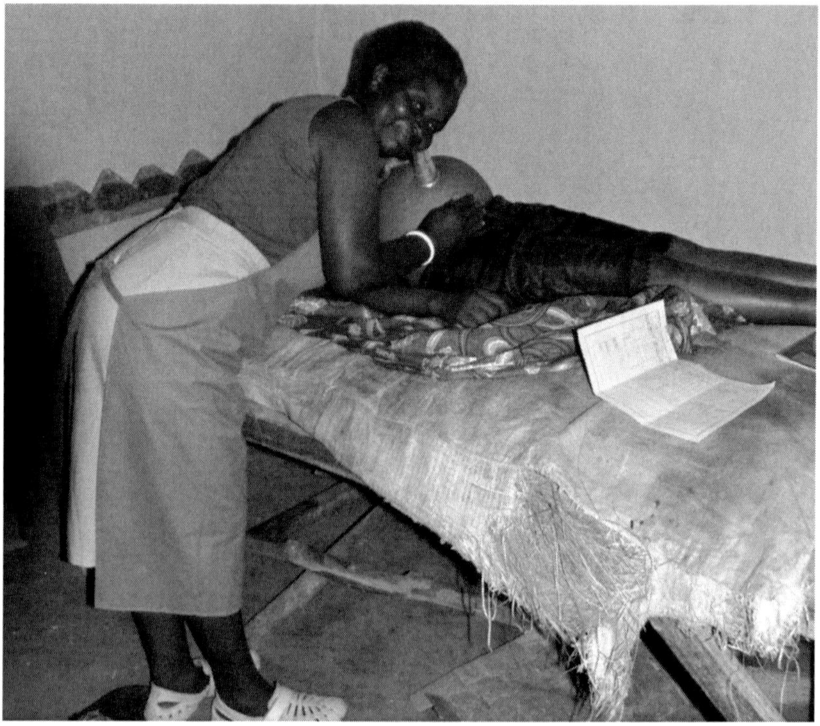

Picture 5: Mothers and their children attending a Mother and Child Health clinic at their local Health Post in Zambia.

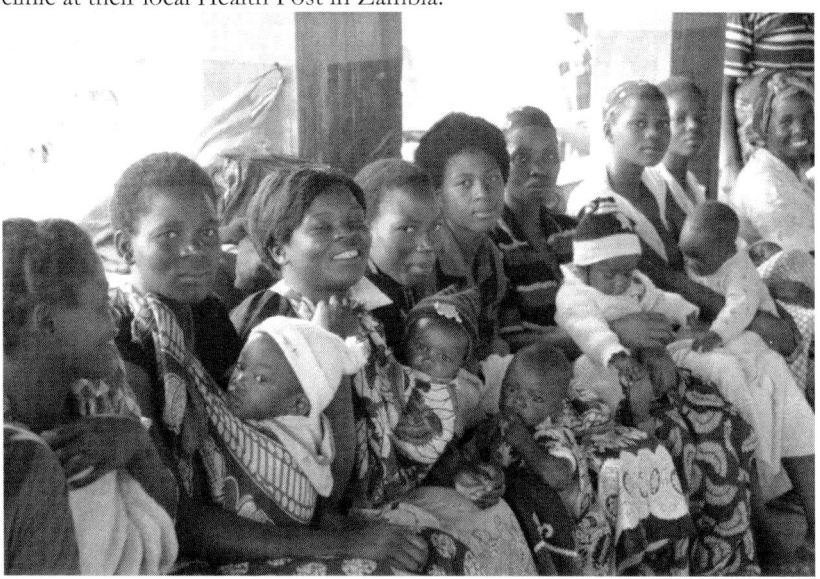

Picture 6: Newly trained Traditional Birth Attendants providing HIV Counseling and Testing services at their Rural Health Post, Zambia.

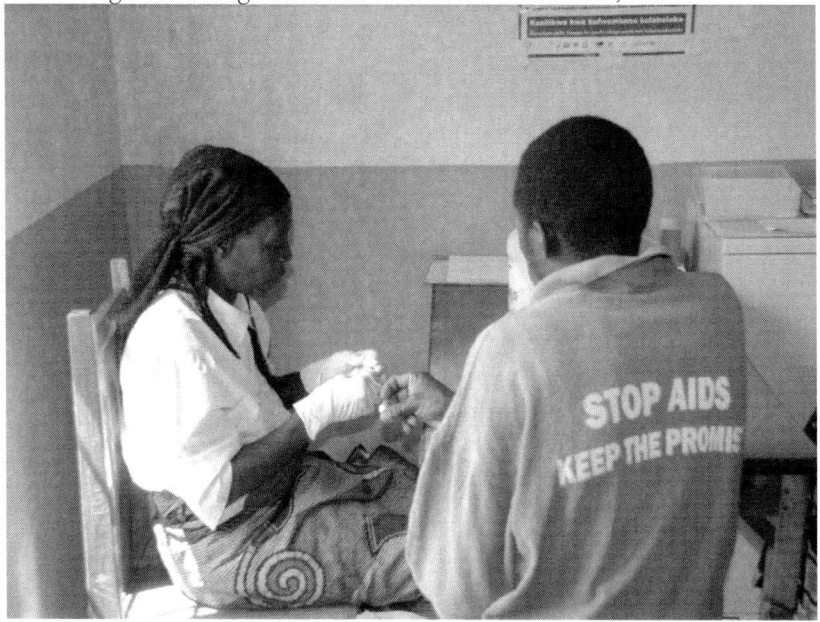

Picture 7: Community volunteers watching an educational video on HIV in their own language, Zambia.

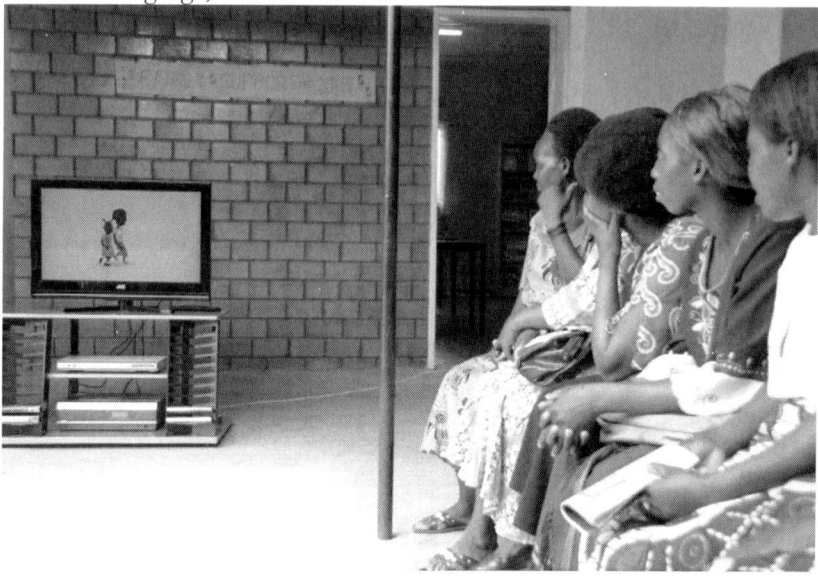

Picture 8: Women use their skills to make and sell baskets to provide for their families, Zambia.

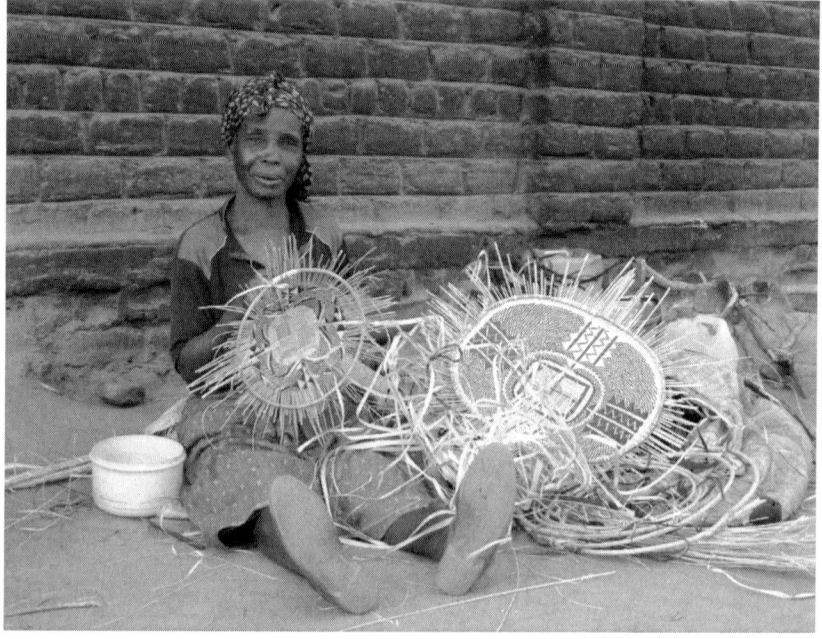

Picture 9: Grandmother with children under her care, Zambia.

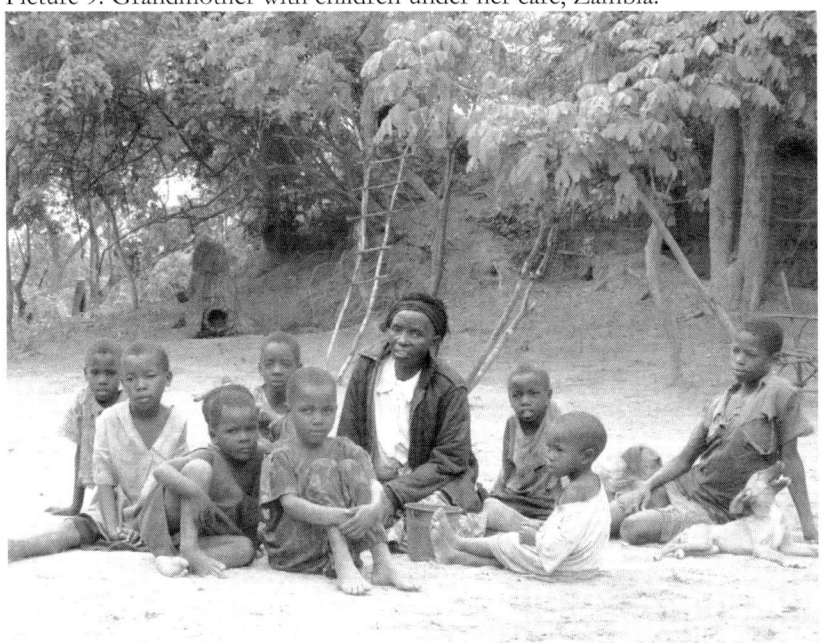

Picture 10: Women as seasonal workers at a Jatropha farm, Zambia.

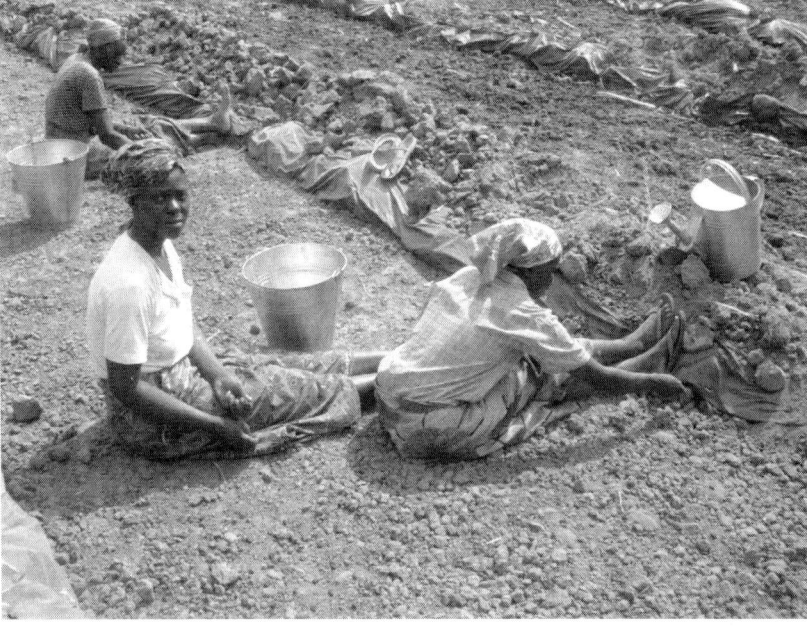

Picture 11: Mushroom harvest, Zambia.

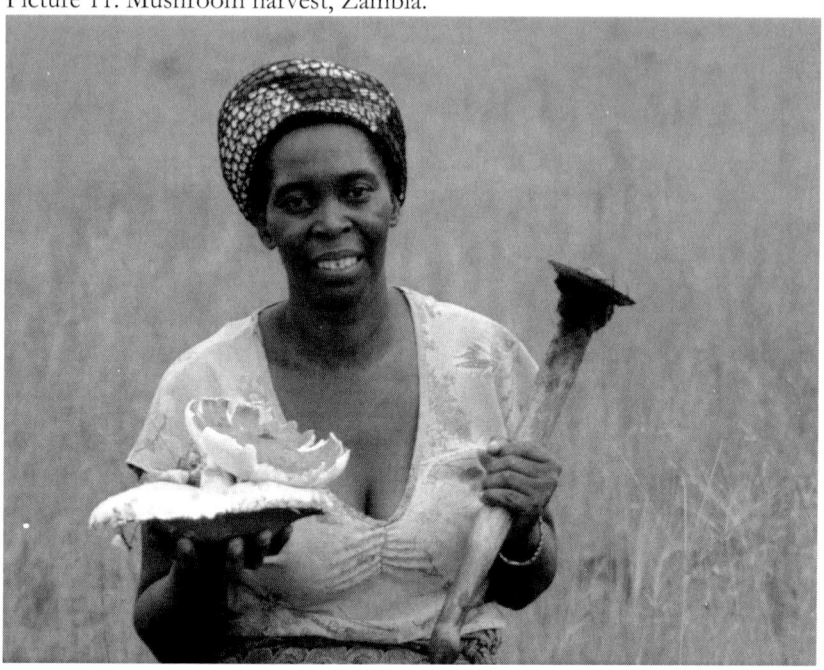

Picture 12: Women selling vegetables at a local market, Zambia.

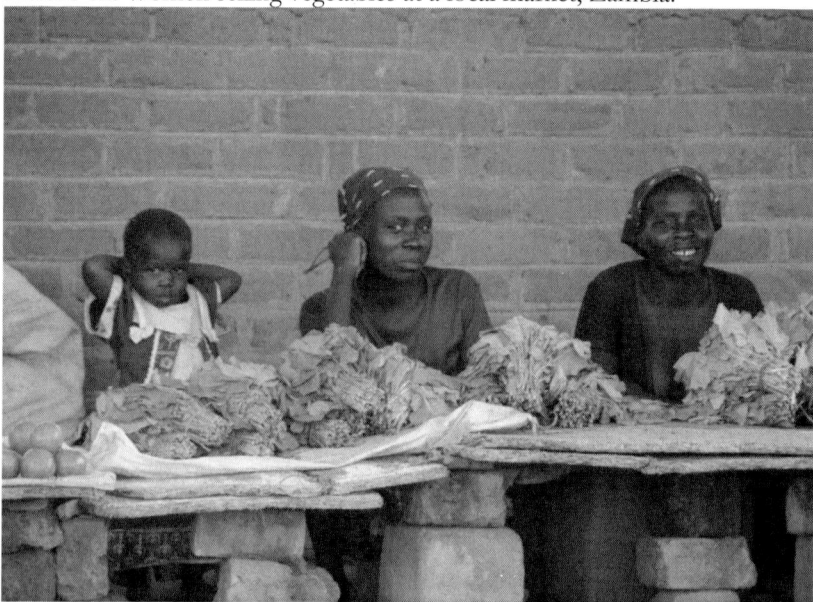

Picture 13: Women fishing in a local river to add variety to the family's diet, and if plenty for sales

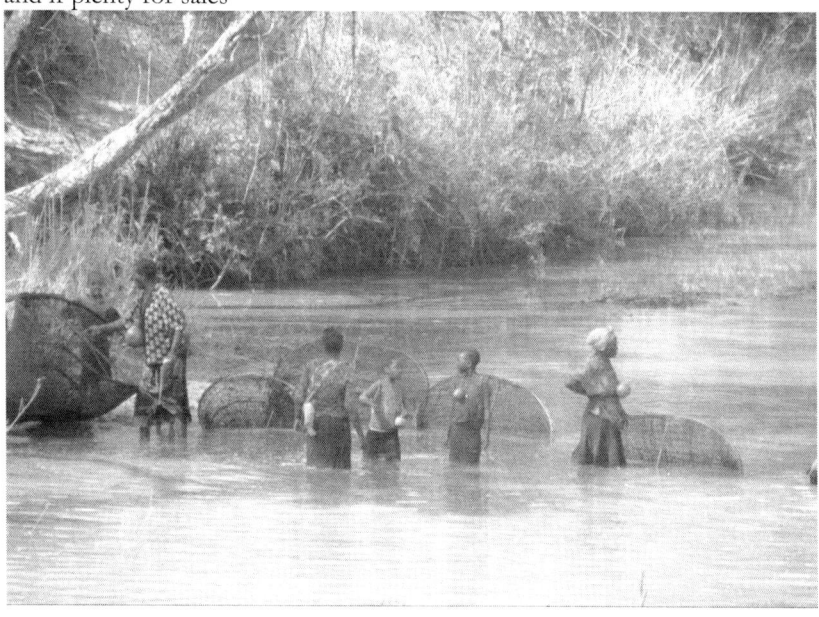

Picture 14: Cooking of Nshima, the staple food in Zambia

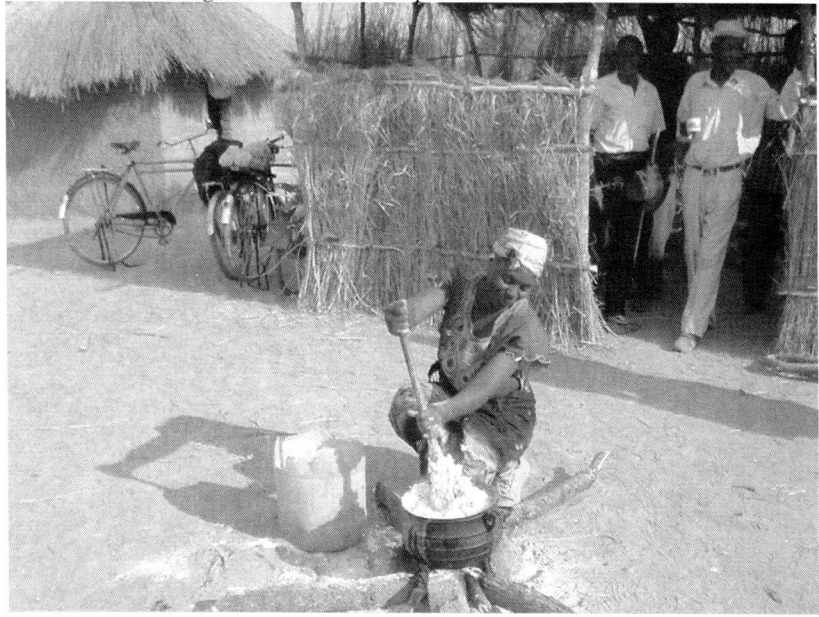

ABOUT THE AUTHORS

Erik BORGMAN, a Lay Dominican, is Professor for Public Theology and holds the Cobbenhagen Chair at Tilburg University, The Netherlands. A systematic theologian by training and a specialist in the history of Twentieth Century Roman Catholic theology, his research concentrates on the public relevance of religion in contexts usually considered secular. He is a member of the Board of Editors of the international theological journal Concilium and chief editor of Dutch Tijdschrift voor Theologie (Journal for Theology).

Ineke BUSKENS is an independent research, facilitation and gender consultant. She is project leader and research director of the GRACE Network, working with 28 research teams in 18 countries. She holds a Masters in Cultural Anthropology. Dutch born Ineke has lived in Ghana, India, Brazil and South Africa where she currently resides. She has published extensively on research methodology, women's health and HIV/AIDS, gender and information communication technology, and open development.

Agnes DINKELMAN is the founder of Stillare, a network that focuses on the human factor in safety and security issues. Agnes has advised the Dutch National Police and the Dutch Army on Intelligence, understanding and community policing. As an analyst, mediator and community builder she worked with complex situations on leadership, gender and conflict in Iraq, Liberia and Ghana. Agnes holds a Bachelor in Social Studies, and has diplomas in conflict management, international relations and strategic public management.

Janneke van DIJK lives in Zimbabwe where she is a Government Medical Officer at Parirenyatwa Hospital in Harare. Previously she worked as a resident doctor in rural Zimbabwe. She also worked as resident doctor and research associate at a hospital in rural Zambia, later becoming the Clinical Research Director of the Macha Research Trust. Janneke holds a PhD from the Erasmus University in Rotterdam and is an advisor to the Tilburg University GAIC programme. Janneke van Dijk is also a photographer.

Selam KIDANE is a systemic psychotherapist trained at the Institute of Family Therapy in London, UK. She works in London as a policy officer on education and children's services for a local authority. She has worked with refugee communities in the UK and has authored practice guides and training manuals in relation to that work. Selam is a human rights activist and a director of Release Eritrea. She is a commentator on Eritrean politics, and contributes to various Eritrean websites as well Eritrean and non-Eritrean media outlets.

Grace KWINJEH is from Zimbabwe. She is a journalist by profession, and a women's rights activist. She chaired the Global Zimbabwe Forum, is a founding member of the Movement for Democratic Change (MDC) and served as the MDC representative to the EU (2001-2005). Since 2007 Grace has lived in exile, in South Africa, Rwanda and Belgium. Grace is a columnist with South Africa based Mail and Guardian and the Canada based Women's International Press. Grace is also a fellow with the Vineyard Institute.

Chikomborero MAFURIRANWA is a women's rights activist living in Harare, Zimbabwe. She holds a Bachelor of Science (Hon) Degree in Psychology. A young woman passionate about defending women's rights in a male-dominated society, her main focus is community-based education for rural women. She currently works with the Association of Women's Clubs (AWC), Zimbabwe.

Obadiah MAILAFIA is Nigerian and a career economist, strategist, banker and international development specialist. He is Chief of Staff of the 79-member African, Caribbean and Pacific (ACP) Group of States based in Brussels. He has held senior positions in the Central Bank of Nigeria and African Development Bank (ADB) Group and has been Special Advisor to the President of Nigeria. He was also Founder/Chairman of the Centre for Policy and Economic Research (CEPER). He holds a PhD from Oxford University.

Stella MARANGA is a Kenyan gender specialist who has worked with women, leadership and governance issues in the Horn and East Africa. As part of UN Women's Kenya Programme she worked with a range of actors to promote women's participation in the 2012 elections, promoting country wide civic and voter education on women's participation and affirmative action. She previously worked with Oxfam GB as a gender advisor. She is a Women Leadership and Gender Specialist at the Coady international Institute.

Pamela MBABAZI is Deputy Vice Chancellor of Mbarara University of Science and Technology (MUST), and Associate Professor in the Institute of Interdisciplinary Training and Research (IITR). She served as Dean of the former Faculty of Development Studies from 1998 to 2009. Pamela is a member of the Makerere University Senate and President/Executive Chair of the Uganda Development Studies Association. She holds a PhD and Masters in Development Studies and in Regional Planning and Management.

ABOUT THE AUTHORS

Clementia Neema MUREMBE is a lecturer in the Institute of Inter-Disciplinary Training and Research (IITR) at Mbarara University of Science and Technology (MUST) where she was former associate dean in the Faculty of Development Studies. She teaches Human Resource Management, Development Practice and Theories. She researches on gender and family relations, women's empowerment and decision making at household level. She has a Masters in Development Studies and is a PhD student at Tilburg University.

Primrose NAKAZIBWE is a lecturer in the Institute of Inter-Disciplinary Training and Research (IITR) at Mbarara University of Science and Technology (MUST) in Uganda. She lectured at the Islamic University in Uganda from 2008 to 2012 and was a Gender Consultant with Child Health Uganda. She has contributed to several gender based curricula. She holds Bachelors and Masters degrees in Development Studies from MUST. She is currently pursuing her PhD studies at Tilburg University.

Angeline NGEUDIEU is Regional Conflict Transformation and Advocacy Advisor for ICCO. Her work includes, training, peer education, managing seed grants for community income generating activities. Angeline has been working on gender issues for 17 years, including with the UN peacekeeping mission in South Sudan. She holds a Masters in political Sciences from the University of Heidelberg-Germany, and a PhD thesis on women's empowerment in the informal sector.

Ruth Ojiambo OCHIENG is Executive Director of Isis-Women's International Cross Cultural Exchange (Isis-WICCE) in Uganda. Isis-WICCE is a feminist women's human rights organisation advocating the rights of women, including in armed conflict settings. She ensured women's voices were included in the Juba Peace talks, and mobilised to engender the Government Peace, Recovery and Development Plan (PRDP). Ruth holds a BSc. in Information and Communication and a Masters in Communication policy Studies.

Antony Otieno ONG'AYO is a Researcher at International Development Studies, Utrecht University (The Netherlands). His PhD examined the contribution of diaspora organisations to countries of destination and origin. He is a member of the GAIC research group at Tilburg University. He has an MSc in Politics and Development. He is a Research fellow at the European Centre for Development Policy Management, African Migration and Development Policy Centre and Transnational Institute.

Betty Achan OGWARO is a Member of the South Sudan Legislative Assembly. She served as a State Minister in Eastern Equatoria State, and as

National Minister of Agriculture, Forestry, Cooperatives and Rural Development. She was a member of the Mediation Team that negotiated the Juba Peace agreement. She campaigns for women's participation, promotion and protection. She spearheaded the formation of the South Sudan Women Parliamentary Caucus. Betty is an Animal Scientist and specialist in Microbiology.

Gerard van OORTMERSSEN is professor at Tilburg University and an independent consultant. His special interest is on how Information and Communication Technology (ICT) is evolving, and how it shapes our world and influences our behaviour. As a consultant he advises public and private organisation on interactions between ICT, organisational culture and personal values. For over a decade he has been active on rural development projects in sub-Saharan Africa and in advising universities.

Mirjam van REISEN is Professor for International Social Responsibility at Tilburg University and chair of the "Globalisation, Ageing, Migration and Care" research group (GAIC). She lectures at Amsterdam University College, is Director of Europe External Policy Advisors (EEPA), and directs Research on Human Trafficking at The Broker. She is a member of the Dutch Government Council on International Relations, and a member of the Supervisory Boards of the Transnational Institute (TNI) and the Dutch Development Organisation (SNV). She is a member of the International Coordinating Committee of Social Watch. She has an MSc from Nijmegen University and a PhD in Social Sciences from the University of Maastricht. She is a member of the Board of Hands of Friendship and a member of the International Commission on Eritrean Refugees (ICER). She advised the Organ for National Healing Reconciliation and Integration (ONHRI) in Zimbabwe. In 2012 Mirjam van Reisen received the Golden Image Award for Peace-Building from President Ellen Johnson Sirleaf of Liberia.

Leena RIKKILÄ-TAMANG is Director for Asia and Pacific at International IDEA (Institute for Democracy and Electoral Assistance). From 2007 to 2013 she managed IDEA's programme on Supporting Constitution Building Process in Nepal. Originally from Finland, Leena has worked in India, Nepal and Vietnam and on Burma/Myanmar. She has published numerous articles about the intersection of gender and political religion in India, as well as on democracy in Nepal and at the global level.

Robyn STOCKER is a DJ and trainee music producer living London. She supports event management company, Cellar Door Promotions and works with Fizz DJ. She works part-time in the service industry to sustain her ambitions. With Fiona Roberts she set up `Girls Make Music` as an online research-based platform, to support and encourage women to pursue a profession in music production and sound engineering. She broadcasts on Astute Radio, an online station supporting women in music. She campaigns for a Living Wage.

Geresu TUFA was born in a village outside Addis Ababa, Ethiopia. As a fourth year management student he was forced to leave Eritrea due to his student activism. He has lived in Nairobi, Kenya and in Asmara, Eritrea as a refugee. He has been active in human right activism, advocating for the rights of the Oromo people. He writes articles on Oromo and Ethiopian issues. Geresu has studied International Business Management in the University of Applied Science. He lives with his family in The Netherlands.

Catherine SCHOOK is an external PhD student at Tilburg University, GAIC programme, in Tilburg, Netherlands. She received her Research Master's degree at the Vrije Universiteit Amsterdam in Lifestyle and Chronic Disorders in 2011. As a native from Portland, Oregon, USA, she completed her bachelor's education in Community Health Education in 2009. She currently works in English proofreading, editing and research with the Amsterdam-based NGO, HealthNet TPO.

Susan SELLARS-SHRESTHA is a copyeditor and author living in Kathmandu, Nepal. A lawyer by training, she holds Bachelor degrees in Law and Commerce, and a Diploma in Publishing and Editing. Her first short story, 'Coffee for Buddha', was published by Central Queensland University Press in 2006. She brings her vast knowledge of international law and development (including constitutional law and European Union policy) to her work as a copyeditor and project manager for clients in Nepal and Europe.

Gertjan van STAM and his family lived in rural Zimbabwe and rural Zambia for 12 years before moving to Harare. His goal is to identify and inspire local talent through community engagement, workforce development and thought leadership. He seeks to identify dynamics of change in rural African communities, enabled by engendered leadership that inspires, initiates, implements, and scales up sustainable progress, and through the use of technology in local communities. He is a PhD student in the Tilburg University GAIC programme.

Sandra TUMWESIGYE is an independent researcher and writer with a specific interest and focus on issues of women, peace and security in conflict and post-conflict countries.

Vickie WAMBURA is founder and Executive Director of Nafisika Trust. Nafisika has become a key partner with the Kenya Prison Service. She was elected an Ashoka Fellow in 2013 and a Mandela Washington Fellow in 2014 (Young African Leaders Initiative by President Obama). She holds a Cambridge International Diploma in Business Management and is an alumnus of the Institute for National Transformation. She graduated as an International Associate of Wagner College in New York.

Syed Manzar Abbas ZAIDI is Counter Terrorism project advisor to the British High Commission in Pakistan. Previously he was Director of the National Counter Terrorism Authority of Pakistan, and a lecturer on Policing and Criminal Investigation at the University of Central Lancashire (UK). He is a Counter Terrorism/Security Preparedness Trainer. Manzar has been published widely. His PhD thesis was on the Transmigration of Radical tendencies from the rural to the urban in the context of the Taliban in Pakistan.

Andre ZAAIMAN is Director of MindSight, a private company providing training in intelligence and security for the South African Government, UN Missions in Africa and the African Union. He he was an ANC underground activist in the 80's and a prominent member of the End Conscription Campaign. He was Director of the Goree Institute in Senegal. Andre provided strategic intelligence support to President Thabo Mbeki. He was a member of a Progressive African Discussion Group of six Africans.

100815-50-1-60